Recent Progress in Pediatric Endocrinology

Proceedings of the Serono Symposia, Volume 12

Edited by

G. Chiumello
Department of Pediatrics, Endocrine Unit,
University of Milan, Italy.

Z. Laron
Institute of Pediatric and Adolescent Endocrinology,
Beilinson Medical Center,
Tel Aviv University, Israel.

1977

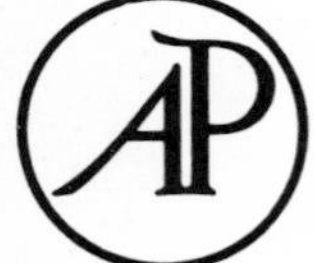

ACADEMIC PRESS London New York San Francisco
A Subsidiary of Harcourt Brace Jovanovich, Publishers

ACADEMIC PRESS INC. (LONDON) LTD.
24-28 OVAL ROAD
LONDON NW1

U.S. Edition published by
ACADEMIC PRESS INC.
111 FIFTH AVENUE
NEW YORK, NEW YORK 10003

Library of Congress Catalogue Card Number: 77 088129
ISBN: 0-12-173250-9

Printed by Photolithography in Great Britain by
Whitstable Litho Ltd, Whitstable, Kent

PREFACE

Pediatric endocrinology is a new discipline which is gaining recognition and independence from adult endocrinology. The increasing number of pediatric endocrinologists, the development of new laboratory methods and availability of new hormones for clinical trial have enabled the accumulation of much new information in the field of childhood endocrinology. Thus it was decided to hold an international Symposium on Recent Progress in this field in Milan in October 1976. The themes chosen were carbohydrate metabolism, abnormal puberty and hypertension. The main lectures were accompanied by short communications relating to the same subject and vivid discussion ended each session.

We hope that the proceedings of this Symposium will transmit to non-participants the highlights of this conference. This Symposium was made possible by the generous support of the Serono Foundation.

G. CHIUMELLO
Z. LARON

CONTENTS

THE HORMONAL CONTROL OF ENERGY METABOLISM

A.L. Drash

Department of Pediatrics University of Pittsburgh, School of Medicine Children's Hospital of Pittsburgh, Pa., USA

Survival of the human organism is dependent upon a continuous supply of energy. Adaptation to intermittent feeding and fasting involves not only mechanisms for control of energy flow, but also highly refined systems to insure the constancy of the internal milieu. Not only must a source of energy be always available, but the concentration of the energy substrates, such as glucose, must be maintained within very narrow limits.

The energy homeostasis system is highly complex, involving close integration of the function of the gastrointestinal tract in digestion and absorption of nutrients, the liver, muscle and adipose tissue as organs of storage, and the endocrine and central nervous systems in the control of the interrelationships of energy storage, retrieval, interconversion and utilization. The absence of complete integration of all these systems will result in maladaptation of energy homeostasis and disease of the organism (Cahill, 1970, 1971, 1976; Havel, 1972).

NUTRIENT SUPPLY

The human organism is extraordinarily adaptable in its ability to utilize extremely variable nutrient sources to meet energy requirements. In Table I are given some examples of this adaptability. The fetus is a particularly interesting example. The figures are estimates as no firm data exist on the changing nutrient mix which traverses the placenta during the course of gestation. It is clear, however, that glucose is the dominant fuel and that the larger fat molecules cross little if at all. The importance of maternally-derived free fatty acids in fetal energy balance is unresolved. At birth there is acute termination of the system of continuous nutrient supply, and immediate activation of a previously untried system to support intermittent feeding. This highly important transition period will be the topic of several discussions to follow.

Table I. Nutrient "mix" in selected populations.

	Fetus	Patients Given Parenteral Alimentation	Less-developed Countries	Eskimo	United States
Protein (%)	25	20	10	55	12
Fat (%)	5	0	10	45	41
Carbohydrate (%)	70	80	80	5	47

The average American diet contains approximately 47% of total calories as carbohydrate, 41% as fat and 12% as protein. Of the carbohydrate calories, 50-60% are derived from starch, 30-40% from sucrose and the remainder from lactose, from milk and other dairy products, and fructose from fruits and vegetables. Fat in the American diet is primarily animal in origin and is highly saturated. Similarly, the protein content is largely of animal origin, particularly beef.

Most of the peoples of the world today, and in the past, consume a diet highly different from that of the affluent West. Naturally occurring carbohydrate, derived from some mixture of grains, corn, rice, potatoes, vegetables and fruits, make up 60-80% of the total calories. Refined sugar, or sucrose, is a minor contributor. Fat makes up a smaller portion of the diet and protein is frequently inadequate, both in terms of total quantity and proper relationship between essential and non-essential amino acids. The Eskimo represents an especially interesting example of Man's capacity to thrive on what we would consider to be an unusual, if not potentially dangerous, nutrient mix. Prior to the intrusion of Western civilization, the Eskimo had essentially no exogenous source of carbohydrate. The diet was derived from fish and animal with about equal portions of fat and protein.

Table II. Fuel stores in the immediate post-absorptive state in a normal 70 kg man.

	Storage Form	Source	Amount	Calories
Glucose	Glycogen	Muscle	.400 kg	1,600
		Liver	.100 kg	400
				2,000
Amino Acids	Protein	Muscle	6.3 kg	25,000
Free Fatty Acids	Triglycerides	Adipose	15 kg	140,000

FUEL STORAGE

Caloric intake in excess of immediate energy needs is stored. The body stores glucose as glycogen in liver and muscle. Amino acids are converted to protein and dietary fat is stored as triglyceride in adipose tissue and liver, and to a lesser extent in other organs. The energy stores present in the theoretical 70 kg man in the post-prandial state are presented in Table II (Ruderman, 1975; Aoki *et al.*, 1975a,b; Felig, 1975a,b).

CARBOHYDRATE STORES

Carbohydrate may be stored in liver and muscle as glycogen. The concentration in the post-prandial state rarely exceeds 5% in liver and 1% in muscle. Consequently the storage capacity is extremely limited. In addition, it is an inefficient storage depot as there are 1 or 2 grams of intracellular water associated with each gram of glycogen, reducing the theoretical 4 calories per g of carbohydrate to approximately one-third of this in terms of tissue storage. In the average 70 kg man there are approximately 400 grams of glycogen available in muscle and 100 grams in liver in the fed state, representing 2000 calories, or just enough to meet the estimated basal energy requirements of 1800 calories for one day.

PROTEIN STORES

There is no specific storage form of protein; all of body protein is committed to structural or functional activity. Dietary protein in excess of these requirements is converted to either glucose (glucogenic amino acids) or fat (ketogenic amino acids). The use of body protein to meet energy needs also requires degradation and conversion to either glucose or fat, an energy-requiring process, making this an inefficient system when compared with the direct oxidation of glucose and FFA.

The great majority of body protein is found in skeletal muscle which makes up approximately 40% of body weight and total oxygen consumption in the resting state. The 70 kg man is estimated to have 28 kg of muscle, 6.3 kg of which is protein, a theoretical caloric reserve of 25,000 calories. It is obvious that there is a limit to the amount of structural protein which can be degraded in situations of prolonged starvation before death occurs. Gluconeogenic amino acids constitute 55% of muscle protein, equivalent to 3.6 kg or 14,400 calories (Krebs, 1964). It is estimated that approximately half of the available protein may be utilized before death occurs from muscular weakness or hypoglycemia.

LIPID STORES

Excess dietary calories from carbohydrate, protein or fat may be stored as triglyceride. The primary storage site is adipose tissue, but appreciable quantities may also be found in liver, muscle and other tissue. Triglyceride is a most efficient form for energy storage, because intracellular lipid has a minimal amount of water. The theoretical value of 9.4 calories per gram of fat is nearly achieved in subcutaneous adipose tissue. Further, the capacity for storage of fat is almost limitless as documented by the extent of obesity to which the human may be subject. In the 70 kg man there are 15 kg of fat which can yield 140,000 calories. Unlike protein, all body fat can be oxidized to meet energy requirements.

ENERGY HOMEOSTASIS AND THE ENDOCRINE SYSTEM

The human is exposed to a great variety of dietary nutrients. In addition, the relationship between quantity and timing of nutrient intake and energy requirements may be extremely diverse. Four areas require special attention:

1) the prandial-immediate post-prandial period most characteristic of our

nutrient status during waking hours;

2) brief fasting, such as occurs daily during 8-10 hours of sleep;

3) prolonged fasting; and

4) exercise.

The homeostatic mechanisms involved in each of these circumstances are similar, but can be most dramatically viewed by the capacity of our 70 kg man to tolerate prolonged starvation. Based upon energy stores totaling 160,000 calories, survival for approximately 100 days should be possible. However, in order to achieve this, metabolic alterations must be promptly made so that hypoglycemia is prevented and glucose utilization is minimized. Protein degradation and gluconeogenesis must be controlled at a rate to meet glucose requirements but to prevent wasteful use of protein for non-essential needs. Lipid oxidation must be maximized in such a manner that acidosis from ketonemia and carbon wastage from ketonuria do not become significant problems. These adaptive biochemical processes result from changes in the secretion of specific hormones.

The major focus of this discussion will be on insulin and the counter-insulin regulatory hormones including glucagon, growth hormone, ACTH, cortisol and the catecholamines. The control by thyroxine of the rate of metabolism, the effect of gonadotropins and sex steroids on growth and sexual maturation, parathyroid hormone on calcium, phosphate and bone metabolism and vasopressin on fluid homeostasis are obviously intimately related to the nutritional and energy status of the organism, but will not be considered in detail here.

INSULIN

Insulin has long been considered the dominant controlling factor in energy homeostasis. It is the hormone of plenty with actions which are predominantly anabolic or synthetic. The primary stimulus for the release of insulin from the beta cells of the pancreas is an increase in the concentration of nutrients, particularly glucose and specific amino acids. Oral administration of nutrients is a more effective mode of stimulating insulin release than is a comparable or higher concentration achieved by intravenous administration (Raptis *et al.*, 1973), indicating the involvement of a gut factor in insulin release. Recently, a number of gastrointestinal polypeptides have been isolated and their physiologic action at least partially defined (Brown *et al.*, 1975; Johnson, 1976; Thomas *et al.*, 1976; Rayford *et al.*, 1976). The importance of the gastrointestinal tract as an endocrine organ is now established. The entero-insular axis is a closed loop feed back system involving gastric inhibitory polypeptide (GIP), gut glucagon, pancreatic glucagon and insulin. The digestion and absorption of food stuffs stimulate the release of these GI factors which augment the effect of nutrient concentration on insulin release.

Suppression of insulin release results from hypoglycemia, food deprivation, malnutrition, exercise and stress. Elevation in the concentration of catecholamines are known to inhibit insulin release and may be the mechanism involved in stress situations (Woods *et al.*, 1974). Growth hormone deficiency is associated with diminished basal and stimulated insulin responses while growth hormone therapy in the hypopituitary patient will return insulin responses to normal (Hopwood *et al.*, 1975). Similar changes occur in glucocorticoid deficiency and replacement therapy.

Insulin has profound effects on many aspects of energy metabolism. Although the precise mode of action of insulin remains incompletely defined, it is clear that attachment to cell membranes, leading to a change in permeability to glucose, amino acids and possibly other metabolites is a primary event. Alteration in the synthesis and activity of a number of enzyme systems is either a primary or secondary reaction to changing concentrations of insulin. Unlike most of the other polypeptide hormones, insulin does not stimulate the generation of cyclic AMP as the intracellular messenger.

The actions of insulin are summarized in Table III. The best known effect of insulin is that of increasing the permeability of the cell membrane to glucose, resulting in an increased rate of glucose translocation from the intra-vascular to the intra-cellular space. This action occurs predominantly in muscle and adipose tissue and is not involved in the movement of glucose into the liver, brain or red blood cells. Quantitatively, this effect is relatively minor in terms of glucose utilization. Qualitatively it is highly important in maintaining the normal cyclic nature of energy flow from glucose and FFA.

Table III. The actions of insulin.

1. Promotion of glucose uptake in insulin-sensitive tissues.
2. Promotion of glycogen synthesis.
3. Inhibition of glycogenolysis.
4. Stimulation of glycolysis.
5. Suppression of gluconeogenesis.
6. Stimulation of lipoprotein lipase activity.
7. Stimulation of lipogenesis.
8. Inhibition of lipolysis.
9. Inhibition of ketogenesis.
10. Promotion of protein synthesis.

Quantitatively of far greater importance is the effect of insulin on hepatic glucose utilization. Glucose from the portal circulation readily enters hepatic cells, based upon the concentration gradient. The biochemical options are shown in Fig. 1. Following phosphorylation to glucose-6-phosphate four major biochemical alternatives are possible; glycogen synthesis and storage, glycolysis through either the Embden-Meyerhof pathway or the hexose monophosphate shunt, or release of free glucose into the general circulation. Insulin, by virtue of its effect on several crucial enzymes promotes the first three reactions and inhibits or minimizes the fourth. The overall effect then is the promotion of glycogen synthesis and storage and the degradation of glucose to meet current hepatic energy requirements or for the production of important intermediates. Glucose release from the liver is minimized but not completely inhibited. A constant basal release is essential to maintain a normal glucose concentration and to meet glucose requirements, primarily of the central nervous system.

The major route of glucose degradation is the Embden-Meyerhof. This is an anaerobic reaction whose end product is pyruvate. An intermediate in this pathway is alpha-glycerol phosphate. Ninty percent of the hepatic glucose oxidation results from pyruvate metabolism through the tricarboxylic acid cycle (TCA) for the generation of high energy phosphate in the form of ATP as illustrated in Fig.

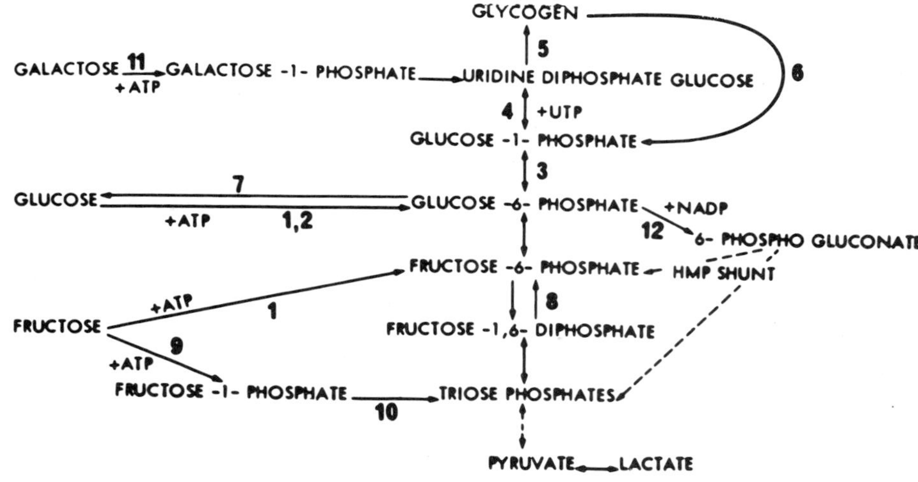

ENZYMES

1. Hexokinase
2. Glucokinase
3. Phosphoglucomutase
4. Uridine diphosphate glucose pyrophosphorylase
5. Uridine diphosphate glucose transglucosylase (glycogen synthetase)
6. Phosphorylase
7. Glucose-6-phosphatase
8. Fructose-1,6-diphosphatase
9. Fructokinase
10. Fructose-1-phosphate aldolase
11. Galactokinase
12. Glucose-6-phosphate dehydrogenase (first step of hexose monophosphate [H.M.P. shunt])

Fig.1 The metabolism of monosaccharides. The major pathways of glucose, galactose and fructose metabolism are illustrated, including glycogen synthesis, glycogenolysis, glycolysis through the Embden-Meyerhof pathway and through the hexose monophosphate shunt. The numbers indicate the enzymes involved in the biochemical reactions.

2. Pyruvate can give rise to both acetyl COA and oxaloacetate. Both may be used as substrate for the TCA cycle while acetyl COA is the basic component of fatty acid synthesis and ketogenesis and oxaloacetate may serve as gluconeogenic substrate.

A quantitatively minor but highly important alternate glycolytic route is the hexosemonophosphate shunt. This is a direct oxidative pathway whose end products are triose phosphates and nicotinamide-adenine dinucleotide phosphate (NADPH). This compound is the hydrogen donor essential for lipid synthesis.

Lipogenesis derived from insulin-mediated glucose metabolism within the liver includes the production of alpha-glycerol phosphate, the "backbone" of triglyceride, NADPH, the hydrogen ion donor for FFA synthesis and the generation of acetyl COA, the basic unit of FFA elongation. Consequently, excess dietary carbohydrate is rapidly and efficiently converted into triglyceride.

Dietary fat circulates as chylomicron, small fat droplets, in the post-prandial period. The circulation is cleared of chylomicron by the action of lipoprotein lipase, an enzyme system located in the capillary bed which splits the chylomicron triglyceride into FFA and glycerol. FFA readily gains entrance to essentially all cells of the body where it may be used as a direct energy source or as substrate for triglyceride synthesis. Lipoprotein lipase is an insulin-sensitive enzyme, the activity increasing with increasing insulin concentration.

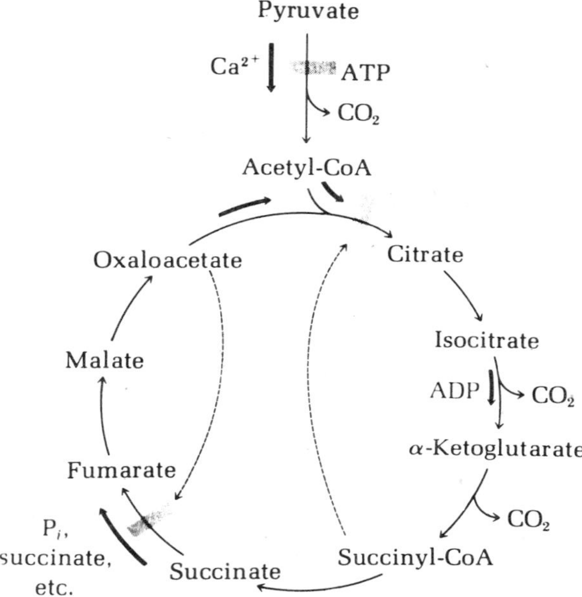

Fig.2 The tricarboxylic acid cycle (TCA or Krebs cycle). The metabolism of pyruvate, the end product of glycolysis, is illustrated. The major pathway is from pyruvate to acetyl COA which may be further oxidized through the cycle or converted to triglyceride or ketone bodies. Additionally pyruvate may be converted to oxaloacetate which is then oxidized through the TCA cycle.

Free fatty acids are a highly compact energy source which circulate loosely bound to serum albumin. The half-life of circulating FFA is very short, owing to its rapid uptake and utilization. FFA present in the circulation is derived from intracellular lipolysis of triglyceride to FFA and glycerol. This process is under the control of a hormone sensitive cyclic AMP-mediated lipase which is directly inhibited by insulin. Ketogenesis, the production of beta hydroxy butyric acid and acetoacetic acid, occurs when there is an increase in substrate, FFA, and impairment of movement of acetyl COA to either lipogenesis or through the TCA cycle (Fig.3). The action of insulin inhibits the release of FFA and insures the metabolism of acetyl COA, thus preventing the production and accumulation of ketone bodies.

Insulin promotes protein synthesis by increasing the rate of cellular uptake of amino acids and the prevention of gluconeogenesis. Insulin and growth hormone are synergistic for growth, both necessary in proper concentration if optimal growth is to occur.

THE COUNTER-INSULIN HORMONES

For many years there has been speculation that energy homeostasis was controlled entirely by insulin; the rate and direction of energy flow relating directly to the circulating concentration of insulin. Under this theory, glucose utilization and anabolic activities occurred in the immediate post-prandial period under the

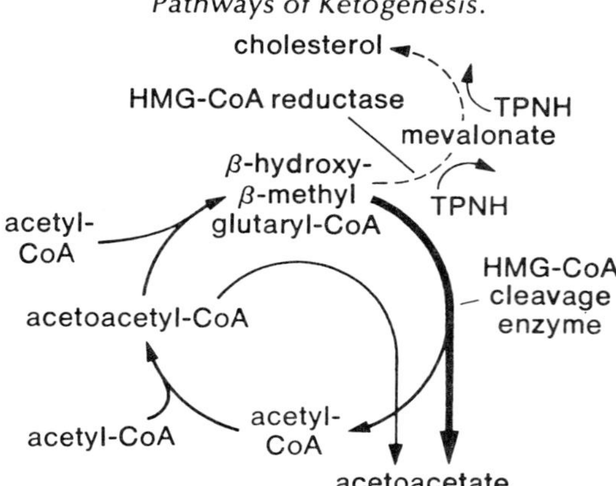

Fig.3 Pathways of ketogenesis. Acetyl COA derived from the beta oxidation of long chain fatty acids is normally oxidized through the TCA cycle. When this route is not available condensation of two acetyl COA units will result in the production of acetoacetyl-COA which may be further converted to acetoacetate or to b-hydroxy butyrate.

direction of high levels of insulin, while FFA utilization and catabolic energy reactions occurred under fasting conditions in the presence of low insulin concentration. The insulin antagonist actions of several hormones could be demonstrated in pharmacologic situations but were considered trivial or of minor importance in the physiologic setting. More recently the physiologic importance of several insulin-antagonistic hormones have been unequivocally documented. In Table IV are listed the insulin antagonist hormones and their apparent modes of action.

Table IV. Insulin antagonist hormone action.

	Glucagon	GH	ACTH	Cortisol	Epinephrine
Insulin Release	↑	↑	—	±	↓
Glucose Uptake	—	↓	—	—	±
Glycogenesis	↓	—	—	—	↓
Glycogenolysis	↑	—	—	—	↑
Gluconeogenesis	↑	±	—	↑	—
Lipolysis	↑	↑	↑	±	↑
Ketogenesis	↑	—	—	↓	±
Proteolysis	—	↓	±	↑	±

↑ increase; ↓ decrease; — no effect; ± equivocal effect.

GLUCAGON

Glucagon, a small polypeptide produced by the alpha cells of the pancreas, has been known for its hyperglycemic properties for many years. However, its importance in energy homeostasis has been only recently appreciated, owing largely to the work of Unger and associates over the past 20 years. This work has been summarized in Unger's Banting Memorial Lecture of 1975 (Unger, 1976).

The present thesis, based on substantial evidence, is that the alpha and beta cells of the pancreas represent a functional unit and that the control of energy flow at any moment in time is the result of the relationship between the concentrations of insulin and glucagon, rather than the absolute concentration of either (Parrilla *et al.*, 1974). The discovery of somatostatin (Brazeau *et al.*, 1973; Vale *et al.*, 1975) and its application in experimental animals (Koerker *et al.*, 1974) and in normal and diabetic humans (Gerich *et al.*, 1975a,b) has verified the physiologic function of glucagon and the validity of the glucagon:insulin ratio concept (Eaton, 1975).

In most, but not all respects, glucagon functions in opposition to insulin, serving a restraining or modulating influence. Glucagon is the hormone of fasting. It is catabolic, promoting degradation of glycogen, protein and fat to meet the requirements of a restricted fuel economy. Factors stimulating the release of glucagon include hypoglycemia, starvation, exercise, stress and catecholamines. Specific amino acids, particularly arginine and alanine, stimulate glucagon release. However, when mixed with glucose or present in the form of a mixed meal, the insulin response dominates and glucagon release is impaired. Glucagon release is inhibited by hyperglycemia and hyperinsulinemia. Glucagon produces its effects by altering the rates of enzyme reactions. This results from a generation of cyclic AMP which functions as the second messenger for glucagon within the cell. Glucagon has no effect on muscle or on cell permeability (Pozefsky *et al.*, 1976). The liver is the primary site of glucagon action with adipose tissue of secondary importance.

The administration of glucagon in pharmacologic amounts leads to prompt increase in the circulating concentration of glucose. This results from activation of the hepatic phosphorylase system, promoting glycogenolysis and glucose release from the liver. This same mechanism undoubtedly occurs in physiologic situations such as stress or exercise (Galba *et al.*, 1975; Bloom, 1973). Under basal conditions glucose production remains at a constant low level. The source of this glucose is both pre-formed glycogen and gluconeogenic substrate, such as alanine, lactate, pyruvate and glycerol. Glucagon has a primary role in increasing the rate of gluconeogenesis by stimulating specific hepatic enzymes. This mechanism is illustrated in Fig.4. It will be noted that in this illustration the gluconeogenetic stimulant is glucocorticoid, the action of which will be discussed later. It appears that glucagon stimulates the same enzymes and is of greater physiologic importance.

Glucagon has two demonstrable actions on fat metabolism. It promotes lipolysis, acutely increasing circulating levels of FFA (Schade and Eaton, 1975a,b). Further, it stimulates ketogenesis. This effect is not simply secondary to the increased availability of FFA. Glucagon specifically alters the "set" of liver enzymes so that ketone production increases out of proportion to the circulating FFA level (McGarry *et al.*, 1975; Grey *et al.*, 1975). The physiologic significance of this biochemical alteration is not clear but probably relates to the CNS adaptation to ketone utilization as an alternate fuel to glucose during prolonged starvation. The administration of pharmacologic doses of glucagon produces a prompt increase in both insulin and glucagon and a delayed increase in growth hormone. The apparent dichotomy of glucagon-stimulated insulin release appears to be physiologically important. The augmentation of insulin release by gastrointestinal absorption of nutrients is at least partially related to the release of glucagon. The apparent glucagon stimulation of growth hormone release results from the fall in

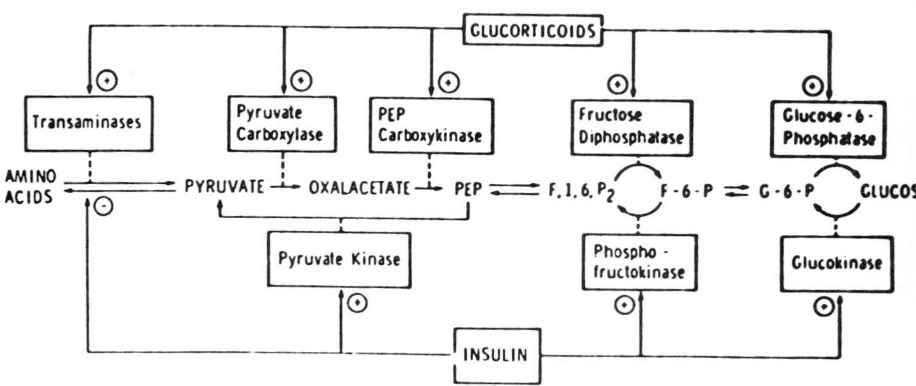

Fig.4 The hormonal control of gluconeogenesis and glycolysis. The figure illustrates the key enzymes involved in gluconeogenesis (movement from left to right) or glycolysis (movement from right to left). Glucocorticoids are known to stimulate the enzymes involved in increasing the rate of gluconeogenesis. Glucagon stimulates the same enzymes. The reversal of this process, glycolysis, is under the influence of enzymes which are responsive to the action of insulin.

blood glucose concentration and has no clear physiologic application.

GROWTH HORMONE

It has long been known that growth hormone excess, as occurs in acromegaly, is regularly associated with carbohydrate intolerance and growth hormone deficiency is frequently associated with hypoglycemia, particularly in the younger child. The demonstrable pharmacologic actions of growth hormone on energy metabolism include antagonism to the action of insulin on cell membrane permeability to glucose and the stimulation of lipolysis. The insulin-synergistic action is the promotion of amino acid uptake and protein synthesis. The mechanisms responsible for stimulation and inhibition of growth hormone release are extraordinarily similar to those for glucagon. Growth hormone is under control of the hypothalamic release (GHRH) and inhibiting (SHRIF or somatostatin) factors. Growth hormone release is inhibited by hyperglycemia and stimulated by hypoglycemia, starvation, exercise and stress. Pharmacologically, growth hormone release follows administration of L-dopa, propranalol (a beta-adrenergic blocker) followed by epinephrine, and glucagon.

The precise mechanism of the hypoglycemia of hypopituitarism remains unclear. There is increased insulin sensitivity and defective lipid mobilization, expected findings. However, there is also evidence suggestive of impaired gluconeogenesis, possibly related to decreased substrate depot (muscle) (Hopwood *et al.*, 1975; Haymond *et al.*, 1976).

ACTH

The actions of ACTH on energy metabolism must be coupled with that of its target organ, the adrenal cortex and its major glucocorticoid, cortisol. Like growth hormone, ACTH has a direct stimulatory effect on lipolysis. Cortisol, long felt to play a major role in glucose metabolism, probably is more important as a permissive agent. This is certainly true for the lipolytic action of ACTH.

The best-described action of cortisol is that on gluconeogenesis and proteolysis. It is quite clear that the pathologic condition, Cushing's syndrome, and the administration of pharmacologic amounts of glucocorticoids result in an increased rate of protein degradation and increased hepatic gluconeogenesis as described earlier. Conversely, cortisol deficiency is associated with a tendency toward fasting hypoglycemia due to deficient gluconeogenesis and glycogenesis. In a somewhat more physiologic situation, prolonged fasting, we found that cortisol secretion rates fell rather than rose (Garces *et al.*, 1968) during a period of active gluconeogenesis. It appears, therefore, that in the physiologic state, the actions of cortisol on energy metabolism are permissive and synergistic with glucagon, growth hormone and ACTH.

THE CATECHOLAMINES

The pharmacologic effects of the major catechol metabolites, epinephrine and nor-epinephrine, include the activation of the phosphorylase enzyme system in both liver and muscle, leading to glycogenolysis, activation of intracellular lipase in adipose tissue leading to very active lipolysis, and suppression of insulin release (Porte *et al.*, 1966; Graber *et al.*, 1976). The physiologic significance of these observations remains to be determined. The importance of the adrenal medulla in acute glucose homeostasis has been placed in doubt by the recent observation that glucose response to intravenous insulin is not different between adrenalectomized and control individuals (Ensinck *et al.*, 1976). Certainly the catecholamine system is involved in the individual's response to stress, including hypoglycemia. The mode of action is through alpha and beta adrenergic receptors located within the central and peripheral nervous systems. It is an area of intense research interest, but beyond the scope of this report. Several comprehensive reviews of the relationship between the central nervous system, adrenergic receptors, the endocrine system and nutrition and energy modulation have recently appeared (Brooks, 1973; Day, 1975; Frohman, 1975a,b; Olson, 1975).

THE INTEGRATION OF ENERGY HOMEOSTASIS

The Post-prandial Period

The average individual ingests his total 24 h caloric intake within 10 to 14 waking hours. The food is a mixture of carbohydrate, fat and protein and is usually ingested in three meals and 2 or 3 between-meal snacks. The time interval between caloric exposure is short, averaging 3-4 h and rarely exceeding 6 h. Consequently, the average individual spends his waking hours cycling between the absorptive and immediate post-absorptive period. An evaluation of the biochemical and hormonal changes is of interest.

The digestion and absorption of foodstuffs leads to the release of gastrointestinal hormones which augments the insulin release stimulated by increased arterial concentration of glucose and amino acids. Some of the changes are illustrated in Fig.5. This figure shows the response of normal children to oral glucose tolerance (Drash, 1973). The ingestion of a mixed meal produces similar changes. Glucose absorption is rapid with peak concentration at 30 min, followed by a linear decline in basal concentration at 3 h. The insulin response curve is similar. Growth hormone is initially suppressed by hyperglycemia, but release stimulated

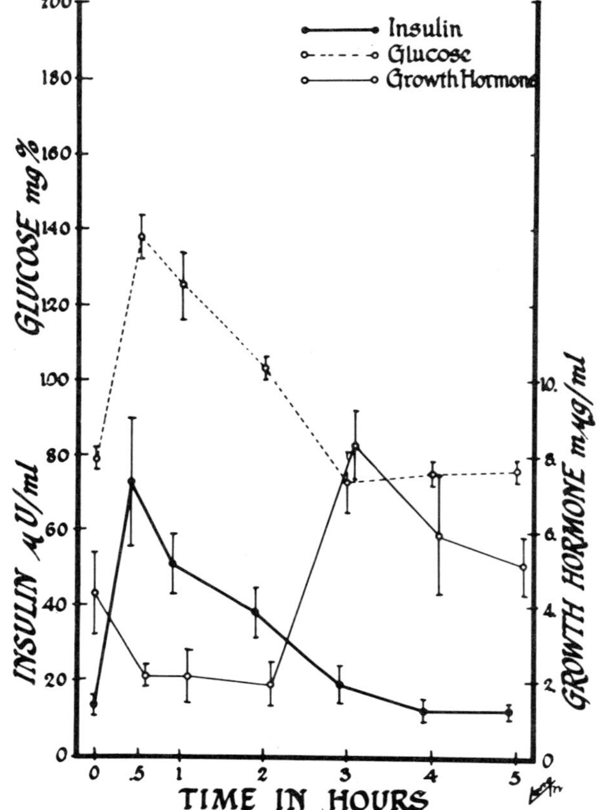

Fig.5 Oral glucose tolerance test. The response of normal children to glucose ingestion showing the variation in glucose, insulin and growth hormone. The values shown are mean ± S.E.M.

between 2 and 3 h post-ingestion during the declining leg of the glucose and insulin curves. Not shown here are the concentration curves for FFA and glucagon. Both are similar to that for growth hormone, initial suppression followed by a rise between 2 and 4 h post-prandially (Lestradet *et al.*, 1976; Sherwin *et al.*, 1976).

The prandial or absorptive period, encompassing the initial 2 to 3 h following food ingestion, is a period of insulin-dominated, glucose metabolism. Basal glucose release from the liver is increased only modestly, leading to the transitory increase in circulating glucose concentration. Based on the studies of Felig *et al.*, (1975c) following oral glucose administration, it appears that only 15% of an oral glucose load reaches the peripheral circulation, the remainder retained, at least initially, within the liver and splanchnic bed. Most of this rise in post-prandial glucose is directed to skeletal muscle to meet the minimal glucose requirements of 10% of basal oxidation, the remainder being derived from FFA (Andres *et al.*, 1956).

Within the liver, insulin directs the metabolism to glycogen and lipid synthesis and storage and glucose oxidation through the TCA cycle to meet current

FASTING MAN

(24 hours, basal : −1800 cal.)

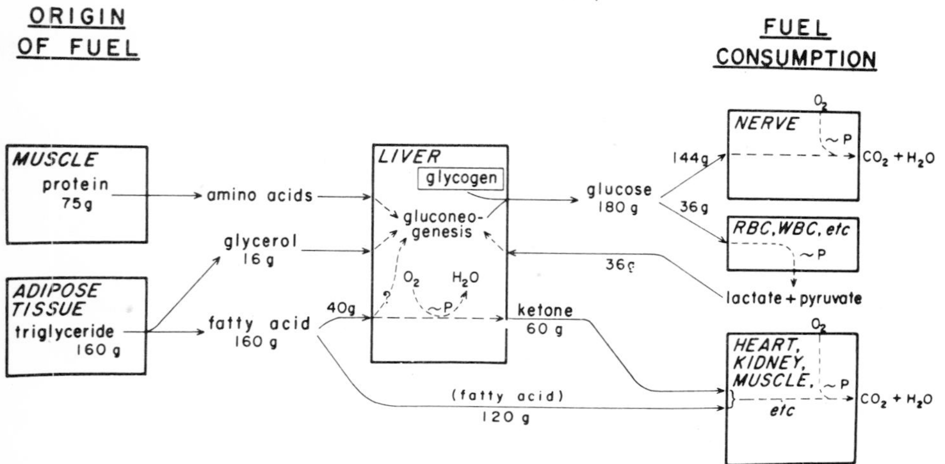

Fig. 6 General scheme of fuel metabolism in a normal fasted man, showing the two primary sources, muscle and adipose tissue, and the three types of fuel consumers, nerve pure glycolyzers (such as the red blood cells and white blood cells) and the remainder of the body composed of heart, kidney and skeletal muscle that use fatty acids and ketones.

energy demands. Peripherally the activation of lipoprotein lipase by insulin insures the clearing of chylomicron with the release of FFA as an immediate energy source or substrate for triglyceride synthesis. The elevation of circulating insulin coupled with the suppression of glucagon and growth hormone provides a situation that maximizes glucose uptake, glycogenesis, glycolysis and lipogenesis while minimizing glycogenolysis, gluconeogenesis, lipolysis and ketogenesis.

At some point between 2 and 3 h post-prandially there is a major change in energy flow. Glucose, which had been the dominant fuel in the prandial period, drops to about 30% and FFA rises to meet 60% of the oxidative requirements. Amino acids remain relatively unimportant as a gluconeogenic source for several hours (Cahill, 1976; Havel, 1972). The process is glucagon (and possibly growth hormone) directed, focusing upon lipolysis to provide FFA for peripheral tissues and glycogenolysis to maintain an adequate glucose production rate in order to meet CNS requirements while stabilizing plasma glucose concentration within normal limits.

Brief Fasting

A period of brief fasting occurs nightly as the interval since the last feeding increases. The transition from the post-absorptive period to early fasting is subtle in terms of both endocrine and biochemical alterations. The declining insulin concentration further removes the brakes on lipolysis, leading to greater than 80% of energy requirements being met by FFA oxidation. The rate of gluconeogenesis increases, resulting from increased protein degradation in muscle, secondary to cortisol increase, and stimulation of the hepatic gluconeogenic enzymes by both glucagon and cortisol. Hepatic glucose production is maintained at the expense of liver and muscle glycogen and muscle protein. The metabolic

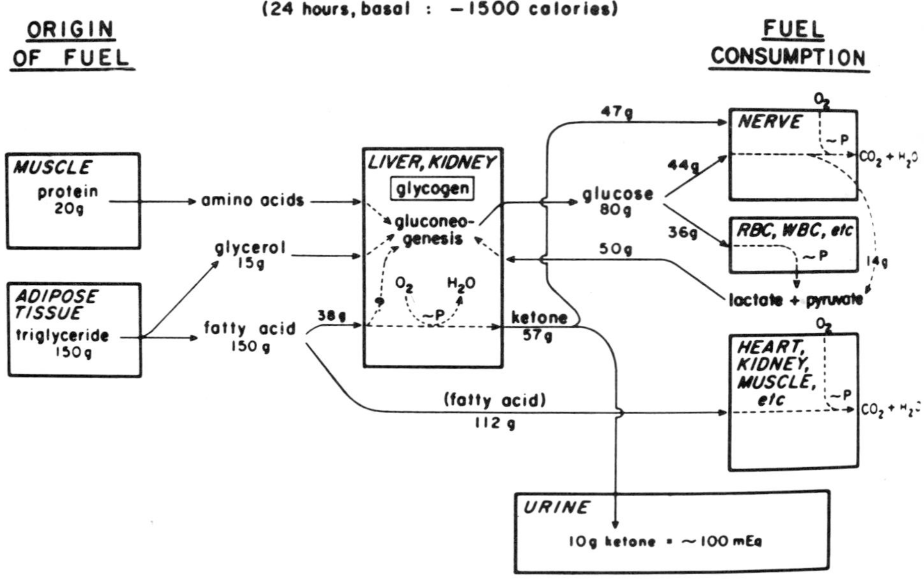

Fig. 7 General scheme of fuel metabolism after five or six weeks of starvation showing the diminished rate of mobilization of muscle protein.

status of early fasting is illustrated in Fig.6 from Cahill (1970).

Prolonged Starvation

Although food deprivation for several days is a rare, if not an unknown event in most of our lives, it is a condition which many of the peoples of the world endure on an ongoing basis. Several major metabolic events occur in the successful adaptation to prolonged starvation as illustrated in Fig.7 from Cahill (1970). Total energy expenditure is reduced. Protein is conserved, the utilization of protein falling from 75 g per day in early starvation to 20 g per day in prolonged starvation. The total utilization of fat decreases modestly, but the proportion of total energy derived from oxidation of fat increases from 85% in early starvation to 95% in prolonged starvation. Hepatic glucose production, derived exclusively from gluconeogenesis, decreases by greater than half. This is possible because CNS utilization of glucose falls dramatically, owing to the highly important cerebral adaptation to ketone oxidation. Further conservation of protein occurs because of increased efficiency of substrate re-cycling through the glucose-alanine cycle (Felig, 1973).

Alanine is the dominant gluconeogenic precursor derived from muscle amino acids despite the fact that alanine comprises no more than 7-10% of the amino acid composition of skeletal muscle (Kominz *et al.*, 1954). The selective "production" of alanine from the muscle amino acid pool is illustrated in Fig.8. The deamination of a number of amino acids, particularly glutamate, can provide the amino group which reacts with pyruvate to form alanine. Pyruvate may be

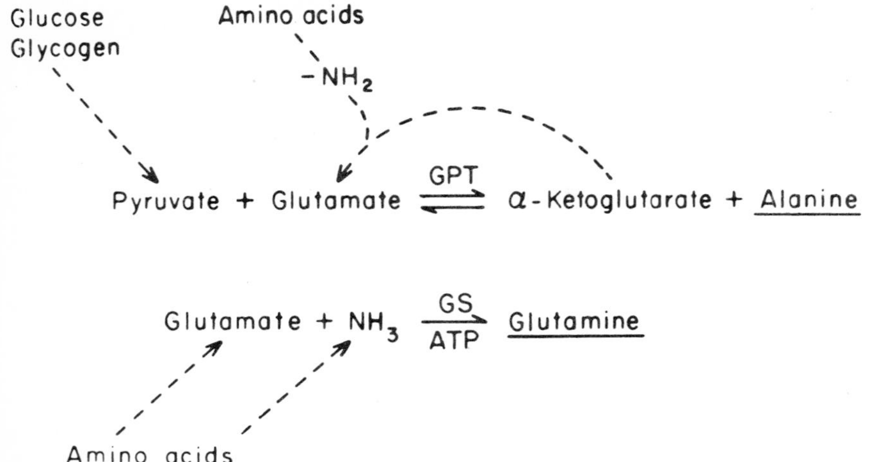

Fig.8 Alanine and glutamine formation in skeletal muscle. GPT equal glutamic pyruvic transaminase; GS equal glutamine synthetase. Alanine formation is favored by an increase in muscle pyruvate or glutamate and glutamine release by an increase in NH_3 or glutamate.

derived from muscle glycogen, circulating glucose or muscle amino acids. The alanine produced in muscle is carried to the liver where the process is reversed, alanine is deaminated to pyruvate which is then used to regenerate glucose. This cycle provides a mechanism for maintaining hepatic glycogen stores while conserving muscle nitrogen. The fact that this occurs is illustrated in Fig.9 (Drash, 1973b). A group of obese adolescents were fasted for two weeks. Some of the patients had mild, asymptomatic carbohydrate intolerance while the remainder had normal carbohydrate metabolism. By converting the change in glucose and insulin following glucagon administration to a single value (glucose in mg/min and insulin in microU/min) it is clear that there is a significant fall in glucose and insulin release after two days on total fasting, but that by 13 days of fasting the responses are essentially back to basal levels, indicating that hepatic glycogen stores have been regenerated.

The conservation of protein which occurs with prolonged starvation results from a declining rate of proteolysis secondary to declining cortisol secretion and to a decrease in effective thyroxine levels (Vagenakis *et al.*, 1975), to increasing efficiency of the glucose-alanine cycle, and to increased lipid mobilization and metabolism.

Exercise

The effects of exercise on energy homeostasis have recently been reviewed by Felig and Wahren (1975). In the resting state less than 10% of the oxygen consumption of muscle is accounted for by glucose oxidation, the remainder resulting from fatty acid oxidation. The changes in muscle metabolism with exercise depend upon the severity and duration of exercise. In the initial phase of exercise preformed muscle glycogen plays a dominant role. As exercise continues beyond ten minutes, blood-borne glucose and fatty acids make up increasing proportions of the energy requirement. Between 40 and 180 min of continuous moderate exer-

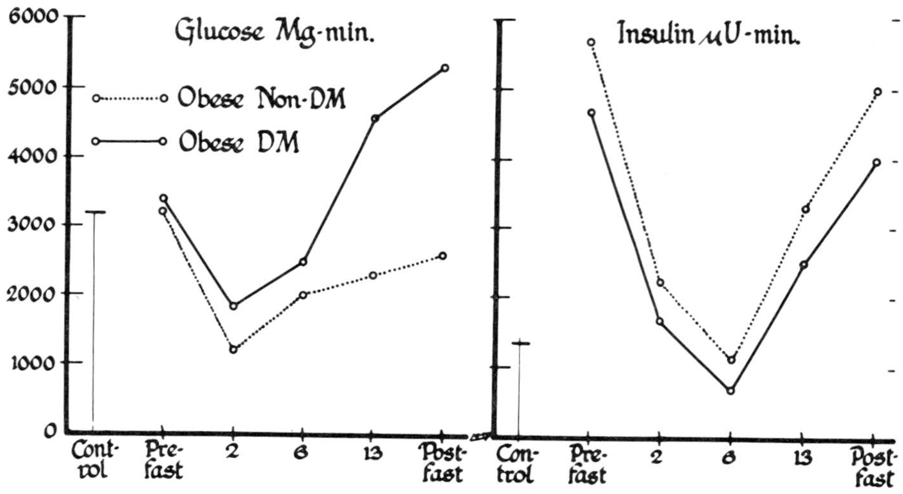

Fig. 9 The effect of intravenous administration of glucagon on plasma glucose and insulin concentration in obese teenagers prior to, during, and after 13 days of total fasting. The incremental changes in glucose and insulin for two hours following glucagon administration are converted by planimetry to single point changes. The incremental changes in glucose and insulin in normal weight adolescent controls are shown at the left of each panel. Initial pre-fast glucose increments in the obese children are similar to controls while the insulin responses are 4-5 times elevated. The dash lines refer to obese, non-diabetic adolescents, while the solid line refers to obese adolescents with mildly symptomatic diabetes mellitus. Glucagon administration was carried out in the pre-fasting state, after 2, 6 and 13 days of total fasting and after three days of re-feeding.

cise there is a linear increase in glucose utilization, achieving a peak of about 40% of total oxygen consumption, after which there is a slow decline in the relative contribution from glucose. Free fatty acid oxidation continues to increase with prolonged exercise, achieving 65% of total oxygen uptake by 4 h.

The glucose uptake by exercise muscle may increase by 20 times that of resting muscle and may reach 90% of total glucose consumption. These changes occur with little or no variation in blood glucose concentration in moderate exercise, a modest increase of 20-30 mg% in severe exercise and some decline in glucose concentration in prolonged exhausting exercise. The stability of glucose concentration under these circumstances results from an increased hepatic glucose production. Under basal conditions hepatic glucose production is about 150 mg per min (2 mg/kg/min), with 75% of the glucose derived from glycogenolysis and 25% for gluconeogenesis. With moderate to severe exercise, hepatic glucose production may increase by 5-fold with almost all of the glucose derived from preformed glycogen. Gluconeogenesis plays a declining role in hepatic glucose production unless exercise is very prolonged. Under these circumstances splanchnic extraction of amino acids and other gluconeogenic substances increases several fold and gluconeogenesis may contribute up to 45% of hepatic glucose production.

The hormonal changes associated with exercise include decline in insulin concentration and increase in the concentration of glucagon, growth hormone, cortisol, epinephrine and nor-epinephrine. The decline in the circulating concentration of insulin releases the "brake" on release of glucose from the liver and FFA from adipose tissue stores. Peripheral glucose uptake, particularly by muscle, increases in spite of the low concentration of insulin because of a factor elaborated by exercising muscle which increases glucose permeability. The effect of increasing levels of glucagon is to promote glycogenolysis from liver and lipolysis from adipose tissue. Glucagon has no demonstrable effect on muscle metabolism. Growth hormone and epinephrine stimulate lipolysis and growth hormone may be involved in the decline in glucose uptake by muscle after 1-2 h of continuous exercise. The stimulation of gluconeogenesis after several hours of exercise is probably controlled by both cortisol and glucagon.

MALADAPTATIONS OF THE ENERGY SYSTEM

It is remarkable that the human organism is readily capable of adapting to variable nutrient sources, intermittent feasting and fasting and extremes of physical exertion. A constant flow of energy is maintained while the concentrations of a number of biochemical factors are controlled within very narrow limits.

The factors responsible for nutrient intake, hunger and satiety, are also at least partially under the control of the endocrine system (Bray and Campfield, 1975). Disorders of the appetite mechanism are common, obesity being one of the most important medical problems of the Western world. Anorexia nervosa, a relatively rare disorder of adolescence, is an excellent example of the relationships between the central nervous system, the endocrine system and the appetite control mechanism.

Malnutrition remains the single most important medical problem in the world today. Chronic malnutrition leads to multiple changes in the endocrine system. These have recently been reviewed by Pimstone (1976) and are beyond the scope of this discussion.

Disorders of energy homeostasis include diabetes mellitus, resulting from insulin deficiency, insulin resistance or excessive production of contra-insulin hormones such as growth hormone, cortisol, glucagon or epinephrine. Hypoglycemic disorders may result from a variety of alterations including hyperinsulinism, deficiencies of growth hormone, cortisol or glucagon, or deficiencies of enzymes essential to glycogenolysis or gluconeogenesis. The hyperlipidemic disorders represent another example of maladaptation of the energy control system.

In the last few years major advances have been achieved in our understanding of the normal physiology of energy control. However, many of the disorders of energy homeostasis remain incompletely defined or are beyond our capability for either cure or adequate control. Further research into the control mechanisms are necessary to improve the diagnosis and management of patients with disorders of energy homeostasis.

ACKNOWLEDGEMENTS

This work was supported by The Renziehausen Fund and U.S. Public Health Service Grant 5M01-RR-0084.

REFERENCES

Andres, R., Cader, C. and Zierler, K.L. (1956). *J. clin. Invest.* **35**, 671-682.

Aoki, T.T., Muller, W.A., Brennan, M.R. and Cahill, G.F. Jr. (1975a). *Am. J. of clin. Nutrit.* **28**, 507-511.

Aoki, T.T., Toews, C.J., Rossini, A.A., Ruderman, N.B. and Cahill, G.F. Jr. (1975b). *Advances in Enzyme Regulation* **13**, 329-336.

Bloom, S.R. (1973). *Postgrad. med. J.* **49**, 607-611.

Bray, G.A. and Campfield, L.A. (1975). *Metabolism* **24**, 99-117.

Brooks, F.P. (1973). *Am. J. clin. Nutrit.* **26**, 291-310.

Brown, J.C., Dryburgh, J.R., Ross, S.A. and Dupre, J. (1975). *Recent Prog. Horm. Res.* **31**, 487-526.

Brazeau, P., Vale, W., Burgus, R., Ling, N., Butcher, M., Rivier, J. and Guillemin, R. (1973). *Science* **179**, 77-79.

Cahill, G.F. Jr. (1970). *New Engl. J. Med.* **282**, 668-675.

Cahill, G.F. Jr. (1971). *Diabetes* **20**, 785-799.

Cahill, G.F. Jr. (1976). *Clinics in Endocrinology and Metabolism* **5**, 397-415.

Day, J.L. (1975). *Metabolism* **24**, 987-996.

Drash, A. (1973a). *Metabolism* **22**, 255-267.

Drash, A. (1973b). *Metabolism* **22**, 337-344.

Eaton, R.P. (1975). *Diabetes* **24**, 523-524.

Ensinck, J.W., Walter, R.M., Palmer, J.P., Brodaws, R.G. and Campbell, R.G. (1976). *Metabolism* **25**, 227-231.

Felig, P. (1975a). *Ann. Rev. Biochem.* **44**, 933-955.

Felig, P. and Wahren, J. (1975b). *New Eng. J. Med.* **293**, 1078-1084.

Felig, P., Wahren, J. and Hendler, R. (1975c). *Diabetes* **24**, 468-475.

Felig, P. (1973d). *Metabolism* **22**, 179-207.

Frohman, L.A. (1975a). *Hospital Practice* 54-67.

Frohman, L.A. and Stachura, M.E. (1975b). *Metabolism* **24**, 211-234.

Galbo, H., Holst, J.J. and Christensen, N.J. (1975). *J. Appl. Physiol.* **38**, 70-76.

Garber, A.J., Cryger, P.E., Santiago, J.V., Haymond, M.W., Pagliara, A.S. and Kipnis, D.M. (1976). *J. clin. Invest.* **58**, 7-15.

Garces, L., Kenny, F., Drash, A. and Taylor, F. (1968). *J. clin. Endocr. Metab.* **28**, 1843-1847.

Gerich, J.E., Lorenzi, M., Hane, S., Gustafson, G., Guillemin, R. and Forsham, P.H. (1975a). *Metabolism* **24**, 175-182.

Gerich, J.E., Lorenzi, M., Bier, D.M., Schneider, V., Tsalikian, E., Karam, J.H. and Forsham, P.H. (1975b). *New Eng. J. Med.* **292**, 985-989.

Grey, N.J., Kane, I. and Kipnis, D.M. (1975). *Diabetes* **24**, 10-16.

Havel, R.J. (1972). *New Eng. J. Med.* **287**, 1186-1192.

Haymond, M.W., Kane, I., Weldon, V.V. and Pagliara, A.S. (1976). *J. clin. Endocr. Metab.* **42**, 846-856.

Hopwood, N.J., Forsman, P.J., Kenny, F.M. and Drash, A.L. (1975). *Am. J. Dis. Child.* **129**, 918-926.

Johnson, L.R. (1976). *Gastroenterology* **70**, 278-288.

Koerker, D.J., Rvch, W., Chideckel, E., Palmer, J., Goodner, C.J., Ensenck, J. and Gale, C.C. (1974). *Science* **184**, 482-483.

Kominz, D.R., Hough, A., Symond, P. and Laki, K. (1954). *Arch. Biochem. Biophys.* **50**, 148-159.

Krebs, H.A. (1964). "Mammalian Protein Metabolism" (H.N. Munro and J.H. Allison, eds) **1**, 125-176. New York, Academic Press.

Lestradet, H., Deschamps, I. and Giron, B. (1976). *Diabetes* **25**, 505-508.

McGarry, J.D., Wright, P. and Foster, D. (1975). *J. clin. Invest.* **55**, 1202-1209.

Olson, R.E. (1975). *Am. J. clin. Nutrit.* **28**, 626-637.

Parrilla, R., Goodman, M.N. and Toews, C.J. (1974). *Diabetes* **23**, 725-731.

Pimstone B. (1976). *Clin. Endocrinol.* **5**, 79-95.

Porte, D., Jr., Graber, A., Kuzuya, T. and Williams, R.H. (1966). *J. clin. Invest.* **42**, 228-236.

Pozefsky, T., Tanenedi, R.G., Moxley, R.T., Dupre, J. and Tobin, J. (1976). *Diabetes* **25**, 128-135.

Raptis, S., Dollinger, H.C., Schroder, K.E., Schleyer, M., Rothenbuchner, G. and Pfeiffer, E.F. (1973). *New Eng. J. Med.* **288**, 1199-1202.
Rayford, P.L., Miller, T.A. and Thompson, J.C. (1976). *New Eng. J. Med.* **294**, 1093-1101.
Ruderman, N.B. (1975). *Ann. Rev. Med.* **26**, 245-258.
Schade, D.S. and Eaton, R.P. (1975a). *J. clin. Invest.* **56**, 1340-1344.
Schade, D.S. and Eaton, R.P. (1975b). *Diabetes* **24**, 502-515.
Sherwin, R.S., Fisher, M., Hendler, R. *et al.* (1976). *New Eng. J. Med.* **294**, 455-461.
Thomas, F.B., Mazzaferri, E.L., Crockett, S.E., Mekhjian, H.S., Gruemer, H.D. and Cataland, S. (1976). *Gastroenterology* **70**, 523-527.
Unger, R.H. (1976). *Diabetes* **25**, 136-151.
Vagenakis, A.G., Burger, A., Portnoy, G.I., Rudolph, M., O'Brien, J.T., Azizi, F., Arky, R.A., Nirod, P., Ingbar, S.H. and Braverman, L.E. (1975). *J. clin. Endocr. Metab.* **41**, 191-194.
Vale, W., Brazeau, P., Rivier, C., Brown, M., Boss, B., Rivier, J., Burgus, R., Ling, N. and Guillemin, R. (1975). *Rec. Prog. Horm. Res.* **31**, 365-392.
Woods, S.C. and Porte, D., Jr. (1974). *Physiol. Rev.* **54**, 596-619.

RELATION OF GLUCAGON SECRETION TO GLUCOSE HOMEOSTASIS IN THE PERINATAL PERIOD

M.A. Sperling

Department of Pediatrics, University of California, Los Angeles School of Medicine, Harbor General Hospital Campus, Torrance, USA

INTRODUCTION

Several important adaptations characterize the orderly transition from intra-uterine to extra-uterine life. Although the subject of considerable research, the factors involved in maintaining glucose homeostasis during this critical period are not entirely understood. In an attempt to gain some insight into glucose homeostasis during perinatal life, we have focused our attention on the potential contribution of hormones, specifically glucagon. This hormone stimulates glycogenolysis (Cahill *et al.*, 1957), gluconeogenesis (Exton, 1972), and also ketogenesis (McGarry *et al.*, 1975) and therefore could be considered a prime candidate in initiating autonomous glucose production following curtailment of nutrient supply via the placenta. Our studies were facilitated by the development of radioimmunoassay systems which permitted measurement of circulating pancreatic glucagon (Sperling *et al.*, 1974a), and through the use of a model, the fetal and newborn lamb. This newborn animal, unlike its adult counterpart, is not a ruminant and, while not ideal has served as a very useful model for studies of perinatal glucose homeostasis (James *et al.*, 1972; Tsoulos *et al.*, 1972; Fiser *et al.*, 1974a; Char and Creasy, 1976a). Where possible we also performed studies in human newborns (Sperling *et al.*, 1974b; Williams *et al.*, 1975a; Fiser *et al.*, 1975; Asch *et al.*, 1975). These studies provided strong presumptive evidence that glucagon does indeed participate significantly in perinatal glucose homeostasis and, supplemented by other published investigations, form the basis of this report.

IN UTERO

A progressive increase in pancreatic glucagon content has been noted by several investigators (Assan and Boillot, 1971; Schaeffer *et al.*, 1973). Similarly, there appears to be progressive maturation of glucagon secretion; in the lamb *in utero* plasma concentrations late in gestation are consistently higher than early in gestation (Fiser *et al.*, 1974b). The infusion of glucose does not suppress plasma glucagon concentration in the fetal lamb, monkey, or rat (Fiser *et al.*, 1974b; Chez *et al.*, 1974; Girard *et al.*, 1974), nor does acute hypoglycemia stimulate secretion (Girard *et al.*, 1974). In contrast, amino acids (Chez *et al.*, 1974; Girard *et al.*, 1974; Wise *et al.*, 1973), prolonged hypoglycemia (Girard *et al.*, 1974), norepinephrine (Girard *et al.*, 1974) and acetylcholine (Girard *et al.*, 1974) are all capable of stimulating glucagon secretion in the fetus. Thus, although glucagon secretion is ongoing and capable of further simulation, plasma concentrations of glucagon do not appear to be affected by acute changes in glucose, the substrate known to exert major control of glucagon secretion in the adult (Unger, 1974). Factors modulating glucagon secretion *in utero* are summarized in Table I. Whether glucagon has any physiological role *in-utero* is unclear. It is known that direct infusion of glucagon into the fetal monkey late in gestation raises plasma glucose concentrations (Chez *et al.*, 1974), implying that glycogenolytic mechanisms can be activated. This effect is mediated via cyclic AMP as demonstrated in explants of rat fetal liver (Sherline *et al.*, 1974). A variety of other effects, including activation of gluconeogenesis from alanine (Schwartz and Rall, 1975), DNA synthesis in the liver (Yeoh and Oliver, 1974), acceleration of the appearance of enzymes involved in gluconeogenesis such as phosphoenolpyruvate carboxykinase and tyrosine aminotransferase have been described (Greengard, 1973; Yeung and Oliver, 1968; Kirby and Hahn, 1974), but only in response to pharmacological, and not physiological doses of glucagon. Thus, the applicability of these findings to physiology is highly questionable.

Table I. Factors modulating fetal glucagon secretion.

Agent	Effect of Glucagon Secretion	Species	Reference
Glucose			
Hyperglycemia	Lack of Suppression	Lamb, Monkey, Rat	Fiser *et al.* (1974b); Chez *et al.* (1974); Girard *et al.* (1974)
Acute Hypoglycemia	Lack of Stimulation	Rat	Girard *et al.* (1974)
Prolonged Hypoglycemia	Stimulation	Rat	Girard *et al.* (1974)
Amino Acid	Stimulation	Monkey, Rat, Human	Chez *et al.* (1974); Girard *et al.* (1974) Wise *et al.* (1973)
Norepinephrine	Stimulation	Rat	Girard *et al.* (1974)
Acetyl Choline	Stimulation	Rat	Girard *et al.* (1974)

Table II. Effect of alanine infusion in mothers during labor on maternal and neonatal glucose and glucagon.

	Glucose, mg/100 ml	Glucagon, pg/ml
Mother		
Control	82 ± 4	96 ± 19
Post-Alanine	93 ± 4*	215 ± 26*
Infant (umbilical vein at delivery)		
Control	56 ± 3	89 ± 14
Post-Alanine	82 ± 14*	231 ± 45*

All values are mean ± SEM. * indicates significant difference from the control when saline was infused. Adapted from Wise, J.K. *et al.* (1973). *J. clin. Endocr.* **37**, 345.

On the other hand, indirect evidence assigns a significant role. In humans at term infusion of alanine to mothers in labor raised maternal as well as neonatal umbilical cord plasma concentrations of glucagon and glucose (Wise *et al.*, 1973) (Table II). And since glucagon does not cross the placenta (Chez *et al.*, 1974; Johnson *et al.*, 1972; Sperling *et al.*, 1973) while amino acids do cross, the findings imply that at term physiological increments in fetal plasma glucagon concentration can rapidly modify plasma glucose concentrations. Further support for an active role of glucagon in glucose homeostasis comes from studies in the immediate post-natal period.

THE IMMEDIATE NEONATAL PERIOD

A. *Humans*

Figure 1 illustrates the spontaneous changes occurring in full-term newborn infants with regard to glucose, glucagon and insulin. In this study (Sperling, 1974b) glucose declined from 77 ± 6 mg/dl (mean ± SEM) to 57 ± 5 mg/dl ($p < 0.02$). Immunoreactive plasma glucagon (IRG) rose from 225 ± 26 pg/ml to 355 ± 52 pg/ml ($p < 0.05$) within 2 h. These reciprocal changes in glucose and glucagon were significantly correlated ($r = -0.73$, $p < 0.01$). Similar changes in humans have been reported by others (Bloom and Johnston, 1972). After 12 h, the changes in IRG shown in Fig.1 reflect glucagon-like immunoreactivity derived presumably from the gut, since in these early studies a non-specific glucagon antiserum was employed. Moreover, when these samples were measured by the more specific antiserum, no significant correlation was evident (Table III). However, in separate sequential studies the early surge in IRG was confirmed and a second rise in IRG identified (Sperling *et al.*, 1974b). This second rise (Fig.2) occurred between day 1 and day 3 of life and was correlated to the restoration of glucose to normal concentrations. It is striking that throughout these first days plasma immunoreactive insulin (IRI) concentrations remain low. This relationship of low IRI with relatively high IRG secretion persists when perturbations are introduced. Thus, amino acids such as arginine or alanine evoke a greater response in IRG than IRI (Sperling *et al.*, 1974b) (Fig.3), and in addition intravenous administration of alanine also evokes a small but significant increment in glucose (Sperling *et al.*, 1974b). In contrast, glucose infusion does not suppress IRG nor does glucose readily promote IRI secretion in normal newborn infants (Luyckx *et al.*, 1972). Consequently, the situation in the newborn vis-à-vis insulin and glucagon

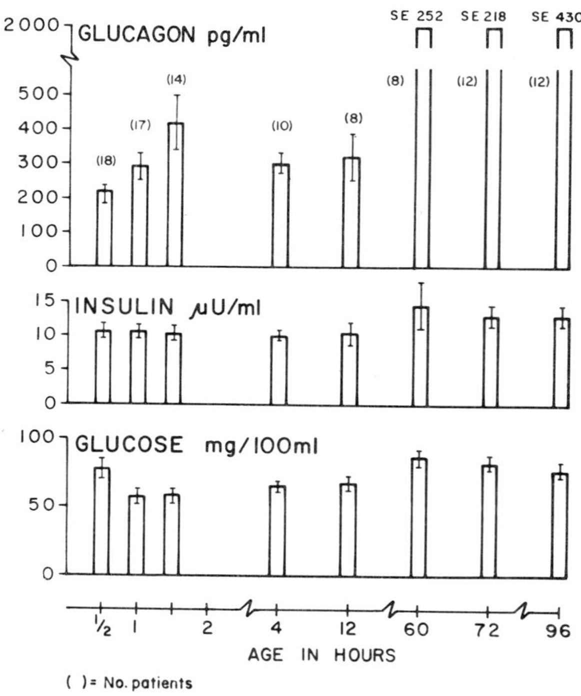

Fig.1 Cross-sectional studies showing the spontaneous changes in immunoreactive glucagon, insulin, and glucose in the postnatal period. The vertical lines indicate 1 SEM. The numbers of patients are in parentheses. From Sperling, M.A. *et al.* (1974b).

interrelations resembles the situation in diabetes mellitus, were relative hyperglucagonemia in the presence of insulinopenia has been considered a major contributing factor to hyperglycemia (Dodds *et al.*, 1975) and also to promote ketogenesis (McGarry *et al.*, 1975; Gerich *et al.*, 1975a). And similar to diabetes, glucose administered concurrently with insulin will suppress IRG in normal infants (Massi-Benedetti *et al.*, 1974). Although this hormonal profile in the newborn is transient, it could be important to augment glycogenolysis and enhance gluconeogenesis, as recently demonstrated in the newborn puppy (Adam *et al.*, 1975).

If the neonatal surge in IRG has significance in maintaining glucose homeostasis, then suppression of IRG secretion should be associated with hypoglycemia. A significant reduction in the spontaneous IRG surge with simultaneously higher plasma IRI levels occurs in infants of diabetic mothers (Fig.4). Moreover, in contrast to normal infants, intravenous alanine does not cause a rise in glucose or glucagon (Fig.5). Since infants of diabetic mothers are prone to hypoglycemia, it seems reasonable to suggest that relative glucagon deficiency contributes to their disordered glucose homeostasis (Bloom and Johnston, 1972; Williams *et al.*,

Table III. **Comparison of total immunoreactive glucagon and pancreatic glucagon concentrations in plasma of ten normal human infants.***

Infant	Hours After Birth	Cross-Reacting Antibody (GL-1)	Specific Antibody (GL-5)
1	1	260	280
2	15	715	435
3	60	2325	400
4	60	3400	100
5	72	3350	87
6	72	2700	450
7	96	2200	480
8	96	5000	600
9	96	5000	600
10	120	5000	305

Coefficient of correlation r = 0.27, p > 0.1. Glucagon in pg/ml. *Infants delivered normally without complications. Neonatal course uneventful.

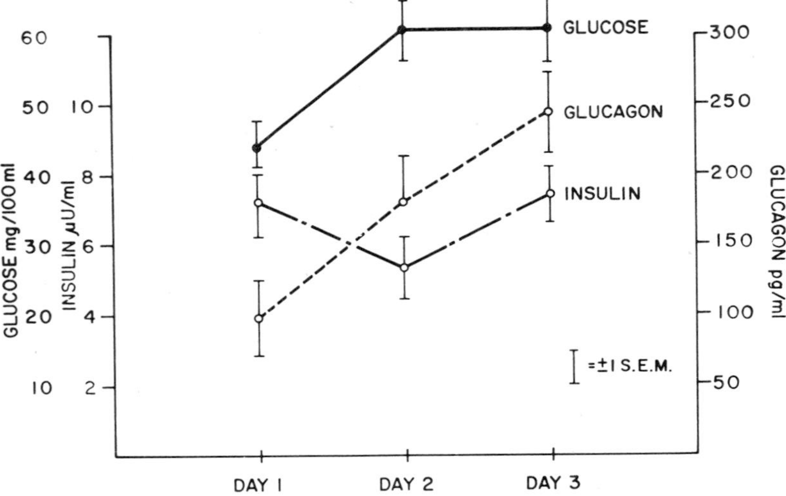

Fig. 2 Sequential changes in glucose, glucagon, and insulin in eight infants each of whom was sampled at approximately 24, 48, and 72 h after birth. The increments in glucose and glucagon are significantly correlated (r = 1.0; p < 0.01). From Sperling, M.A. *et al.* (1974b).

1975b). Moreover, the obtunded rise in IRG in infants of diabetic mothers during the first hours of life occurs despite a greater fall in glucose during this time. And infusion of glucose to infants of diabetic mothers causes further suppression of IRG with stimulation of IRI (Luyckx *et al.*, 1972). Thus in humans, presumptive evidence assigns a significant role for the neonatal glucagon surge in maintenance of glucose homeostasis. More direct evidence is provided from animal experiments.

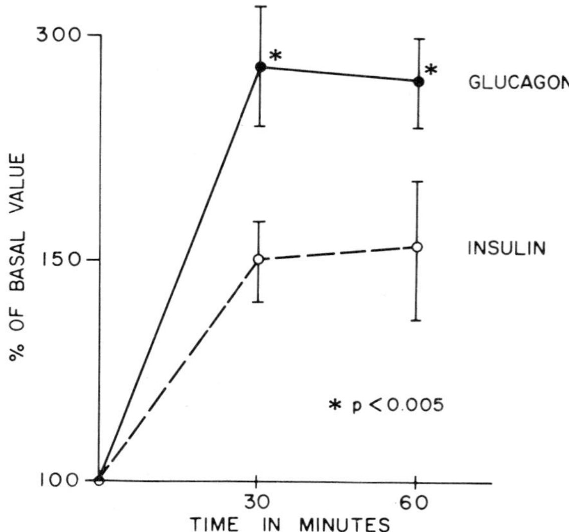

Fig.3 Effect of intravenous infusion of arginine on plasma insulin and glucagon concentrations in newborn babies less than 6 h of age. Infused and sampled via an umbilical vein catheter. From Sperling, M.A. *et al.* (1974b).

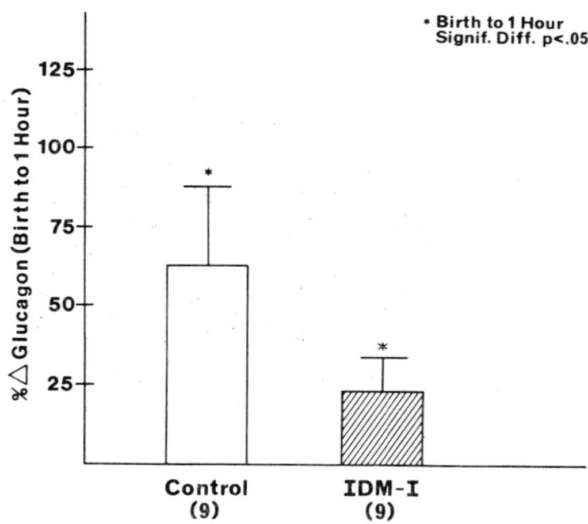

Fig.4 The change in plasma glucagon at one hour of life expressed as the percent of the value at birth in umbilical vein blood in normal full-term infants (control) and infants born to insulin-dependent diabetic mothers (IDM-I). From Williams *et al.* (1975b).

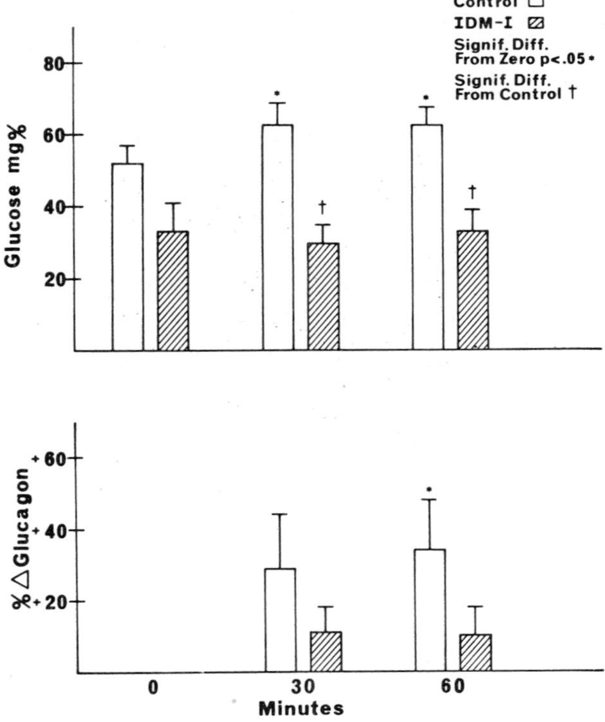

Fig.5 The effect of infusing alanine (1 mM/kg) at one hour of life (0 time) on subsequent plasma glucose and glucagon in normal full-term infants (control) and infants of insulin dependent diabetic mothers (IDM-I). From Williams *et al.* (1975b).

B, Animals

A dramatic, four-fold surge in immunoreactive glucagon occurs in newborn rabbits and rats (Assan, 1974). Similarly we have shown that a surge in IRG also occurs following delivery in the newborn lamb (Fig.6). It should be noted that it is separation of the cord rather than delivery and removal from the intra-uterine environment that is followed within minutes by increased plasma concentrations of IRG. Since the placental space represents approximately one half the distribution volume, simple redistribution could account for only a doubling of plasma concentrations rather than the observed four-fold increase. Therefore increased secretion must be taking place shortly after delivery.

The stimulus to this newborn surge in IRG is not entirely clear. Because the newborn rise in IRG is associated with a fall in blood glucose in the human (Sperling *et al.*, 1974b) and rat (Assan *et al.*, 1974; Girard *et al.*, 1973), it was suggested that hypoglycemia was the dominant stimulus. However, in newborn lambs, plasma glucose does not fall during this period, and free fatty acids (FFA) rise (Fig.7). Therefore, unless a nutrient other than glucose or FFA, for example acetate (Char and Creasy, 1976b) is a major source of fuel *in utero*, so that interruption in its transplacental supply after cord cutting stimulates IRG, a different mechanism must be invoked as the major stimulus. Activation of catecholamine

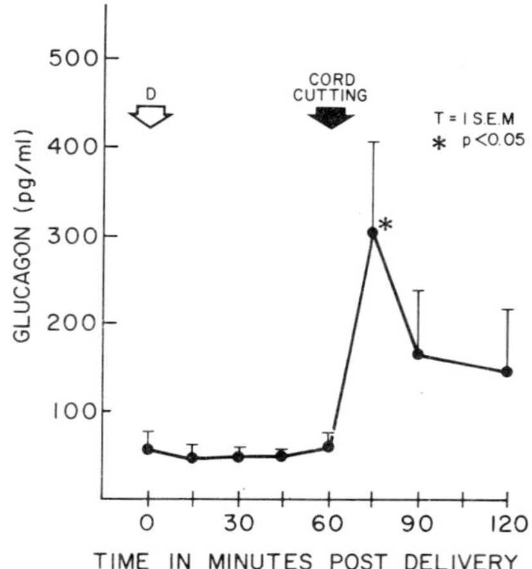

Fig. 6 Effect of delivery (D) and umbilical cord cutting on plasma glucagon concentration in newborn lambs.

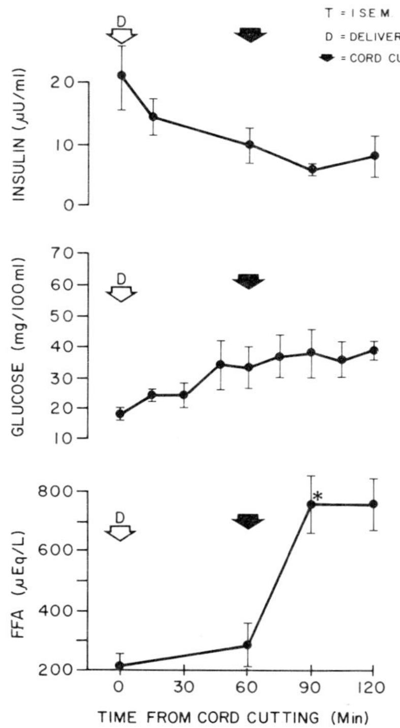

Fig. 7 Effect of delivery (D) and umbilical cord cutting on plasma insulin, glucose and free fatty acids (FFA) in newborn lambs. Note there is no fall in glucose, whereas FFA rise rapidly following cord cutting. Adapted from Sack *et al.* (1976).

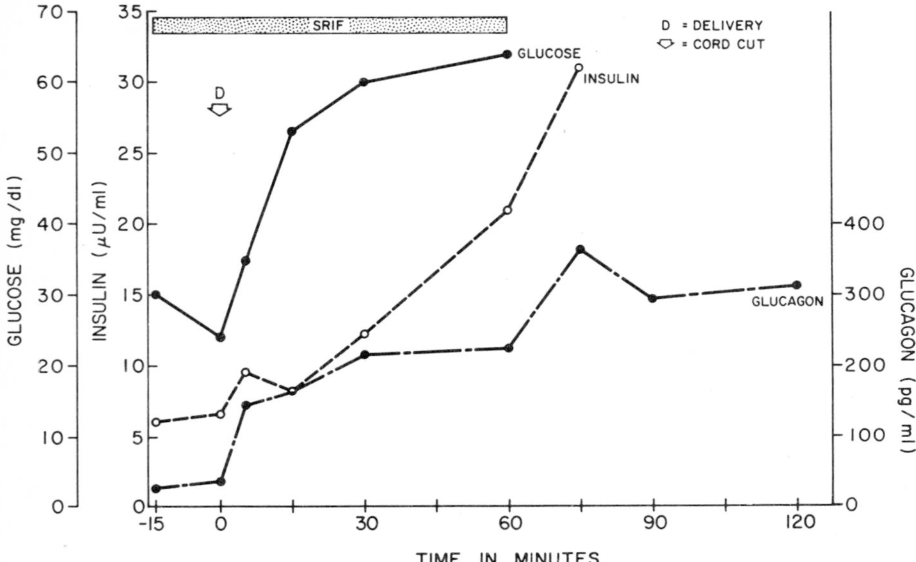

Fig. 8 Changes in glucose, insulin and glucagon in newborn lambs following delivery and immediate umbilical cord cutting. Note that a rise in glucagon is not prevented by somatostatin (SRIF) infusion begun *in utero.* Moreover, insulin and glucose rise in contrast to the normal (see Figs 6 and 7).

secretion consequent upon cord cutting could be such a stimulus (Sack *et al.*, 1976). Epinephrine and norepinephrine are capable of stimulating glucagon, suppressing IRI via stimulation of alpha-adrenergic receptors and mobilizing FFA (Woods and Porte, 1974). Since the hypothalamic peptide somatostatin (SRIF) when given in doses sufficient to inhibit growth hormone secretion will not prevent catecholamine secretion (Christensen *et al.*, 1975), we infused SRIF into fetal lambs *in utero* prior to delivery, and for one hour after delivery by Caesarean section. The glucagon surge was not prevented, and it was not significantly less than the spontaneous surge without SRIF (Fig.8).

The availability of SRIF, an inhibitor of the secretion of a number of hormones including insulin and glucagon (Vale *et al.*, 1975), provides a tool with which to explore the significance and contribution of each hormone in glucose homeostasis (Gerich *et al.*, 1975b). By infusing SRIF the effects on glucose when both insulin and glucagon are suppressed can be examined, re-infusion of either hormone at doses designed to achieve physiological concentrations in plasma while SRIF infusion continues permits examination of the contribution of that hormone. We have used this approach in fasting newborn lambs aged 24 to 72 h. Figure 9 and Table IV demonstrate that infusion of SRIF as a bolus of 50 μg followed by 200 μg per hour for 2 h caused a prompt and sustained fall in the plasma concentration of IRG and IRI, as long as only SRIF was infused. With the concentrations of both hormones suppressed, plasma glucose fell. Re-infusion of glucagon (Table IV) restored plasma glucose toward normal. Thus, glucagon appears to be critically important for maintaining fasting glucose

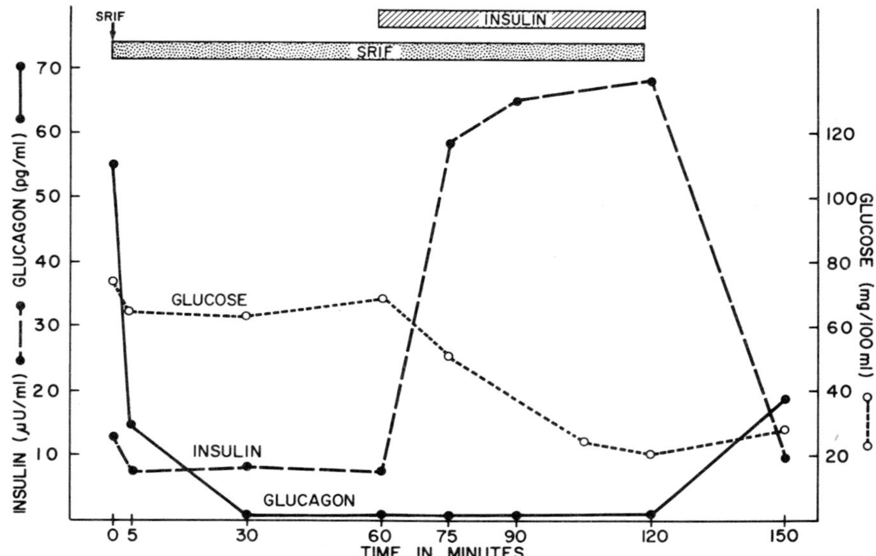

Fig.9 Effect of SRIF on plasma glucose, insulin and glucagon in fasting lambs aged one to three days. Note that all parameters fall during infusion of SRIF only. Re-infusion of insulin (0.1 U/kg/h) results in profound hypoglycemia when insulin peaks at 70 μU/ml and glucagon remains suppressed.

Table IV. Changes during SRIF and glucagon infusion.

Minutes	0–5	0–30	0–60	60–90	60–120	120–150
ΔGlucagon, pg/ml	–43	–46	–52	342	292	–105
± SEM	8	9	8	92	123	40
	(7)	(7)	(6)	(7)	(7)	(7)
	**	**	**	**		*
ΔInsulin, uU/ml	–9.0	–11.7	–7.8	6.8	19.7	11.2
± SEM	2	2	3	4	7	7
	(8)	(8)	(7)	(8)	(7)	(8)
	**	**	*		*	
ΔGlucose, mg/dl	–6.3	–3.3	–9.0	10.4	13.0	–16.5
± SEM	3.4	7.6	3.5	6.3	9.6	4.25
	(7)	(7)	(6)	(7)	(7)	(6)**

( ) number of animals. * $p < 0.05$. ** $p < 0.01$. Studies in fasting lambs aged one to three days. SRIF was infused as a bolus of 50 μg followed by 200 μg/h from 0 to 120 min. Glucagon was infused at 5 ng/kg/min from 60 to 120 min. Note the change (Δ) in each parameter is recorded.

concentration since a suppressed plasma concentration of IRI would be expected to result in hyperglycemia, as occurs in diabetes mellitus (Dobbs *et al.*, 1975). Cessation of glucagon and SRIF infusion at 2 h resulted in a fall in plasma IRG concentration and a rebound in plasma IRI concentration (Table IV). This reversal in the relation of IRI and IRG concentrations is again associated with a significant fall in plasma glucose. When insulin was infused during the second hour, while IRG remained suppressed, profound hypoglycemia resulted (Fig.9). Recovery of glucose occurred only when infusion ceased, plasma IRI concentration fell and IRG rose.

These results provide compelling evidence that glucagon participates significantly in maintaining fasting plasma glucose concentrations and that the prevailing ratio of insulin and glucagon modulate glucose concentration in the newborn lamb. The universality of the observed spontaneous surge in plasma IRG following delivery, while insulin remains suppressed, also suggests that these phenomena are important adaptive events permitting the initiation of normal glucose homeostasis. A theoretical but highly likely chain of events following delivery would depend on the release of catecholamines. These would stimulate glucagon, suppress insulin and mobilize FFA. As a result, glycogenolysis would proceed and gluconeogenesis would be initiated. Low insulin concentrations would limit peripheral glucose utilization making it available for brain where glucose metabolism is insulin-independent. The availability of FFA and the prevailing hormone concentrations would stimulate hepatic ketogenesis and provide fuel for muscle metabolism. Glucagon would thus play a key role in neonatal glucose homeostasis. And disturbances in any of the above steps could result in abnormal glucose homeostasis. One additional maturational step involves the hepatic receptor for glucagon. As recently demonstrated in the rat (Blazquez *et al.*, 1976), the binding of glucagon and generation of cyclic AMP by liver membranes increases in the postnatal period. This observation would explain the apparent increased effectiveness of a given dose of glucagon on day 3 as opposed to day 1 of life (Reisner *et al.*, 1973).

ACKNOWLEDGEMENT

This work was supported by Research Career Development Award 1K04 HD 00029 from the United States Public Health Service.

REFERENCES

Adam, P.A.H., Glazer, G. and Rogoff, F. (1975). *Pediat. Res.* **9**, 816-820.

Asch, M.D., Leake, R., Sperling, M.A., Fiser, R.H., Oh, W. and Moore, T.C. (1975). *Ann. Surg.* **182**, 62-65.

Assan, R., Boillot, J. (1971). *In* "Metabolic Processes in the Fetus and Newborn Infant", pp. 218-219. Williams and Wilkins Company, Baltimore.

Assan, R., Attali, J.R., Ballerio, G., Girard, J.R. *et al.* (1974). *In* "Diabetes" (W.J. Malaisse and J. Pirart, eds) pp.144-179. Excerpta Medica, Amsterdam.

Blazquez, E., Rubalcava, B., Montesano, R., Orci, L.K. and Unger, R.H. (1976). *Endocrinology* **98**, 1014.

Bloom, S.R. and Johnston, D.K. (1972). *Br. med. J.* **4**, 453-454.

Cahill, G.F., Jr., Zottu, S. and Earle, A.L. (1957). *Endocrinology* **60**, 265.

Char, V.C. and Creasy, R.K. (1976a). *Pediat. Res.* **10**, 231.

Char, V.C. and Creasy, R.K. (1976b). *Am. J. Physiol.* **230**, 357.

Chez, R.A., Mintz, D.H., Epstein, M.F. (1974). *Am. J. Obstet. Gynec.* **120**, 690-696.

Christensen, N.J., Christensen, S.E., Hansen, A.P. and Lundbaek, K. (1975). *Metabolism* **24**, 1267.

Dobbs, R., Sakurai, H., Sasaki, H., Faloona, G., Valverde, I., Baetens, D., Orci, L. and Unger, R. (1975). *Science* **187**, 544-547.

Exton, J.L. (1972). *Metabolism* **21**, 945.

Fiser, R.H., Jr., Phelps, D.L., Williams, P.R., Sperling, M.A., Fisher, D.A. and Oh, W. (1974a). *Am. J. Obstet. Gynec.* **120**, 944-950.

Fiser, R.H., Erenberg, A., Sperling, M.A. and Fisher, D.A. (1974b). *Pediat. Res.* **8**, 951-955.

Fiser, R.H., Williams, P.R., Fisher, D.A., DeLamater, P.V., Sperling, M.A. and Oh, W. (1975). *Pediatrics* **56**, 78-81.

Gerich, J.E., Lorenzi, M., Bier, D.M., Schneider, V., Tsalikian, E., Karam, J.H. and Forsham, P.H. (1975a). *New Engl. J. Med.* **292**, 985-989.

Gerich, J.E., Lorenzi, M., Hame, S., Gustafson, G., Guillemin, R. and Forsham, P.H. (1975b). *Metabolism* **24**, 175.

Girard, J.R., Cuendet, G.S., Marliss, E.B., Kervran, A., Rieutort, M. and Assan, R. (1973). *J. clin. Invest.* **52**, 3190.

Girard, J.R., Kervran, A., Soufflet, E. and Assan, R. (1974). *Diabetes* **23**, 310-317.

Greengard, O. (1973). *Clin. Pharmacol. Ther.* **14**, 721-726.

James, E.J., Raye, J.R., Gresham, E.L., Makowski, H.L., Meschia, G. and Battaglia, F.C. (1972). *Pediatrics* **50**, 361.

Johnston, D.I., Bloom, S.R., Greene, K.R. and Beard, R.W. (1972). *Biol. Neonate* **21**, 375-380.

Kirby, L. and Hahn, R. (1974). *Pediat. Res.* **8**, 37-41.

Luyckx, A.A., Massi-Benedetti, F., Falorni, A. and Lefebvre, P.H. (1972). *Diabetologia* **8**, 296-300.

Massi-Benedetti, F., Falorni, A., Luyckx,,A. and Lefebvre, P. (1974). *Horm. Metab. Res.* **6**, 392-396.

McGarry, J.D., Wright, P.H. and Foster, D.W. (1975). *J. clin. Invest.* **55**, 1202.

Reisner, S.H., Aranda, J.V., Colle, E. *et al.* (1973). *Pediat. Res.* 7, 184-191.

Sack, J., Beaudry, M., DeLamater, P.V., Oh., W. and Fisher, D.A. (1976). *Pediat. Res.* **10**, 169.

Schaeffer, L.D., Wilder, M.L. and Williams, R.H. (1973). *Proc. Soc. exp. Biol. Med.* **143**, 314-319.

Schwartz, A.L. and Rall, T.W. (1975). *Diabetes* **24**, 650-657.

Sherline, P., Eisen, H. and Glinsman, W. (1974). *Endocrinology* **94**, 935-939.

Sperling, M.A., Erenberg, A., Fiser, R.H., Oh, W. and Fisher, D.A. (1973). *Endocrinology* **93**, 1435-1438.

Sperling, M.A., DeLamater, P.V., Fiser, R.H., Fisher, D.A. and Kazenelson, M. (1974a). *Clin. Chem.* **20**, 566-570.

Sperling, M.A., DeLamater, P.V., Phelps, D., Fiser, R.H., Oh, W. and Fisher, D.A. (1974b). *J. clin. Invest.* **53**, 1159-1166.

Tsoulos, N.G., Colwill, J.R., Battaglia, F.C., Makowski, E.L. and Meschia, G. (1972). *Am. J. Physiol.* **221**, 234.

Unger, R.H. (1974). *Metab. (Clin. Exp.)* **23**, 581-593.

Vale, W., Brazeau, P., Rivier, C., Brown, M., Boss, B., Rivier, J., Burgus, R., Ling, N., Guillemin, R. (1975). *Rec. Prog. Horm. Res.* **31**, 365-397.

Williams, P.R., Fiser, R.H., Sperling, M.A. and Oh, W. (1975a). *New Eng. J. Med.* **292**, 612-614.

Williams, P.R., Sperling, M.A. and Racasa, Z. (1975b). *Diabetes* **(Suppl.2) 24**, 411.

Wise, J.K., Hendler, R. and Felig, P. (1973). *J. clin. Endocr. Metab.* **37**, 345-348.

Woods, C. and Porte, D., Jr. (1974). *Physiol. Rev.* **54**, 596.

Yeoh, G.C.T. and Oliver, I.T. (1974). *Eur. J. Biochem.* **34**, 474-478.

Yeung, D. and Oliver, I.T. (1968). *Biochem. J.* **108**, 325-331.

REGULATION OF INSULIN AND GH SECRETION IN HUMAN FOETUS AND NEWBORN

G. Reitano*, S. Grasso**, G. Distefano*, A. Messina†, G. Palumbo†† and R. Vigo*

**Department of Pediatrics, **Morbid Anatomy, †General Pathology, ††Obstetrics and Gynecology, University of Catania, Italy*

FOETAL INSULIN SECRETION DURING EARLY GESTATION

After the 10th week of gestation the human foetal pancreas contains insulin, which rises during pregnancy to much above adult level, being 12.7 ± 3.2** U/g between 34 and 40 weeks of gestation whereas in the adult it is 2.1 ± 0.33** U/g (Steinke and Driscoll, 1965; Rastogi *et al.*, 1970a). Van Assche (1970) calculated that the relative amount of islet tissues of 40 normal foetuses, 20 weeks old or more is 5.1 ± 1.6%* (range from 1.9 to 9.8) which is considerably higher than the mean value of 1.5% of the human adult pancreas. The average ratio of beta cells in the same foetuses is 40 ± 7%* (range from 27 to 57) and is lower than that of normal adults. Plasma insulin can be detected by the 14th or 16th week of gestation. Neither maternal nor foetal insulin cross the placenta (Adam *et al.*, 1969; Sabata *et al.*, 1970).

Insulin secretion *in utero* has been studied at hysterotomy between 13 and 26 weeks of gestation. Plasma insulin, taken 5–10 min after the injection of glucose (300 mg to 1 g according to the foetal size) into foetuses of 15 to 20 weeks of gestation remained unaltered (Adam *et al.*, 1969) but foetal hyperglycemia resulting from maternal infusion of glucose (6 mg/kg body weight/min) for 3 h caused a small rise in plasma insulin at the same stage (Obenshain *et al.*, 1970). On the other hand, Thorell (1970) saw no change in foetal plasma insulin (gestational age of 15–26 weeks), despite the hyperglycemia, after infusing glucose to the mothers in a dose of 15 g, 25 g, or 50 g; or the oral administration of 100 g of glucose

* = S.D.; ** = S.E.M.

1 to 50 min before the evacuation of the uterus. Turner *et al.* (1971) showed that prolonged elevation of the foetal plasma glucose levels (gestational age of 20—24 weeks) as a result of 24 h maternal glucose (300 g) infusion did not affect the foetal plasma insulin levels. King *et al.* (1971) demonstrated that a maternal administration of arginine (0.5 g/kg body weight/30 min) during hysterotomy between 13—18 weeks of gestation caused no significant change in plasma insulin.

The fact that glucose is a poor stimulant of insulin secretion early in gestation has been confirmed by *in vitro* studies using human foetal pancreas (Espinosa *et al.*, 1970; Milnes *et al.*, 1971; Fujimoto and Williams, 1972; Leach *et al.*, 1973).

An explanation of these *in vivo* and *in vitro* results remains uncertain even if it has been suggested that the low effectiveness of glucose in human foetal pancreas could be due to an inadequate intracellular accumulation of cyclic AMP within the beta cell. In the pre-term infant theophylline and glucagon, agents known to increase cyclic AMP in the beta cells, stimulate insulin release (Grasso *et al.*, 1970). *In vitro* with foetal organ culture glucose becomes a powerful stimulant in the presence of methylxantines or of glucagon (Fujimoto and Williams, 1972; Milner *et al.*, 1971) while methylxantines also stimulate insulin secretion in a glucose-free media (Milner *et al.*, 1971). Even if this has been confirmed in animals both *in vitro* (Lambert *et al.*, 1976; Heinze and Steinke, 1972) and *in vivo* (Mintz *et al.*, 1969) studies, there is contrasting evidence for a deficient cyclic AMP system in the B cell of foetal and newborn animals and humans. Direct measurements comparing basal cyclic AMP in the islets from rat foetus at term and their mothers, however, failed to demonstrate diminished levels of the cyclic nucleotide in the foetus (Mintz *et al.*, 1973). On the other hand, Grill *et al.* (1975) found no effect of glucose on cyclic AMP in one-day old rats. Contrastingly, in adult rats cyclic AMP accumulation was significantly enhanced after sixty minutes incubation in a high glucose concentration.

Milner *et al.* (1971) showed that between the 16th and 24th week of foetal life the B cell of the human foetal pancreas is capable of secreting insulin *in vitro* when incubated with potassium, sodium, calcium or oubain.

FOETAL INSULIN IN SECRETION AT TERM

At term, after the maternal infusion of glucose, or arginine, the foetal insulin secretion has been studied at various intervals, by using capillary scalp blood (Saling, 1963).

After an intravenous glucose load (25 g in 2—3 min) during labor, Paterson *et al.* (1968) found no change in foetal insulin at 15 and 60 min. However, after giving a rapid glucose infusion (1 g/kg body weight/10 min) to normal women in labor, Cordero *et al.* (1970a,b) observed a delayed increase in foetal serum insulin and an increase in foetal blood glucose that declined slowly. The highest foetal insulin values were reached approximately 60 min after the glucose peak. Similar delayed insulin response was obtained by Bossart *et al.* (1969) after a double maternal intravenous glucose load (0.3 g/kg body weight) and Oakley *et al.* (1972) after maternal intravenous injection of glucose (23 g to 90 g) for 70 min. On the other hand, Coltart *et al.* (1969) showed that the rapid infusion of 25 g of glucose to 8 normal women before the onset of labor caused a rise in insulin five mintues after the glucose injection in four foetuses, in one foetus a gradual rise, maximum at 70 min, and in 3 either no rise or only a small one. The infusion of arginine

(25 g/30 min) to pregnant women prior to the onset of labor caused a small but significant increase in foetal plasma insulin.

At term foetal insulin secretion has also been studied by infusing glucose, arginine, or leucine with or without glucose to the mother and taking a blood sample from the umbilical cord after delivery. Milner and Hales (1965) gave an acute glucose load to mothers during labor and demonstrated elevated plasma levels in umbilical cord blood only when the glucose was administered 61 to 100 min before delivery. Wolf *et al.* (1970) infused glucose (12 to 15 mg/kg body weight/min) to mothers for 18 to 100 min prior to delivery and noted elevated plasma insulin levels in the umbilical cord blood. Tobin and his associates (1969) reported a slight but significant increase of plasma insulin in the foetus 47 min after an acute glucose load (0.5 g/kg body weight/3 min) to normal mothers during labor. The infusion of arginine (20 to 45 g/27–60 min) to pregnant women at term during active labor did not cause any significant serum insulin rise in their foetuses (King *et al.*, 1971).

We have studied the foetal insulin response *in utero* by infusing glucose, leucine with or without glucose to normal pregnant women at term during cesarean section (Grasso *et al.*, 1976). Leucine was chosen as it is an insulinogenic amino acid in the adult. The infusion lasted 30 or 60 min and was synchronized so that birth occurred 10 min after it ended. Venous blood samples were taken from the mother throughout the infusion and simultaneously at delivery from both maternal and umbilical veins.

The pregnant women were neither obese nor had history or evidence of diabetes mellitus and underwent cesarean section for pelvic disproportion. They were chosen because the foetuses did not undergo the stress of labor. The results of these studies are shown in Tables I and II.

Leucine (15 g) with glucose (50 g) administered for 30 min to the mothers markedly stimulated maternal and foetal insulin secretion while the infusion of glucose (50 g) caused a lower response. When infusing glucose alone we noted that the duration rather than the degree of hyperglycemia determined the foetal insulin response. In fact, when glucose was given to the mother for 60 min the foetal insulin response was higher than when the same dose was infused for 30 min. Maternal infusion of leucine (15 g) for 30 min elicited a very slight increase of insulin secretion in the mother and no change in the foetus.

INSULIN SECRETION IN PRE-TERM AND FULL-TERM INFANTS

After birth the insulin response to glucose varied markedly which seems to depend, to some extent, on the technique of glucose administration, the timing of blood sampling, the glucose dose, and also on the gestational age of the infant, its birthweight *etc.* (Persson, 1975).

After a rapid injection of glucose 0.5 g (Isles *et al.*, 1968), 1 g (Gentz *et al.*, 1969; Mølsted-Pedersen and Jørgensen, 1972; Le Dune, 1972; Falorni *et al.*, 1974), or 1.5 g (Edström, 1975) per kg of body weight to normal infants the insulin concentration in plasma shows two peaks with the maximum value at 60 min. The first peak can be easily missed if samples are not obtained within 5 min after the injection of glucose (Levy *et al.*, 1971). These findings have been reported by using blood from the portal, umbilical or peripheral veins. However, Gentz *et al.* (1969) on studying low birth weight infants showed three kinds of

Table I. Comparison of maternal and foetal blood glucose, serum insulin and HGH (Mean ± S.E.M.) in pregnant women at term infused for 30 min with saline, glucose, leucine, or glucose with leucine.

MATERNAL INFUSION OF SALINE (n = 12)				
	Mother		Delivery	Umbilical Vein
	0′	30′	40′	
Blood Glucose (mg/100 ml)	79 ± 3	84 ± 3	85 ± 3	61 ± 3
Serum Insulin (μU/ml)	8 ± 1	7 ± 1	8 ± 1	9 ± 2
Serum HGH (ng/ml)	6 ± 0.3	6 ± 0.3	6 ± 3	15 ± 2

MATERNAL INFUSION OF GLUCOSE (50 g) (n = 11)				
	Mother		Delivery	Umbilical Vein
	0′	30′	40′	
Blood Glucose (mg/100 ml)	84 ± 7	333 ± 5	293 ± 9	236 ± 6
Serum Insulin (μU/ml)	9 ± 2	70 ± 14	59 ± 10	26 ± 6
Serum HGH (ng/ml)	6 ± 0.5	6 ± 0.5	7 ± 0.7	20 ± 3

MATERNAL INFUSION OF LEUCINE (15 g) (n = 4)			
	Mother		Umbilical Vein
	0′	30′	
Blood Glucose (mg/100 ml)	82 ± 5	88 ± 5	70 ± 2
Serum Insulin (μU/ml)	9 ± 2	18 ± 2	15 ± 2
Serum HGH (ng/ml)	7 ± 2	7 ± 2	24 ± 5

MATERNAL INFUSION OF GLUCOSE (50 g) WITH LEUCINE (15 g) (n = 17)				
	Mother		Delivery	Umbilical Vein
	0′	30′	40′	
Blood Glucose (mg/100 ml)	74 ± 3	242 ± 8	187 ± 7	157 ± 5
Serum Insulin (μU/ml)	16 ± 4	202 ± 25	165 ± 30	88 ± 15
Serum HGH (ng/ml)	8 ± 0.6	8 ± 0.6	9 ± 0.8	22 ± 4

Table II. **Comparison of maternal and foetal blood glucose, serum insulin and HGH (Mean ± S.E.M.) in pregnant women at term infused for 60 min with saline or glucose.**

MATERNAL INFUSION OF SALINE (n = 10)					
	Mother			Delivery	Umbilical Vein
	0′	30′	60′	70′	
Blood Glucose (mg/100 ml)	72 ± 3	77 ± 4	82 ± 4	84 ± 4	64 ± 3
Serum Insulin (μU/ml)	16 ± 3	12 ± 2	13 ± 2	12 ± 2	12 ± 2
Serum HGH (ng/ml)	7 ± 0.5	7 ± 0.4	7 ± 0.4	7 ± 0.3	26 ± 4
MATERNAL INFUSION OF GLUCOSE (n = 10)					
	Mother			Delivery	Umbilical Vein
	0′	30′	60′	70′	
Blood Glucose (mg/100 ml)	77 ± 3	194 ± 9	237 ± 9	207 ± 11	187 ± 13
Serum Insulin (μU/ml)	17 ± 3	70 ± 12	82 ± 13	55 ± 11	46 ± 8
Serum HGH (ng/ml)	6 ± 0.7	6 ± 1	6 ± 0.7	8 ± 1	23 ± 4

serum insulin response to a rapid glucose administration. Some responded with a double peak, some with an early single peak curve while others showed no appreciable insulin response. Mølsted-Pedersen and Jorgensen (1972) have shown that in normal newborns the insulin response to a rapid glucose infusion in the first day of life is significantly greater in infants weighing over 3,500 g. We have observed that in premature infants receiving 2.5 g of glucose for 30 min the serum insulin rose slightly, but if an infusion of glucose administered for 120 min (total dose 920 mg) precedes the acute injection of glucose, the latter injection became a potent stimulus of insulin secretion. Serum insulin rose from a value of 15.6 ± 2.3** to 93.6 ± 23,8** μU/ml at 60 min (Grasso *et al.*, 1975) (Fig.1).

Completely the opposite to glucose, we have noted that a mixture of essential amino acids is a potent stimulus of insulin release in the pre-term infant (Grasso *et al.*, 1968). In fact, the infusion of 2.5 g of this mixture for 30 min caused a rapid rise of serum insulin from a control value of 14 ± 2** μU/ml to a peak value of 100 ± 16.9** μU/ml at 30 min (Fig.2). We have also seen that the simultaneous administration of an ineffective dose of amino acids (1.25 g) with glucose (1.25 g) caused a rapid and marked increase in serum insulin levels with serum insulin rising from a control level of 8 ± 1** μU/ml to a peak of 58 ± 9** μU/ml at 60 min (Grasso *et al.*, 1973) (Fig.3). A similar synergism was observed between glucose (1.25 g) and arginine (1.25 g) in the pre-term infant (Reitano *et al.*, 1971). Arginine (0.5 g/kg body weight/30 min) given alone to pre-term (Ponté *et al.*, 1972) and term infants (King *et al.*, 1974; Sperling *et al.*, 1974;

** = S.E.M.

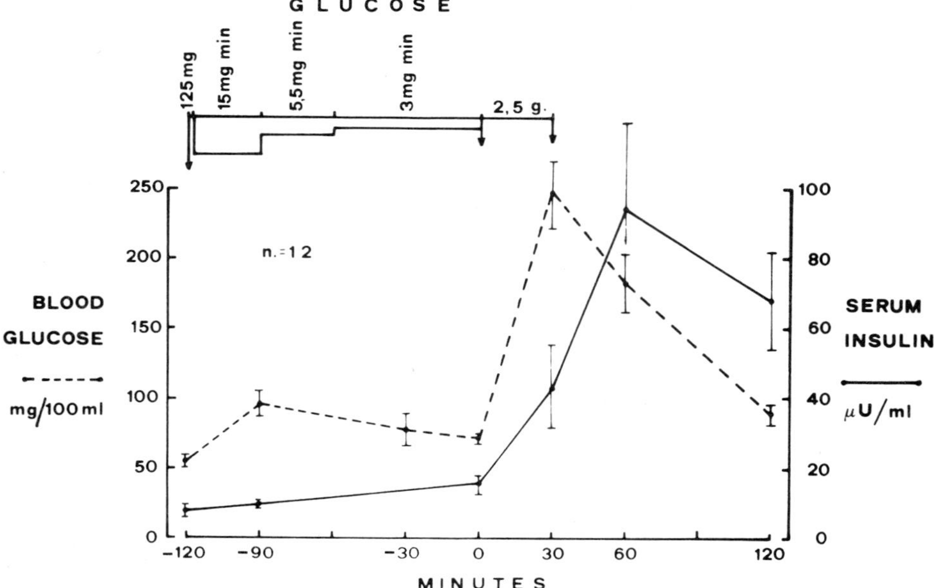

Fig. 1 Effect of a preinfusion of saline or glucose on a 30 min infusion of glucose.

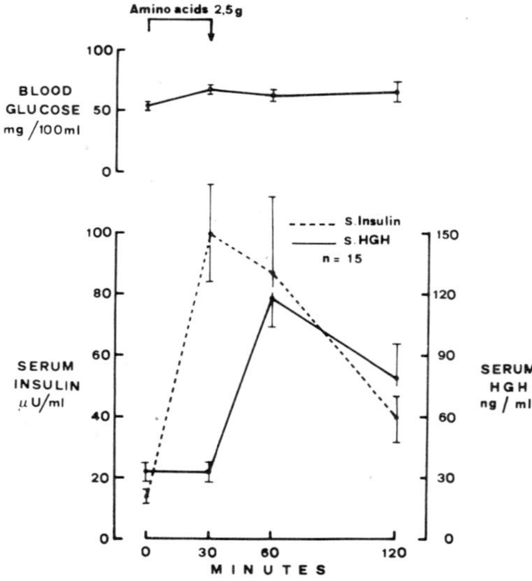

Fig. 2 Levels of blood glucose, serum insulin and HGH in the pre-term infant following a 30 min infusion of a mixture of amino acids.

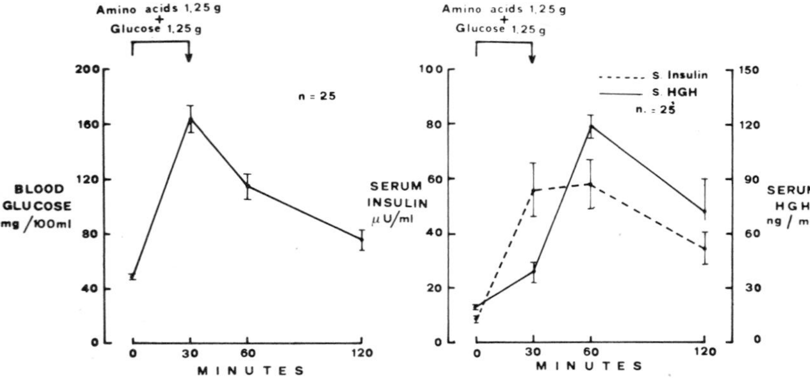

Fig.3 Levels of blood glucose, serum insulin and HGH in the pre-term infant following a 30 min infusion of amino acids and glucose.

Falorni *et al.*, 1975) caused a modest rise of insulin levels. Furthermore recently we have observed that the insulin response to glucose infusion is markedly enhanced by the prior administration for 120 min of a mixture of essential amino acids. Serum insulin rose from a value of 15 ± 5** μU/ml to 93 ± 24** μU/ml at 30 min (Reitano *et al.*, 1976) (Fig.4).

The injection of glucagon in the pre-term infant (300 μg in 5 min)(Grasso *et al.*, 1970) and term infants [300 μg (Milner and Wright, 1967) or 30 μg/kg body weight (Reisner *et al.*, 1972) or 1 μg rapidly (Hunter and Isles, 1972)] caused a rise in serum insulin by the end of the injection, but when given in the pre-term infant as an infusion of 400 μg/min for 1 h (total dose 24 μg) it had no effect on serum insulin (Grasso *et al.*, 1970). The combination of 400 μg of glucagon and 0.5 mg of theophylline/min for 1 h, neither of these agents being stimulatory alone, also caused a large and progressive rise in serum insulin levels (Grasso *et al.*, 1970). The intravenous administration of tolbutamide (20 mg/kg body weight/ 3 min) in full term infants (Velasco and Paulsen, 1969) or pre-term infants (50 mg/ 5 min) caused a slight rise in serum insulin. However, the simultaneous administration in the pre-term infants of tolbutamide (50 mg) and glucose (2.5 g) caused a marked increase in serum insulin.

It is known that insulin is synthesized as a single chain polypeptide, proinsulin, most of which being converted to insulin within the beta cell (Steiner and Oyer, 1967). Proinsulin has also been seen in adult human blood. Gorden and Roth (1969) and Gorden *et al.* (1972) have shown that the immunoreactive portion of serum insulin can be resolved by gel filtration into 2 components. One component is indistinguishable by crystalline pancreatic insulin (insulin component or little insulin); the second component, with higher molecular weight, may closely resemble proinsulin (proinsulin-like component or big insulin). Many questions concerning the extrapancreatic significance of proinsulin, in terms of biological activity, remain unanswered. As yet little information has been obtained about these components in the pancreas and in the blood of the newborn.

** = S.E.M.

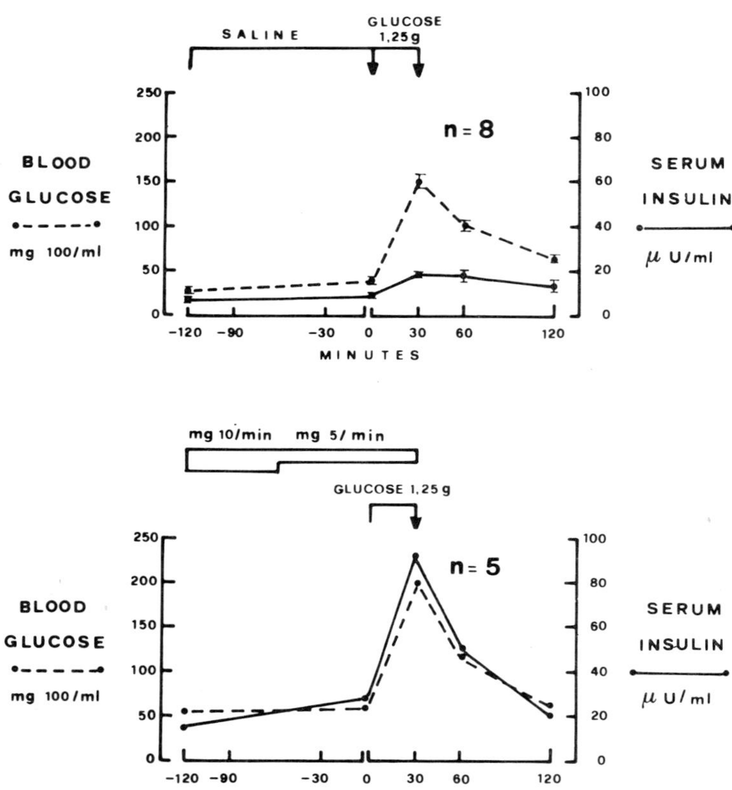

Fig.4 Effect of a preinfusion of saline or a mixture of essential amino acids on a 30 min infusion of glucose.

Rastogi *et al.* (1970b) found the amount of proinsulin in 16 pancreases of human foetuses (aged 11-24 weeks) to vary from 0.26 to 1.6% of the total immunoreactive insulin.

We have analyzed blood samples taken from 4 pre-term infants at the end of a 120 min infusion of glucose with glucagon (Table III). The two components were separated using the method of Gorden and Roth (1969) and assayed for immunoreactive insulin by a double-antibody technique (Hales and Randle, 1963) using human insulin standards and antiserum against human insulin. Serum concentration of insulin was high (from 73.8 to 527.4 μU/ml) and the percentage of proinsulin varied from 3.8 to 8.3%. From this it is clear that the beta cell of the pre-term infant can release a large amount of insulin under the appropriate stimulus and that the proinsulin-insulin converting system functions adequately.

Table III. **Percentage of "big insulin" after a 120 min infusion of glucose (4 g) plus glucagon (250 μg) in the pre-term infant during the first 24 h of life.**

	Total Insulin	"Little Insulin"	"Big Insulin"	%
1.	343.8	329.0	14.8	4.3
2.	527.4	507.2	20.2	3.8
3.	201.5	178.0	13.5	6.7
4.	73.8	67.7	6.1	8.3

FOETAL HGH SECRETION

The human pituitary gland secretes HGH early in gestation which is immunologically and physicochemically similar to that in the child and adult (Kaplan *et al.*, 1972). In fact acidophyle cells have been observed in the anterior or hypophysis by the 9th week of gestation (Conklin, 1969) and explants of the human pituitaty synthesize and store HGH and other polypeptide hormones at the same stage (Gitlin and Biasucci, 1969; Silver-Kodr *et al.*, 1974). As early as 8–9 weeks of gestation HGH has been measured in human foetal pituitary and its content increases up to birth. In 117 human foetal pituitary glands Kaplan *et al.* (1972) found that the HGH increases from 0.44 ± 0.2** ng at 10–14 weeks gestation to 675 ± 122* ng at 35–40 week. HGH has been detected in the foetal blood as early as the 10th week. Gitlin *et al.* (1965), Laron *et al.* (1966) and King *et al.* (1971b) have all shown, using isotope stuides, that HGH does not cross the placenta. In Table IV are our data regarding serum HGH in spontaneously aborted foetuses, pre-term and full-term infants and they are compared with Kaplan's results. It can be seen that the foetal serum HGH increases to a peak level of 20–24 weeks of gestation and then decreases sharply. At term the serum HGH in the cord blood was 23 ± 2** ng/ml, similar to the value seen by Joassin *et al.* (1967) (25 ± 19* ng/ml, n = 21), Cramer *et al.* (1971) (23.8 ± 14.8* ng/ml, n = 440), Aubert *et al.* (1971) (21.5 ± 0.81** ng/ml, n = 227). Similarly, the blood HGH in foetuses from 28 women, measured after surgical induction of labor, was 32 ± 14* ng/ml, before contraction had started (Turner *et al.*, 1973). In contrast Spellacy *et al.* (1973) reported a mean value of 63.6 ± 4.9* ng/ml in the umbilical artery at the birth of 126 infants. We have found non-significant difference in the HGH levels of cord blood between pre-term and full-term infants.

Little is known about the secretion of this hormone *in utero*. The stress of delivery does not seem to influence the fetal HGH level as in our experience the concentration of serum HGH of infants delivered by cesarean section (23.09 ± 1.2* ng/ml, n = 146) was similar to that of spontaneously delivered newborn (23.10 ± 1.9** ng/ml, n = 83). However, higher levels of HGH have been observed in foetuses with foetal distress or in small-for-date infants (Aubert *et al.*, 1971). Aubert *et al.* (1971) found that at term the foetal serum HGH remained unaltered throughout a maternal double glucose load while Turner *et al.* (1973) observed that maternal glucose infusion was associated with a fall in foetal HGH level even if a small rise in foetal HGH concentration followed maternal arginine infusion. Contrastingly, we have seen that at term the maternal infusion of glucose (50 g)

* = S.D.; ** = S.E.M.

Table IV. **Serum HGH (mean ± S.E.M.) at different gestational age.**

Gestational Age	Kaplan *et al.* (1972)	Reitano *et al.* (1976)
10–14 wks	65.2 ± 7.6	—
15–19 wks	114 ± 12	—
20–24 wks	119 ± 19.8	110 ± 12 (n = 14)
25–29 wks	72 ± 11.5	73.5 ± 23 (n = 4)
30–33 wks	—	31.6 ± 4.2 (n = 29)
34–37 wks	—	28.4 ± 3 (n = 96)
38–42 wks	33.5 ± 4.2	23 ± 2 (n = 146)

with and without leucine given for 30 or 60 min does not influence the foetal HGH (Grasso *et al.*, 1976).

At birth the serum HGH levels are high varying from subject to subject and declining to lower levels after the first weeks of life (Cornblath *et al.*, 1965; Westphall, 1968; Schueren-Lodeweyckx *et al.*, 1972). Insulin induced hypoglycemia gives rise to a net increase of plasma HGH both in full term and pre-term infants although the increase is less pronounced in the full term infants aged five to six days (Cornblath *et al.*, 1965; Westphall, 1968).

Table V. **Blood glucose and serum HGH (mean ± S.E.M.) in pre-term infants at the 1st, 4th and 6th day of life following a 30 min infusion of a mixture of amino acids (1.25 g) with glucose (1.25 g).**

		Time in minutes			
		0′	30′	60′	120′
Blood Glucose mg/100 ml	1st day (n = 15)	37 ± 2	156 ± 6	98 ± 6	68 ± 7
	4th day (n = 6)	68 ± 6	211 ∓ 25	126 ± 26	58 ± 4
	6th day (n = 6)	81 ± 9	163 ± 14	77 ± 6	62 ± 4
Serum HGH ng/100 ml	1st day (n = 12)	29 ± 7	80 ± 8	123 ± 23	76 ± 9
	4th day (n = 6)	30 ± 6	48 ± 9	50 ± 10	28 ± 8
	6th day (n = 6)	16 ± 3	15 ± 3	10 ± 3	14 ± 4

Arginine [(0.5 g/kg body weight) in the pre-term infant (Pontê *et al.*, 1972) and full term infant (Falorni *et al.*, 1975) or 1.25 g in the pre-term infant (Reitano *et al.*, 1971)] ; a mixture of essential amino acids (2.5 g in the pre-term infant; Grasso *et al.*, 1973, Fig.2), as well as glucagon (300 μg/kg body weight/ 3 min; Milner, 1967) are potent stimuli and induce a marked increase of serum HGH on the first day of life. Unlike in older children and adults where the HGH is decreased by hyperglycemia, the intravenous injection of glucose (Cornbath *et al.*, 1965; Westphall, 1968; Reitano *et al.*, 1971) or a mixture of essential amino acids (1.25 g) with glucose (1.25 g) stimulated the secretion of HGH (Fig.3). This paradoxical increase of HGH to hyperglycemia reverts to adult type on the 6th day of life (Table V; Vigo *et al.*, 1972).

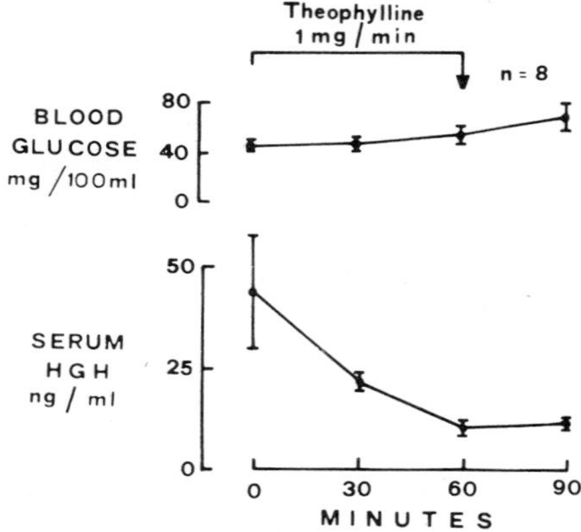

Fig.5 Levels of blood glucose and HGH in the pre-term infant following a 60 min infusion of theophylline.

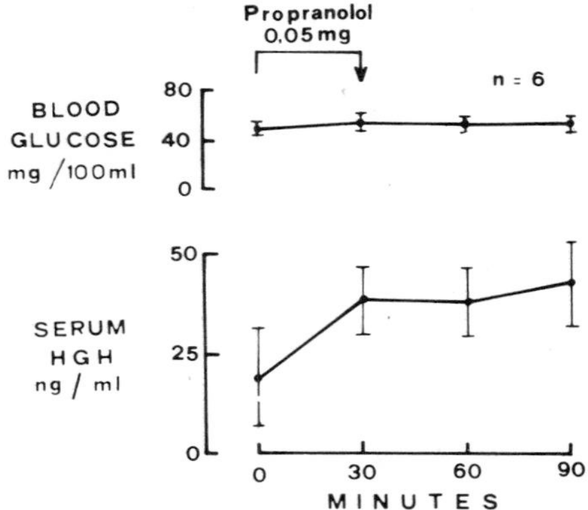

Fig.6 Levels of blood glucose and HGH in the pre-term infant following a 30 min infusion of propranolol.

Vigneri and D'Agata (1971) have noted the absence of sleep-induced HGH secretion in the human neonate during the first 3 months of life.

In the adult, evidence indicates that the hypothalamus secretes a neurohormone called Growth Hormone Releasing Factor (GH-RF) which controls HGH release by the anterior pituitary (Pecile *et al.*, 1955; Frohman, 1972). The chemical structure and the mechanism of secretion of GH-RF remains obscure. Recent evidence indicates that an adrenergic mechanism is involved in the relase of GH-RF (Imura *et al.*, 1971). It has also been stated that this control is not exerted in the newborn at the time of birth but comes into force a few days later (Bassett *et al.*, 1970). But preliminary studies carried out in our laboratory have proved this is probably not the case. In these experiments we have used theophylline, which is a substance that mimics the β-adrenergic stimulating agents (Ensinck *et al.*, 1970; Grasso *et al.*, 1976) and propanolol which is a β-adrenergic blocking agent. We have noted that these substances act in the same way as in the adult (Imura *et al.*, 1971). The former depresses HGH secretion from 44.9 ± 14.1** to 10.3 ± 2.3** ng/ml, while the latter increases it from 18 ± 5** to 44 ± 12 ng/ml at 90 min (Reitano *et al.*, 1973) (Figs 5 and 6)

These data could suggest that the alpha and beta adrenergic receptors in the hypothalamic nuclei of the pre-term infant modulate HGH secretion in the same way as in the adult. From this we assume that the hypothalamic-pituitary system is operant in the premature infant. In fact the hypophyseal portal system develops in the human foetus around the middle of the foetal period (Räihä *et al.*, 1957), neuro-secretory material has been stained in the foetal period as the 20th week of gestation (Rinne *et al.*, 1962), and both vasopressor and oxytocic activity has been detected in the pituitary of foetuses from 70 to 110 days old.

REFERENCES

Adam, P.A., Teramo, K., Räihä, N., Gitlin, D. and Schwartz, R. (1969). *Diabetes* **18**, 409-416.

Aubert, M.L., Sistex, J., Chabot, V. and Bossart, H. (1971). *Schwiez. med. Wschr.* **101**, 1102-1107.

Bassett, J.M. and Thornburn, G.D. (1971). *J. Endocr.* **50**, 59-74.

Bossart, H., Sistex, J., Chabot, V. and Felber, J.P. (1969). *Schwiez. med. Wschr.* **99**, 1350-1354.

Coltart, T.M., Beard, R.W., Turner, R.C. and Oakley, N.W. (1969). *Br. med. J.* **4**, 17-19.

Conklin, J.L. (1968). *Anat. Rec.* **160**, 79-92.

Cordero, L., Yeh, S., Grunt, J.A. and Anderson, G.G. (1970a). *Am. J. Obstet. Gynec.* **107**, 295-302.

Cordero, L., Grunt, J.A. and Anderson, G.G. (1970b). *Am. J. Obstet. Gynec.* **107**, 560-564.

Cornblath, M., Parker, M.L., Reisner, S.H., Forbes, A.E. and Daughaday, W.H. (1965). *J. clin. Endocr.* **25**, 209-218.

Cramer, D.W., Beek, C.H. and Makowsky, E.L. (1971). *Am. J. Obstet. Gynec.* **109**, 649-655.

Edström, K., Cerasi, E., Luft, R., Persson, B. and Thalme, B. (1975). *Acta Endocr.* **78**, 44-53.

Ensinck, J.W., Stoll, R.W., Gale, C.C., Santen, R.J., Touber, J.L. and Williams, R.H. (1970). *J. clin. Endocr.* **31**, 153-161.

Espinosa, M.M.A., Driscoll, S.G. and Steinke, J. (1970). *Science* **168**, 1111-1112.

Falorni, A., Fracassini, F., Massi-Benedetti, F. and Maffei, S. (1974). *Diabetes* **23**, 172-178.

Falorni, A., Massi-Benedetti, F., Gallo, G. and Trabalza, N. (1975). *Biol. Neonate* **27**, 271-278.

Fujimoto, W.Y. and Williams, R.H. (1972). *Endocrinology* **91**, 1133-1136.

Frohman, L.A. (1972). *New Engl. J. Med.* **286**, 1391-1397.

Gentz, J.C.H., Warner, R., Persson, B.E.H. and Cornblath, M. (1969). **58**, 481-490.

Gitlin, D., Kumate, J. and Morales, C. (1965). *J. clin. Endocr.* **25**, 1599-1608.

Gitlin, D. and Biascucci, A. (1969). *J. clin. Endocr.* **29**, 926, 935.

Gorden, P. and Roth, J. (1969). *J. clin. Invest.* **48**, 2225-2234.

Gorden, P., Roth, J., Freychet, P. and Kahn, R. (1972). *Diabetes* **21 (Suppl.2)** 673-677.

Grasso, S., Saporito, N., Messina, A. and Reitano, G. (1968). *Lancet* **2**, 755-757.

Grasso, S., Messina, A., Saporito, N. and Reitano, G. (1970). *Diabetes* **19**, 837-842.

Grasso, S., Messina, A., Distefano, G., Vigo, R. and Reitano, G. (1973). *In* "Diabetes, Proc. 8th Congr. Intern. Diab. Fed." (W.J. Malaisse and J. Pirart, eds) pp.489-498.

Grasso, S., Messina, A., Distefano, G., Vigo, R. and Reitano, G. (1973). *Diabetes* **22**, 349-353.

Grasso, S., Distefano, G., Messina, A., Vigo, R. and Reitano, G. (1975). *Diabetes* **24**, 291-294.

Grasso, S., Palumbo, G., Messina, A., Mazzarino, C. and Reitano, G. (1976). *Diabetes* **25**, 545-549.

Grill, V., Asplund, K., Hellerstrom, C. and Cerasi, E. (1975). *Diabetes* **24**, 746-752.

Hales, C.N. and Randle, P.J. (1963). *Biochem. J.* **88**, 137-146.

Heinze, E. and Steinke, J. (1972). *Horm. Metab. Res.* **4**, 234.

Hunter, D.J.S. and Isles, T.E. (1972). *Biol. Neonate* **20**, 74-80.

** = S.E.M.

Imura, H., Kato, Y., Ikeda, M., Morimoto, M. and Yawata, M. (1971). *J. clin. Invest.* **50**, 1069-1079.
Isles, T.E., Dickson, M. and Farquhar, J.W. (1968). *Pediat. Res.* **2**, 198-208.
Joassin, G., Parker, M.L., Pildes, R.S. and Cornblath, M. (1967). *Diabetes* **16**, 306-311.
Jørgensen, K.R., Deckert, T., Mølsted-Pedersen, L. and Pedersen, J. (1966). *Acta Endocr.* **52**, 154-167.
Kaplan, S.L., Grumbach, M.M. and Shepard, T.H. (1972). *J. clin. Invest.* **51**, 3080-3093.
King, K.C., Buth, J., Raivio, K., Räihä, N., Roux, J., Teramo, K., Yamaguchi, K. and Schwartz, R. (1971a). *New Engl. J. Med.* **285**, 607-612.
King, K.C., Adam, P.A.J., Schwartz, R. and Teramo, K. (1971b). *Pediatrics* **48**, 534-539.
King, K.C., Adam, P.A.J., Yamaguchi, K. and Schwartz, R. (1974). *Diabetes* **23**, 816-820.
Lambert, A.E., Jeanrenaud, B., and Renold, A.E. (1967). *Lancet* **1**, 819-820.
Laron, Z., Pertzelan, A., Mannheimer, S., Goldman, J. and Gutman, S. (1966). *Acta Endocr.* **53**, 687-692.
LeDune, M.A. (1972). *Arch. Dis. Child.* **47**, 111-114.
Leach, F.N., Ashworth, M.A., Barson, A.J. and Milner, R.D.G. (1973). *J. Endocr.* **59**, 65-79.
Levy, J.M., Segura, N., Klein, F., Grunewald, C., Thierry, R. and Peter, M.O. (1971). *Arch. Franç. Ped.* **28**, 133-146.
Milner, R.D.G. and Hales, C.N. (1965). *Br. med. J.* **1**, 284-286.
Milner, R.D.G. and Wright, A.D. (1967). *Clin. Sci.* **32**, 249-255.
Milner, R.D.G., Barson, A.J. and Ashwort, M.A. (1971). *J. Endocr.* **51**, 323-332.
Milner, R.D.G., Ashwort, M.A. and Barson, A.J. (1972). *J. Endocr.* **52**, 497-505.
Mintz, D.H., Chez, R.A., Horger, E.O. (1969). *J. clin. Invest.* **48**, 176-186.
Mintz, D.H., Levy, G.S. and Schenk, A. (1973). *Endocrinology* **92**, 614-617.
Mølsted-Pedersen, L. and Jørgensen, K.R. (1972). *Acta Endocr.* **71**, 115-125.
Oakley, N.W., Beard, R.W. and Turner, R.C. (1972). *Br. med. J.* **1**, 466-469.
Obenshain, S.S., Adam, P.A.J., King, K.C., Teramo, K., Raivio, K.O., Räihä, N. and Schwartz, R. (1970). *New Engl. J. Med.* **283**, 566-570.
Paterson, P., Taft, P. and Phillips, L. (1968). *J. Obstet. Gynaec. Br. Commonw.* **75**, 917-921.
Pecile, A.E., Müller, E., Falconi, G. and Martini, L. (1965). *Endocrinology* **77**, 241-246.
Persson, B. (1975). *In* "Carbohydrate Metabolism in Pregnancy and the Newborn" (H.W. Sutherland and J.M. Stowers, eds) pp.106-126. Churchill Livingstone, Edinburgh, London and New York.
Ponté, C., Gaudier, B., Deconinck, B. and Fourlinnie, J.C. (1972). *Biol. Neonate* **20**, 262-269.
Räihä, N. and Hyelt, L. (1957). *Acta Paediat. Scand.* **46**, 610-616.
Rastogi, G.K., Letarte, J. and Fraser, T.R. (1970a). *Diabetologia* **6**, 445-446.
Rastogi, G.K., Letarte, J. and Fraser, T.R. (1970b). *Lancet* **1**, 7-9.
Reisner, S.H., Aranda, J.V., Colle, E., Schiff, D., Scriver, C. and Stern, L. (1972). *Israel J. Med. Sci.* **8**, 791.
Reitano, G., Grasso, S., Distefano, G. and Messina, A. (1971). *J. Endocr.* **33**, 924-928.
Reitano, G., Grasso, S., Distefano, G., Messina, A. and Vigo, R. (1974). *In* "Atti XII Giornata di Nipiologia Internazionale – Riva del Garda – 2/VI/1973" (W. Tangheroni and A. Falorni, eds) **Vol.II**, pp.33-44.
Reitano, G., Distefano, G., Vigo, R. and Grasso, S. (1976). *(In preparation).*
Rinne, U.K., Kivalo, E., Talanti, S. (1962). *Biol. Neonate* **4**, 351-364.
Sabata, V., Frerichs, H., Wolf, H. and Stubbe, P. (1970). *J. Obstet. Gynaec. Br. Commonw.* **77**, 121-128.
Saling, E. (1963). *Arch. Gynecol.* **197**, 108-122.
Schueren-Lodeweyckx, M.V.D., Eggermont, E. and Eeckels, R. (1972). *Acta Pediat. Bel.* **26**, 241-253.
Siler-Khodr, T.M., Morgenstern, L.L. and Greenwood, F.C. (1974). *J. clin. Endocr.* **39**, 891-905.
Spellacy, W.N., Facog, W.C.B., Bradly, B. and Holsinger, K.K. (1973). *Obstet. Gynec.* **41**, 323-331.
Steinke, J. and Driscoll, S.G. (1965). *Diabetes* **14**, 573-578.
Steiner, D.F. and Oyer, P.E. (1967). *Proc. natn. Acad. Sci. U.S.A.* **57**, 473-480.
Sperling, M.A., DeLamater, P.V., Phelps, D., Fiser, R.H., Oh, W. and Fisher, D.A. (1974). *J. clin. Invest.* **53**, 1159-1166.
Thorell, J.L. (1970). *Acta Endocr.* **63**, 124-140.

Tobin, J.D., Roux, J.F. and Soeldner, J.S. (1969). *Pediatrics* **44**, 668-671.
Turner, R.C., Schneeloch, B. and Paterson, P. (1971). *Acta Endocr.* **66**, 577-586.
Turner, R.C., Oakley, N.W. and Beard, R.W. (1973). *Biol. Neonate* **22**, 169-176.
Van Assche, F.A. (1970). "The Fetal Endocrine Pancreas. A Quantitative Morphological Approach." Thesis Katholicke Universiteit, Leuven, Belgium.
Velasco, M.S.A. and Paulsen, E.P. (1969). *Pediatrics* **43**, 546-558.
Vigneri, R. and D'Agata, R. (1971). *J. clin. Endocr.* **II**, 561-563.
Vigo, R., Distefano, G., Messina, A. and Grasso, S. (1972). *Riv. Ped. Sci.* **28**, 658-661.
Westphal, O. (1968). *Acta Paediat. Scand.* **(Suppl.182)** 57, 63-80.
Wolf, H., Stubbe, P. and Sabata, V. (1970). *Pediatrics* **45**, 36-42.

PROLACTIN (PRL), GH AND TSH RESPONSE TO TRH IN THE NEWBORN

G.C. Mussa, G. Bona, E. Madon and G. Rapetti
Department of Pediatrics, University of Turin, Italy

As arranged with the moderator, we shall summarize the features of PRL, GH and TSH secretion in the foetal and neonatal period on the basis of the data so far reported and the results of our research at the 1st Department of Puericulture, University of Turin.

Electrophoretic separation of GH from PRL in human hypophysis extracts suggested that the latter might not be present in man (Hodges and McShane, 1970). Improved biological and immunological methods, however, have since offered increasing specific evidence of the existence of a protein with high prolactin activity, and distinct from GH, in both serum and hypophysis extracts (Frantz and Kleimber, 1970; Forsyth *et al.*, 1971). It has also become clear that the synthesis and release of PRL are quite independent of GH (Pasteels, 1972).

Herland's tetrachromatic staining method and immunofluorescence techniques have provided microscopic evidence of specific cells that secrete GH and PRL independently of each other (Haugen and Beck, 1969; Herbest and Hayashida, 1970). The latter appear between the 3rd and 4th month of pregnancy. Their number is higher in the newborn and even more so in the adult. They are first found in the circumference of the anterior lobe and gradually invade its mediosagittal part, whereas GH-secreting cells mainly appear in its lateral bulbs. PRL-secreting cells increase in number until one week after birth, when above-normal levels can still be seen.

REGULATION OF PRL SECRETION

A. *Hypothalamic Inhibition*

A prolactin-inhibiting factor (PIF), the nature of which has not yet been established, has been identified in the neurons at the base of the hypothalamus. It has been shown to pass through the hypothalamus-hypophysis system to the

PRL-secreting cells (Fournier *et al.*, 1974). It is thought that the release of PIF is enhanced and inhibited by a variety of factors acting on the hypothalamic fibres responsible for the release of dopamine, which acts as a direct factor on the release of PIF. Since PIF activity in hypothalamic extracts is apparently located among the catecholamines, it has been suggested that PIF itself is a catecholamine (Takahara *et al.*, 1974; Shaar and Clemens, 1974).

Parson and Nicoll (1971) have shown that PIF inhibits PRL secretion by hyperpolarization of the cells through changes in their cytoplasmic membrane Ca/K balance.

B. Hypothalamic Stimulation

Most workers refuse to accept the existence of a PRL releasing factor (PRF). It has, however, been shown that TRH (pyroglutamyl-histidyl-prolinamide) greatly increases PRL levels in both males and females (Kaplan *et al.*, 1972; L'Hermite *et al.*, 1972; Snyder *et al.*, 1972; Tyson *et al.*, 1972). This increase is 2-3 times greater in women. Furthermore, Sulman (1971) and Jacobs *et al.* (1972) have suggested that TRH and PRF are the same. Since TRH also acts on isolated hypophyseal cells, they argue that its action on the hypophysis is not mediated by a PRF. It is well to remember that, in the case of PRL, since there is no direct hormone response in the breast, a special type of "short" feedback enables it to act on the hypothalamus directly, and restrict its own stimulation by means of a hypothalamic neurohormonal stimulus (Motta *et al.*, 1969; Kanematsu and Mikami, 1969). It may be supposed that PRL influences the hypothalamus via a two-way flow into the hypophyseal portal system that allows it to act on the medial eminence (Torok, 1964). L-dopa has recently been postulated as the mediator of the short feedback between PRL and PIF.

PRL LEVELS DURING PREGNANCY

During pregnancy, PRL (313 ± 195 μU/ml) begins to rise about the 8th week. At term, values are 10-20 times higher than in non-gravids (Hwang *et al.*, 1971; L'Hermite, 1972; Robyn, 1973) (Fig.1). Levels remain very high immediately after childbirth and at the commencement of lactation, but then fall rapidly even if breast-feeding is continued (Fig.2). Franchimont *et al.* (1975), for example, observed values of 4000 μU/ml on the 1st day, 5500 μU/ml on the 2nd day, and a rapid fall to 2000 μU/ml on the 6th day in 30 women. Values returned to normal some 3-7 weeks after childbirth.

It has recently been shown that some foetal endocrine functions are not dependent on those of the mother in the ruminant (Liggins, 1969; Hopkins and Thorburn, 1972; Nathanielsz *et al.*, 1973; Eremberg and Fisher, 1973). Sheep placenta is a barrier to labelled TSH (Dussault, 1972). That it is also a barrier to PRL can be argued from the failure of TSH and PRL to response in either partner when TRH is administered to the other (Fig.3). Thomas *et al.* (1975) have shown maternal-foetal gradients of about 6:1 for PRL and a little less than 1:1 for TSH in the sheep on the 132nd day of gestation. Injection of 200 μg TRH into the mother increased these figures to 20:1 and 3:1 respectively. It would thus appear that the foetal hypothalamo-hypophyseal axis is at no stage dependent upon the mother's secretions.

Serum PRL is rather high in the newborn at term, though lower than in the mother. Values exceed those in the adult until the 3rd and 6th month (Fournier

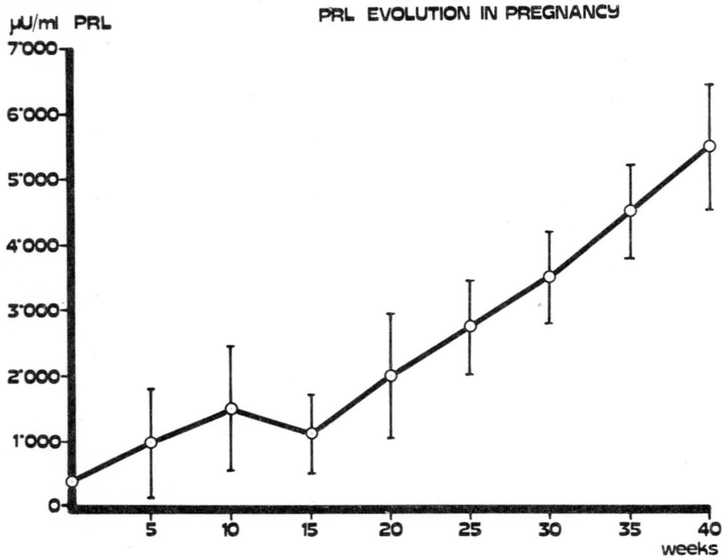

Fig. 1 PRL evolution in pregnancy.

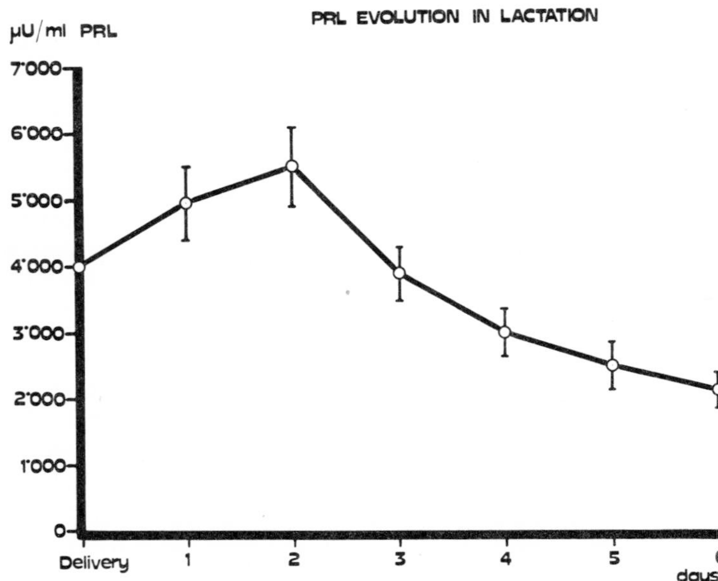

Fig. 2 PRL evolution in lactation.

et al., 1974). Thomas (1975) observed a rapid increase in both TSH (8.3 ± 3.2 μU/ml) and PRL (95.3 ± 2.2 ng/ml) 15 min after injecting 50 μg TRH into the jugular vein of a sheep 5 h after birth. The part played by PRL in the neonate and

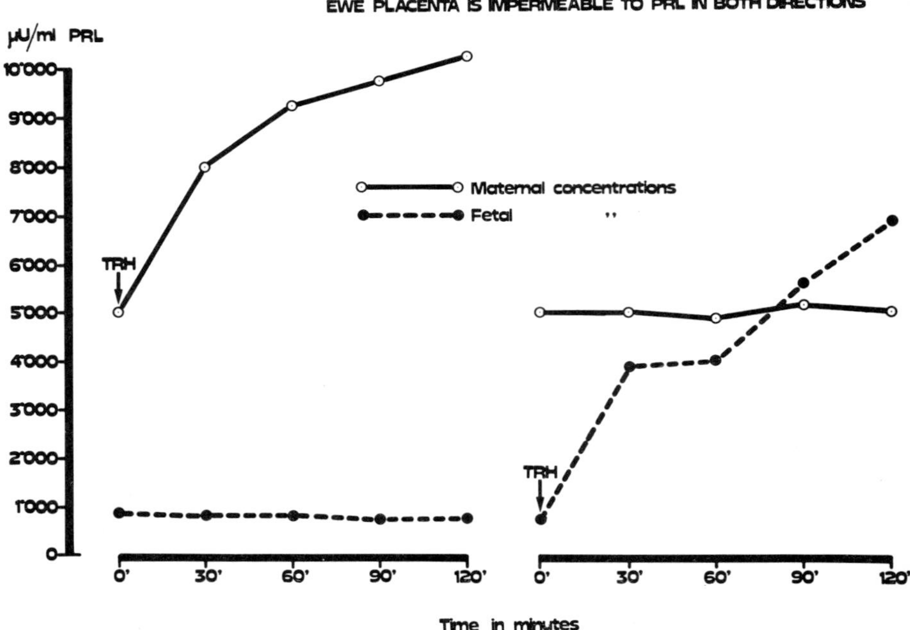

Fig.3 Ewe placenta impermeability to PRL in both directions.

the amniotic fluid is not known. It may be responsible for witch's milk.

PERSONAL RESEARCH

Hypophyseal response to synthetic TRH in the newborn has been examined in the light of the changes in serum TSH, PRL and GH. It must be stressed that TRH appears to affect the secretion of GH, as well as that of TSH and PRL. Kaplan (1972) attributes this to partial similarity between the structure of TRH and that of the GH.RF.

Five male and 5 female newborns weighing 2900—3800 g were examined during the first 5 days after eutocic birth at the 38th-42nd week of pregnancy. After fasting, serum PRL, GH and TSH values were determined radioimmunologically, using kits supplied by SORIN, Saluggia, under basal conditions and 15, 30, 60, 90 and 120 min after stimulation with 200 μg synthetic TRH i.v.. PRL values were expressed in μU/ml and GH and TSH values in ng/ml. Triiodothyronine levels were also determined. No difference in values (ng%ml) was noted at any time after the injection of TRH.

RESULTS

Tables I—IV give the values observed in each case and the respective means are shown on the graphs.

Table I. PRL levels in μU/ml.

Case	Sex	Age	Weight	Time in Minutes					
		days	g	0′	15′	30′	60′	90′	120′
1	F.	1	3260	4800	4820	4600	4000	4000	4200
2	M.	1	3790	5000	5800	4800	4600	4600	5200
3	F.	1	3130	7600	5600	8400	6800	5880	6400
4	F.	2	3960	3300	4550	4200	4000	4000	3800
5	F.	2	3750	9000	9000	9000	8500	9000	8500
6	M.	2	2980	5000	8000	7000	5800	7000	6000
7	M.	3	3520	6800	5880	7600	7500	7000	7500
8	F.	3	2920	2400	3240	3200	3200	3680	3200
9	M.	3	2950	3800	8000	8000	6600	6400	6000
10	M.	5	3950	1800	3000	6000	8000	6000	6000
Mean				**4950**	**5780**	**6280**	**5900**	**5756**	**5680**
SD ±				2505	2010	2005	1880	1700	1625
Range				1800/9000	3000/9000	3200/9000	3200/8500	3680/9000	3200/8500

Table II. GH levels in ng/ml.

Case	Sex	Age	Weight	Time in Minutes					
		days	g	0′	15′	30′	60′	90′	120′
1	F.	1	3260	4.2	6	3.9	7.8	7.8	7.5
2	M.	1	3790	3.3	3.9	3.6	5.2	4.4	4.7
3	F.	1	3130	31.5	30	27.6	19.0	39	49.5
4	F.	2	3960	7	5.2	5.4	5	4.8	4
5	F.	2	3750	37.5	39	24.5	32.7	20.1	34.5
6	M.	2	2980	20.4	20.7	18	11	5.4	7.5
7	F.	3	2920	17.4	21.6	21.6	25.2	19	18
8	M.	3	3520	30	25.8	18.8	24	28	29.5
9	M.	3	2950	22.2	22.2	24.6	18.6	18	19.8
10	M.	5	3950	6.3	3.9	3.3	1.5	1.5	3.0
Mean				**17.98**	**17.83**	**15.13**	**15**	**14.80**	**17.80**
SD ±				12.45	12.4	9.9	10.4	12.2	13.7
Range				3.3 – 37.5	3.9 – 39	3.3 – 27	1.5 – 33	1.5 – 39	3.0 – 49.5

Table III. TSH levels in ng/ml.

Case	Sex	Age	Weight	Time in Minutes					
		days	g	0′	15′	30′	60′	90′	120′
1	F.	1	3260	5.5	8.3	10.7	9.5	10.6	12.8
2	M.	1	3790	2.9	4.2	5.4	5	6.3	7.2
3	F.	1	3130	2.4	4.5	4.6	3.7	3.9	3.6
4	F.	2	3960	0.3	2.2	1.8	3.5	2.8	3.4
5	F.	2	3750	2.1	5.6	6.7	7.1	6.3	9.6
6	M.	2	2980	2.5	3.8	5.6	5.7	4.6	6.7
7	F.	3	2920	1	3.3	3.3	3.2	5.3	5.5
8	M.	3	3520	1.1	5	4.5	3.0	2.7	4.8
9	M.	3	2950	1.9	4.8	5.2	4.2	4.7	5.1
10	M.	5	3950	2.7	6.7	6.0	8.0	10.7	9.7
Mean				**2.24**	**4.84**	**5.38**	**5.29**	**5.79**	**6.84**
SD ±				1.4	1.7	2.2	2.3	2.8	3
Range				0.3/5.5	2.2/8.3	1.8/10.7	3 –9.5	2.7/10.7	3.4/12.8

Table IV. Triiodothyronine levels in ng%ml.

Case	Sex	Age	Weight	Time in Minutes					
		days	g	0′	15′	30′	60′	90′	120′
1	F.	1	3130	400	315	435	350	400	560
2	F.	1	3260	336	450	640	616	616	672
3	M.	1	3790	552	520	640	600	572	672
4	M.	2	2980	270	190	305	305	305	935
5	F.	2	3750	425	575	600	800	500	850
6	F.	2	3960	616	486	484	734	866	800
7	F.	3	2920	120	125	165	180	220	180
8	M.	3	2950	205	210	250	235	290	315
9	M.	3	3520	310	255	250	280	380	400
10	M.	5	3950	375	300	275	325	300	325
Mean				**360.9**	**342.6**	**404.4**	**442.5**	**445.2**	**520.9**
SD ±				150	159	179	224	196	225
Range				120 – 616	125 – 575	165 – 640	180 – 800	220 – 866	180 – 850

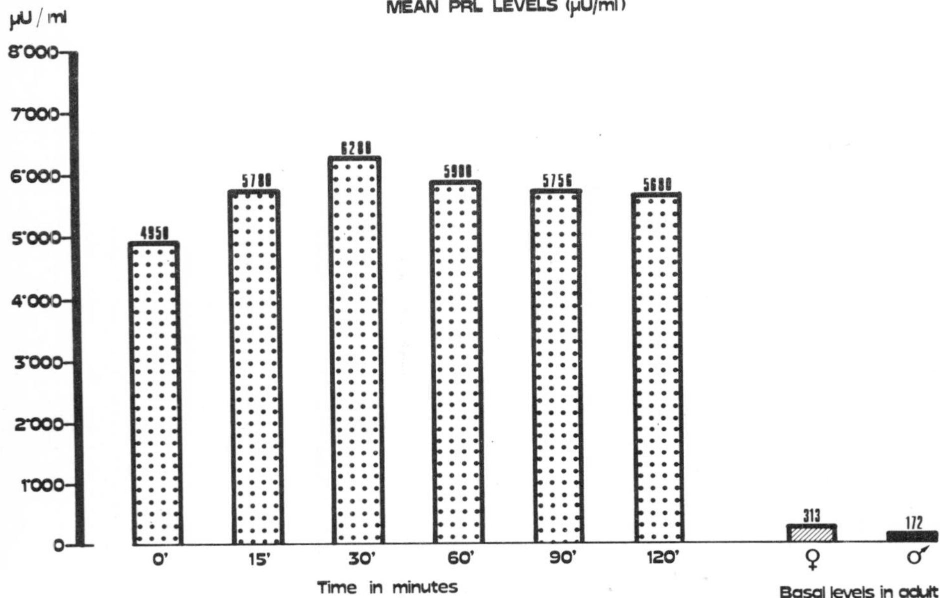

Fig. 4 Mean PRL levels in newborn after TRH.

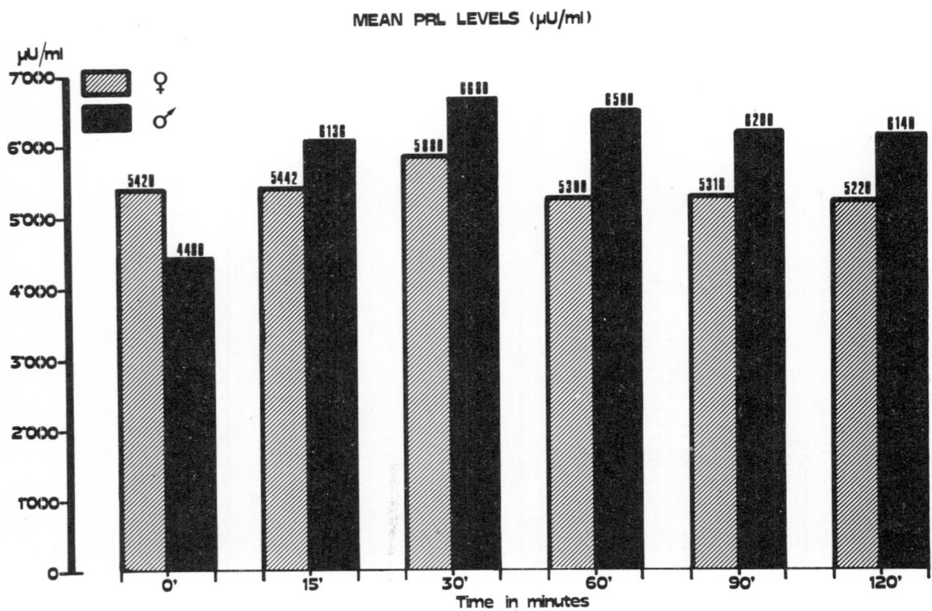

Fig. 5 Mean PRL levels in newborn after TRH — males and females comparison.

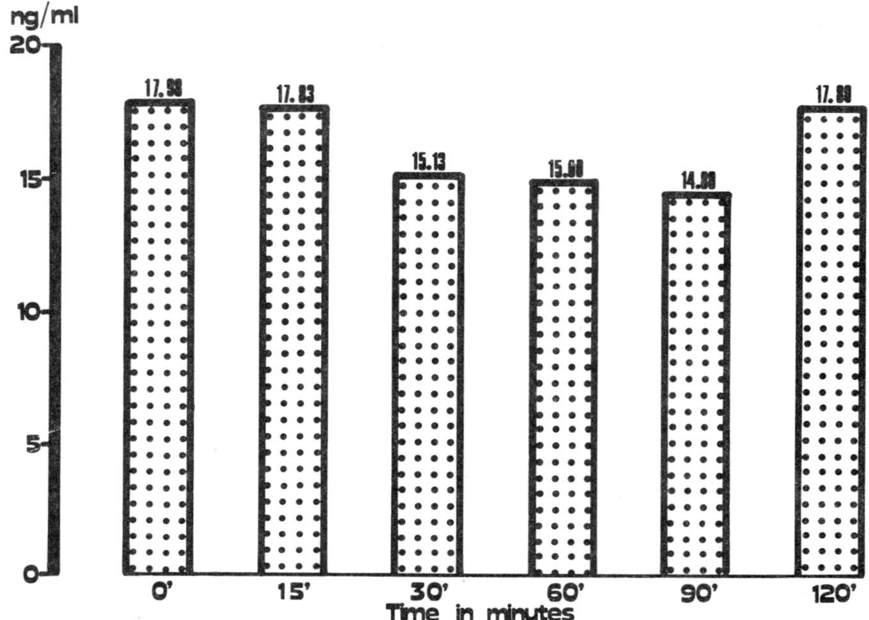

Fig. 6 Mean levels of GH in newborn after TRH.

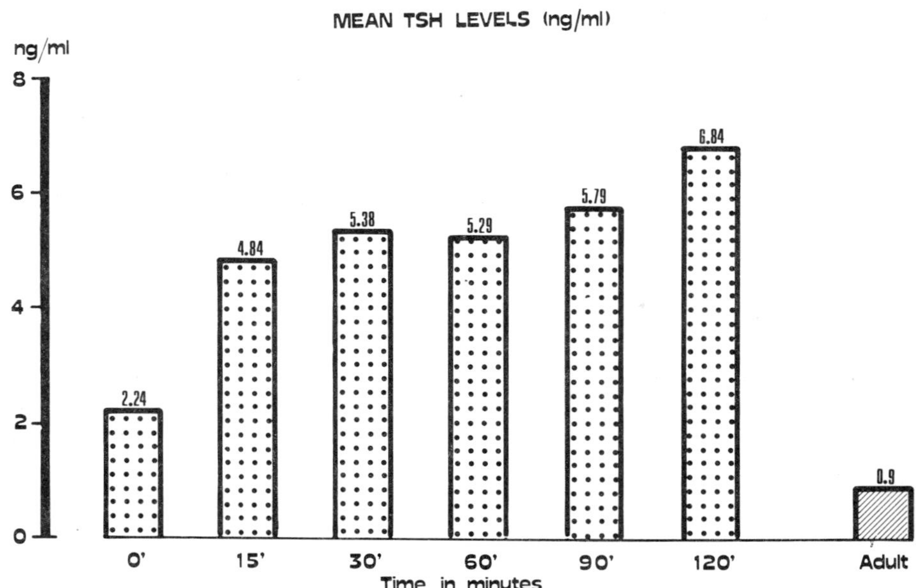

Fig. 7 Mean levels of TSH in newborn after TRH.

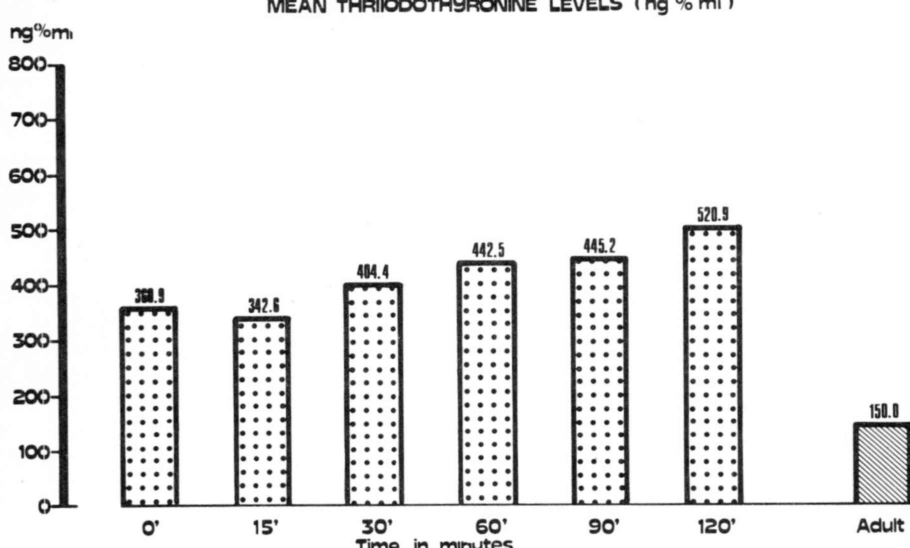

Fig. 8 Mean triiodothyronine levels in newborn after TRH.

PRL (Table I and Fig.4)

1) Basal values (1800–9000 μU/ml; mean 4950 ± 2505) were much higher than in children and adults.

2) All subjects showed a good response to TRH, with a mean increase of 1650 μU/ml ± 2040.

3) The response peak occurred after 15–30 min.

Comparison between males and females (Fig.5) showed a significant difference between the two basal means (4450 and 5420 μU/ml), though the males displayed a more marked response to TRH with a mean increase of 2000 μU/ml and a 6680 μU/ml peak, as compared with 460 μU/ml and 5880 μU/ml in the females.

GH (Table II and Fig.6)

1) As reported by other workers, basal values were much higher than those observed later in life (mean 17.98 ± 12.45 ng/ml), with an extensive range of individual values (3.3 to 37.5 ng/ml).

2) After TRH, all curves fell paradoxically by 6.5 ng/ml initially and then returned to the baseline after 120 min.

TSH (Table III and Fig.7)

1) Basal values (0.3 – 5.5 ng/ml; mean 2.24 ± 1.4) were significantly higher than in older children and adults.

2) All subjects showed a good response to TRH, with a mean increase of 4.9 ng/ml ± 1.4.

3) The response peak occurred after 15–30 min.

4) In 7/10 subjects, there was a second peak after 120 min.

Triiodothyronine (Table IV and Fig.8)

1) Basal values (mean 360.9 ± 150 ng%ml) were significantly higher than in older children and adults (150 ng%ml).

2) All subjects showed a good response to TRH, with a mean increase of 176.6 ± 110 ng%ml and a peak at 120 min, as compared with the 15 min to 30 min peak observed for TSH. This suggests that close control of thyroid performance on the part of the hypothalamus and hypophysis commences soon after birth.

CONCLUSIONS

The literature data and our findings in 0–5-day-old healthy neonates born at term enable the following conclusions to be drawn.

GH, TSH and PRL first appear in the 9th, 11th and 18th weeks of pregnancy respectively. Serum PRL in the neonate at term are lower than in the mother (4000 μU/ml). They are, however, higher than those observed in the normal adult and remain so until the 3rd-6th month. After TRH, values rise still further, with a peak at 15–30 min. Basal values are higher in females, whereas males display both a higher response to TRH and a higher peak value. Neonatal GH values are significantly higher than in older subjects over a short period and in the absence of any apparent stimulation. Injection of TRH initially led to a paradoxical increase of 6.5 ng/ml in GH (mean value), with a return to start levels after 120 min. Since the effect of stress had been avoided by implanting the needle some hours before, as advised by Cornblath *et al.* (1965) and Falorni *et al.* (1972), it may be supposed that this increase was caused by increased glucose utilization, leading to a fall in the sugar quota available for protein synthesis, and hence a decrease in circulating GH. The same effect is produced by insulin before term. The second stage of the response is comparable with the pattern observed after stimulation with prednisone and glucose, and may be attributable to direct TRH stimulation of the hypophysis acidophile cells, on the one hand, as in the case of the second TSH peak (Thomas, 1975), and to an indirect response mediated by hyperglycaemia due to massive secretion of TSH, and thus of thyroid hormones, with a well-known hyperglycaemizing effect.

TSH values at birth were higher in the neonate than in the mother, and increased rapidly at first. They fell to the birth levels after 3–4 days, and were comparable with those of the normal adult after 1 year. In all subjects, basal TSH increased still more (4.9 ng/ml) after TRH, with a peak between 15 min and 30 min. In 7/10 cases, this peak was followed by a second at 120 min. Thomas *et al.* (1975) have shown that this second peak can be suppressed by the simultaneous administration of cycloheximide in lambs and calves, since this substance blocks protein synthesis without interfering with the first peak. If correct, this suggests that TRH first releases the hormone preformed in the hypophysis, and then stimulates the production of more hormone.

Triiodothyronine at birth was lower in the newborn (50 ng%ml) than in the mother (154 ng%ml). This difference was significant. Values began to rise after 24 h, presumably in response to TSH. Levels of 419 ng%ml were noted on the 3rd–4th day. By the 30th day, they had fallen to 180–200 ng%ml and were comparable with those noted in the adult at the end of the first year.

TRH led to a gradual increase, with a peak at 120 min. Seen in the light of the other data, this suggests that thyroid performance is closely controlled by the hypothalamus and hypophysis soon after birth. Lastly, it may be stressed that the further rise in PRL at birth over the already high levels found in the foetus – adult values are not reached until the 3rd–6th month after birth – is certainly not without purpose.

Bern and Nicholl (1971) are of the opinion that foetal PRL. whether of hypophyseal or placental origin, plays a variety of possible roles in animals and man. The same view has been expressed by Sinha *et al.* (1972). Their experiments in the mouse, in fact, indicate that PRL has a somatotrophic effect in both the foetus and the newborn. It also seems that PRL influences the embryonal and foetal hydro-saline balance, since very low values are noted in 1/3 patients with hydramnion (2000 μU/ml as opposed to the 40,000 μU/ml found in the amniotic fluid of the normal gravid at term) (Fournier *et al.*, 1974). These workers also report a direct action on the breast, liver, adrenal glands and kidneys in the course of experiments with radioreceptors on the rat, and a direct, though as yet undetermined, effect on these tissues may be supposed. Lastly, Buckman *et al.* (1973) noted that a rapid fall and an increase in serum osmolarity in man depressed and enhanced PRL levels respectively.

SUMMARY

Prolactin (PRL), Growth Hormone (GH), Thyroid Stimulating Hormone (TSH) and Triiodothyronine (T_3) under basal conditions and after stimulation with i.v. 200 μg. Thyrotropin Releasing Hormone (TRH) was determined in 10 fasting eutocic newborns aged 0–5 days weighing 2.9–3.8 kg and born between the 38th and 42nd week of pregnancy. Withdrawals were made after 15, 30, 60, 90 and 120 min. PRL was expressed in μU/ml, GH and TSH in ng/ml, and T_3 in ng%ml.

Basal PRL was very high. Further increases were noted, with a peak between 15 and 30 min. Basal GH was significantly higher than in older children. After stimulation, all curves fell paradoxically and then returned to the baseline after 120 min. Basal TSH was also high. The increase after TRH displayed a peak between 15 and 30 min. The T_3 were also significantly higher than in older children as the TSH, but the peak after TRH is at 120 min. These results show that initially elevated neonatal PRL, TSH, and T_3 levels are further increased by stimulation with TRH. This bears out the view that close hypothalamic-hypophyseal control is present and a meaningful pituitary response can be mounted in the first hours of extrauterine life.

REFERENCES

Bern, H.A. and Nicol, C.S. (1968). *Rec. Progr. Horm. Res.* **24**, 681-713.

Brien, T.C., Fay, J.A. and Griffin, E.A. (1974). *Arch. Dis. Child.* **49**, 225-227.

Buckman, M.T., Kaminsky, N. and Conway, M. (1973). *Clin. Res.* **21**, 486.

Camanni, F., Massara, F., Losana, O., Messina, M., Belforte, L., Isaia, G.C., Molinatti, G.M. and Müller, E.E. (1976). *Proc. XVI National Congress Endocrinology*, Bari 18-21 May, pp.63-85 (Abstr.).

Cornblath, M., Parker, M.L., Reismen, S.M., Forbes, A.E.,and Daughaday, W.M. (1965). *J. clin. Endocr.* **25**, 209.

De Matteis, F., Spennati, G.F. and Persichetti, B. (1974). *Min Ped.* **26**, 409-416.

Dubois, P. (1968). *C.R. Soc. Biol.* **162**, 689.

Dussault, J.H., Hobel, C.J., Distefano, J.J., Eremberg, A. and Fisher, D.A. (1972). *Endocrinology* **90**, 1301-1308.

Eremberg, A. and Fisher, D.A. (1973). *Proceedings of the Sir Joseph-Barcroft Centenary Symposium*, pp.508-526. Cambridge University Press, London.
Eremberg, A., Phelps, D.L., Lam, R., Delbert, A. and Fischer, D.A. (1974). *Pediatrics* **53**, 2, 215.
Everett, J.W. (1956). *Endocrinology* **58**, 786.
Falck, B., Hillarp, N.A., Thieme, G. and Torp, A. (1962). *J. Histochem. Cytochem.* **10**, 348.
Falin, L.I. (1961). *Acta Anat.* **44**, 188.
Falorni, A., Fracassini, F., Massi-Benedetti, F., Amici, A. and Maffei, S. (1972). *Min Ped.* **21**, 27.
Fisher, D.A. and Odell, W.D. (1969). *J. clin. Invest.* **48**, 1670-1677.
Forsyth, I.A. (1972). *In* "Lactogenic Hormones" (G. Wolstenholme and J. Knight , eds), p.151. Oxford University Press, Edinburgh.
Fournier, P.J.R., Desjardins, P.D. and Friesen, H.G. (1974). *Am. J. Obstet. Gynec.* **118**, 337-343.
Franchimont. P.. Reuter, A.M. and Gevaert, Y. (1975). *(In preparation).*
Frantz, A.G. and Kleimberg, D.L. (1970). *Science* **170**, 745.
Frantz, A.G., Kleimberg, D.L. and Noel, G.L. (1970). *In* "Lactogenic Hormones" (G. Wolstenholme and J. Knight, eds). Oxford University Press, Edinburgh.
Freeman, M.C. and Neill, J.D. (1972). *Endocrinology* **90**, 1292.
Friesen, H.G., Guyda, H.,and Hwang, P. (1972). *J. clin. Invest.* **51**, 706
Frohman, L.A. and Stachura, M.E. (1975). *Metabolism* **24**, 211.
Fuxe, K., Kökfelt, T., Jonsson, G. and Löfstiöm, A. (1973). *In* "Neurosecretion. The Final Neuroendocrine Pathway." (F. Knowles and L. Vollrath, eds) pp.269-280. Springer-Verlag, Berlin.
Fuxe, K. and Jonsson, G. (1974). *In* "Serotin New Vistas" (E. Costa, G.L. Gessa and M. Sandler, eds) pp.1-26. Raven Press, New York.
Gitlyn, D. and Biasucci, A. (1969). *J. clin. Endocr. Metab.* **29**, 926.
Greemberg, A.H., Czernichoy, P., Reba, R.C., Tyson, J. and Blizzard, M. (1970). *J. clin. Invest.* **49**, 1790.
Greenwood, F.G., Bryant, G.D., Siler, T.M., Morgenstern, L.L., Robyn, C., Rubinont, P.O. and Pasteels, J.L. (1971). *In* "Radioimmunoassay Methods" (K.E. Kirkham and W.M. Hunter, eds) pp.218-232. Churchill, London.
Grosvenor, C.Z. and Mena, F. (1967). *Endocrinology* **80**, 840.
Guyda, H.J., Hwang, P. and Friesen, H.G. (1971). *J. clin. Endocr. Metab.* **32**, 120.
Hopkins, P.S. and Thorburn, G.D. (1972). *J. Endocrinol.* **54**, 55-56.
Hökfelt, T., Fuxe, K., Goldstein, M. and Johansson, O. (1974). *Brain Res.* **66**, 235.
Haugen, O.A. and Beck, J.S. (1969). *J. Pathol.* **98**, 97.
Herbert, D.C. and Hayashida, T. (1970). *Science* **169**, 378.
Hodges, D.R. and McShan, W.H. (1970). *Acta Endocr.* **63**, 378.
Hwang, P., Guyda, H. and Friesen, H.G. (1972). *J. biol. Chem.* **247**, 1955.
Iwagaky, H., Kato, K., Takakura, I., Harayama, N., Oumura, J., Shimizu, M. and Ouyama, K. (1974). *Proc. XIV International Congress of Pediatrics*, Buenos Aires, 9 October. **(Abstr.)**.
Jacobs, L.S., Mariz, J.K. and Daughaday, W.H. (1972). *J. clin. Endocr. Metab.* **34**, 484.
Kanematsu, S. and Mikami, S.I. (1969). *Endocr. Jap. Suppl.* **1**, 75.
Kaplan, S., Grumbach, M. and Friesen, H. (1972). A Serono Foundation Conference, Acapulco 29 July, pp.37-49. **(Abstr.)**.
Kaplan, S.L., Grumbach, M.M.,and Shepard, T.H. (1972b). *J. clin. Invest.* **51**, 3080.
Koch, Y., Chow, Y.F. and Meites, J. (1971). *Endocrinology* **89**, 1303.
Kwa, H.G., Feltkamf, C.A., Van der Gugten, A.A. and Verhofstad, F. (1970). *J. Endocrinol.* **48**, 299.
Laron, Z. and Pertzelan, A. (1969). *Lancet* **1**, 680.
L'Hermite, M., Stacric, V. and Robyn, C. (1972). *Acta Endocr. Suppl.* **159**, 37.
Li, C.H. (1957). *J. biol. Chem.* **229**, 157.
Li, C.H. (1972). *In* "Lactogenic Hormones" (G. Wolstenholme and J. Knight, eds) pp.7-28. Oxford University Press, Edinburgh.
Liggins, G.C. (1969). *In* "Foetal Autonomy", *CIBA Foundation Symposium* (G. Wolstenholme and J.F. O'Connor, eds) pp.218-230. Churchill, London.
Makler, M.T. (1968). *Nature* **217**, 1149.
McCann, S.M. and Moss, R.L. (1975). *Life Sci.* **16**, 833.

Meites, J. (1966). *In* "Neuroendocrinology" (L. Martini and W.F. Ganong, eds) p.669. Academic Press, New York and London.

Mishkinsky, J., Khazen, K. and Sulman, F.G. (1968). *Endocrinology* **82**, 611.

Motta, M., Fraschini, F. and Martini, L. (1969). *In* "Frontiers in Neuroendocrinology" (W.F. Ganong and L. Martini, eds) pp.6, 211-253. Oxford University Press.

Mussa, G.C., Martini-Mauri, M., Bacolla, D. and Bona, G. (1974). *Proc. I Symposium Perinatal Endocrinology*, L'Aquila, 26-27 October. (**Abstr.**).

Mussa, G.C., Martini,-Mauri, M., Bacolla, D. and Bona, G. (1976). *Min Ped.* **28**, 18, 1172-1184.

Nathanielsz, P.W., Comline, R.S., Silver, M. and Thomas, A.L. (1973). *J. Endocrinol.* **58**, 535-546.

Nicoll, C.S., Fiorindo, R.P., McKenneee, C.T. and Parsons, J.A. (1970). "Assay and Chemistry" (J. Meites, ed) pp.115-128. Williams and Wilkins, Baltimore.

Nokin, J., Vekemans, M., L'Hermite, M. and Robyn, C. (1972). *Br. med. J.* **3**, 561-562.

Parson, J.A. and Nicoll, C.S. (1971). *Neuroendocrinology* **8**, 213.

Pearse, A.G.E. (1953). *J. Path. Bact.* **65**, 355.

Pasteels, J.L., Gausset, P., Danguy, A., Ectors, F., Nicoll, C.S. and Varavudhi, P. (1972). *J. clin. Endocr. Metab.* **34**, 959.

Polleri, A., Barreca, T., Cicchetti, V., Gianrossi, R., Masturzo, P. and Rolandi, E. (1976). *Chronobiology* **3**, 27-33.

Rasmussen, H. (1970). *Science* **170**, 404.

Reitano, G. (1976). *Min Ped.* **28**, 18, 1107-1111.

Reuter, A.M., Kennes, F., Gevaert, Y. and Franchimont, P. (1975). *J. Nucl. M.B. (to be published).*

Rinne, U.K., Kivalo, E. and Talanti, S. (1962). *Biol. Neonate* **4**, 351.

Sano, M. (1962). *J. Cell Biol.* **15**, 85.

Sassin, J.F., Frantz, A.G., Kapen, S. and Weitzman, E. (1973). *J. clin. Endocr.* **37**, 436-440.

Sinha, Y.N., Lewis, U.J. and Vanderlaan, W.P. (1972). *J. Endocrinol.* **55**, 31.

Sinha, Y.N., Selby, F.W., Lewis, U.J. and Vanderlaan, W.P. (1973). *J. clin. Endocr. Metab.* **36**, 509.

Snyder, P., Jacobs, L., Utiger, R. and Daughaday, W. (1972). A Serono Foundation Conference, Acapulco, 29 July, pp.52-71. (**Abstr.**).

Sulman, F.G. (1971). "Hypothalamic Control of Lactation". Springer-Verlag, Berlin—Heidelberg—New York.

Talwalker, P.K., Ratner, A. and Meites, J. (1963). *Am. J. Physiol.* **205**, 213.

Thomas, A.L., Jack, P.M.B., Manns, J.G. and Nathanielsz, P.W. (1975). *Biol. Neonate* **26**, 109-116.

Torok, B. (1964). *Acta Anat.* **59**, 84.

Tyson, J., Friesen, H.G. and Anderson, M.S. (1972). *Science* **177**, 897.

Valverde, C., Chieffo, V. and Reichlin, S. (1974). *Endocrinology* **91**, 982-993.

Vigneri, R., Papalia, D. and Motta, L. (1969). *J. Nucl. Biol. Med.* **13**, 151-159.

Vigneri, R., Pezzino, V., Filetti, S., Squatrito, S. and Polosa, P. (1976). *Proc. XVI National Congress Endocrinology*, Bari 18—21 May, pp.87-101. (**Abstr.**).

Vignola, G., Barreca, T., Gianrossi, R. and Nizzo, M.C. (1976). *Boll. Soc. Ital. Biol. Sper.* **51**, 759-761.

Wallace, A.L.C., Stacy, B.D. and Thorburn, G.D. (1973). *J. Endocrinol.* **58**, 89-95.

Wilson, D.W., Pierrepoint, C.G. and Griffiths, K. (1973). *Biochem. Soc. Trans.* **1**, 172-175.

Wurtman, R.J. (1971). *Neur. Res. Progr. Bull.* **9**, 41-54.

METABOLIC AND ENDOCRINE RESPONSES TO FEEDING IN THE HUMAN NEWBORN

A. Aynsley-Green, S.R. Bloom**, D.H. Williamson* and R.C. Turner*

**University Department of Pediatrics and the Nuffield Department of Clinical Medicine, University of Oxford*
***The Royal Postgraduate Medical School, Hammersmith Hospital London, England*

ABSTRACT

Little is known on the metabolic and endocrine responses to feeding in the human neonate. We have measured the levels of several hormones and key intermediary metabolites in arterial blood after the first feed of 5 ml/kg breast milk in a group of infants (n = 12) suffering from mild respiratory distress. A significant rise in blood glucose occurred within 25 min of the feed (mean peak increment at 55 min being 0.84 mmol/l) but no change occurred in lactate, pyruvate, alanine or ketones. Significant increases in plasma insulin (fasting 6.8 + 1.3 μU/ml, 55 min: 15.3 + 3.2 μU/ml, $p < 0.01$), gastrin (fasting 10.9 ± 1.3 fmol/ml, 55 min: 26.1 ± 1.9 fmol/ml, $p < 0.01$), G.H. (fasting 17.7 ± 3.2 ng/ml, 55 min: 27.8 ± 5.4 ng/ml, $p < 0.05$) and enteroglucagon (fasting 145.1 ± 30.0 fmol/ml, 55 min: 305.5 ± 64.8 fmol/ml, $p < 0.05$) occurred after the feed, but no change in pancreatic glucagon was seen.

Several hormone systems are functionally active at birth and are stimulated by the first feed of milk. These changes may be important in the process of adaptation to extrauterine life.

INTRODUCTION

At birth, the continuous supply of nutrients which the fetus has received across the placenta is interrupted, and the neonate has to adapt to a new environment of intermittent feeding and fasting. There is evidence that some of the changes in hepatic enzyme activity occurring during this process of metabolic adaptation are due to changes in plasma hormone concentrations, particularly in those of insulin and glucagon (Adam, 1971; Shelley *et al.*, 1975). There is further evidence from animal studies that insulin release in response to glucose increases with the introduction of feeding (Asplund, 1972; Gentz *et al.*, 1971), whilst in man, the urinary excretion of insulin does not increase until feeding is established (Lowy and Schiff, 1968). In view of the known interrelation of hormones of the 'entero-insular axis' in adults, this raises the possibility that neonatal changes in pancreatic insular hormone secretion, and thus hepatic metabolism, are influenced by developmental changes in gastrointestinal hormone secretion during the establishment of feeding. This hypothesis is supported by the studies of Rogers *et al.* (1974, 1975) who noted higher levels of gastrin, enteroglucagon and secretin on the fourth day of life than at birth. There is, however, no information on the development of the dynamic response of gastrointestinal hormones to the stimulus of feeding and their relation to pancreatic insular hormone levels and changes in circulating intermediary metabolites. We are studying this problem, and wish to report our results from one aspect of the study, namely the endocrine and metabolic response to the first feed of breast milk.

The very first feed given to a newborn infant is an event of considerable significance. Substantial amounts of amniotic fluid are swallowed by the fetus and can be utilized (Bradley and Mistretta, 1973), but it is not known how effective this is in preparing the gut for post-natal milk feeding. The first feed challenges the competence of several physiological systems, including the contractile and digestive function of the gut and the integration of hepatic metabolism and hormone secretion to ensure the smooth delivery of substrates to the periphery.

In order to provide information of clinical relevance, we have measured the concentrations of several hormones and key intermediary metabolites before and after the first feed of breast milk, as routinely given in our Special Care Unit, to a group of infants suffering from moderately severe respiratory distress.

METHODS

Patients

Twelve infants were studied with the approval of the Ethical Committee. All had been admitted to the Special Care Baby Unit, and all had indwelling umbilical arterial catheters for clinical monitoring purposes. They were nursed in infant incubators at an environmental temperature appropriate for their weight and gestation (Hey and Katz, 1970). None had a rectal temperature less than 36°C at the time of the study. The mean birth weight was 2945 g (range 2110–3940 g) and mean gestational age 37.8 weeks (range 37–39 weeks). Nine of the infants were suffering from moderately severe respiratory distress requiring enriched inspired oxygen concentrations. Of the other 3, one was a breech delivery with severe birth asphyxia and 2 had lesser degrees of birth asphyxia requiring transient endotracheal intubation, oxygen and alkali therapy. None had an arterial pH less than 7.25, and the inspired oxygen concentration was adjusted to maintain the PaO_2 in the range 60–90 torr. No change in inspired oxygen concentration was required during the study period and the clinical condition of the infants did not change.

Feeding Procedure

The first feed was given between 4 and 6 h of age. Nasogastric tubes were inserted and the stomach contents aspirated 30 min before the feed. Where the stomach contents were copious, tenacious or heavily stained with meconium, 5–10 ml of 0.9% saline at 37°C were used to irrigate the stomach, the contents being re-aspirated. The infants were then given 5 ml/kg pooled mature expressed breast milk (EBM), which is the volume necessary to give 60 ml/kg/24 h with a two-hourly feeding regime. The feed was given by gravity over 2–4 min, the infants lying on the right side with the head of the mattress elevated. The infants were not disturbed during the study period. At the end of the test, the stomach contents were re-aspirated and in no case was more than 25% of the original feed volume returned. Regurgitation of the feed did not occur in any instance.

Blood Sampling

Blood samples, each of 1.0–1.4 ml were drawn from the aorta via the umbilical artery catheter immediately before the feed and at 5, 25 and 55 min after the feed. Immediately on withdrawing, blood (0.4 ml) was added to 4 ml ice-cold 5% perchloric acid for assay of metabolites; 0.1–0.2 ml blood was added to a heparinised tube for insulin and growth hormone assay; 0.5–0.9 ml blood was added to 0.1 ml aprotinin (Trasylol 1000 KIU) containing 50 mM E.D.T.A. for the assay of the other hormones.

Assay Methods

Concentrations of glucose, lactate, pyruvate, alanine, acetoacetate and β-hydroxybutyrate in whole blood were determined enzymatically (Bergmeyer, 1963). Plasma gastrin was measured by a radioimmunoassay using an antiserum raised against synthetic human gastrin 1 which measured big gastrin (G34) and little gastrin (G17) equally, but which did not react significantly with big big gastrin, little little gastrin (G14), or cholecystokinin pancreozymin. Standards (MRC 68–439) were made up in gastrin-free plasma and individual differences of 2.5 fmol/ml plasma could be detected with 95% confidence. Plasma N-terminal reactive glucagon-like immunoreactivity (enteroglucagon, or intestinal glucagon) and plasma C-terminal reactive glucagon-like immunoreactivity (pancreatic glucagon) were measured as described previously (Bloom, 1974). Plasma Gastric-Inhibitory-Peptide (GIP) was measured by conventional radioimmunoassay techniques using an anti-serum raised to pure natural porcine GIP and pure porcine GIP standards. Changes of 10 fmol/ml plasma could be detected with 95% confidence. Plasma insulin was measured using charcoal phase separation (Albano *et al.*, 1972) with simultaneous growth hormone assay (Albano *et al.*, 1972). The precision (± 1 S.D.) was 1.4 μU/ml plasma insulin, and 1.5 ng/ml plasma growth hormone. Results were assessed for statistical significance by means of the Student *t* test.

RESULTS

1. *Blood Glucose and Other Metabolites*

Mean fasting blood glucose concentration was 3.67 ± 0.22 mmol/l (± S.E.M.); a significant rise occurred after the feed, the mean increment at 55 min being 0.84 mmol/l, or 15 mg/100 ml (Fig.1). This increment, even though it was so small, does imply that the first feed had been at least partially digested and absorbed, and the products released as glucose. From a practical point, it means that

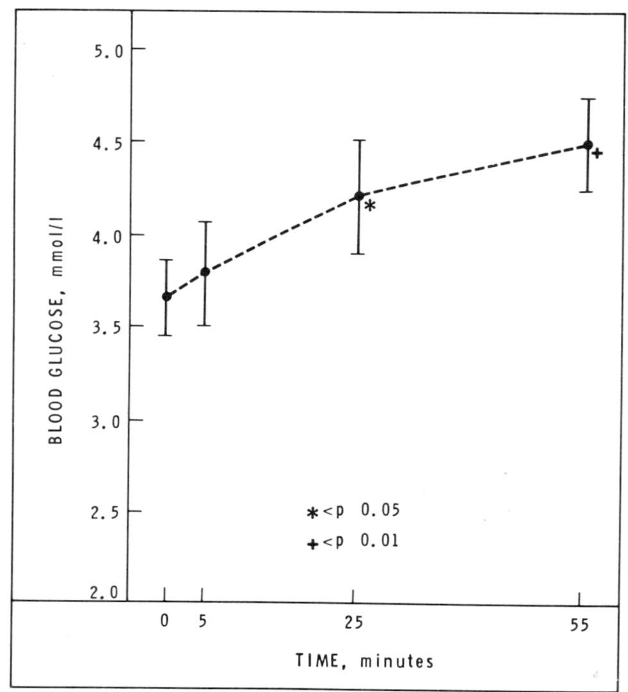

Fig. 1 The effect of the first feed of E.B.M. on blood glucose concentration (n = 12) (± S.E.M.).

Table I. The effect of the first feed of E.B.M. on blood metabolite concentrations (n = 12, ± S.E.M.) (mmol/l).

	Time (Min) 0	5	25	55
Lactate	2.37 (± 0.71)	1.73 (± 0.34)	2.02 (± 0.43)	1.80 (± 0.31)
Pyruvate	0.19 (± 0.04)	0.17 (± 0.02)	0.17 (± 0.03)	0.17 (± 0.03)
Alanine	0.37 (± 0.10)	0.32 (± 0.07)	0.32 (± 0.07)	0.33 (± 0.07)
Ketones	0.25 (± 0.04)	0.28 (± 0.05)	0.29 (± 0.05)	0.32 (± 0.05)

the feed of 5 ml/kg of EBM can be expected to cause a rise in blood glucose in the order of 15 mg/100 ml within 55 min of giving the first feed. Table I shows the values obtained for four intermediaries; lactate, pyruvate and alanine represent the major precursors for gluconeogenesis, total ketone bodies (the sum of acetoacetate and 3-hydroxybutyrate) being alternative fuels for glucose. It can be seen that the concentrations of none of these substances alter after the feed. It is remarkable that the feed does not cause a change in the levels of any of these important substances. The significance of this lack of effect must remain unclear until we have information on the effect of this stimulus in older infants and adults.

2. *Plasma Hormones*

The mean fasting plasma insulin concentration was 6.8 ± 1.3 μU/ml, and a significant rise occurred after the feed, reaching a peak value of 15.3 ± 3.2 μU/ml

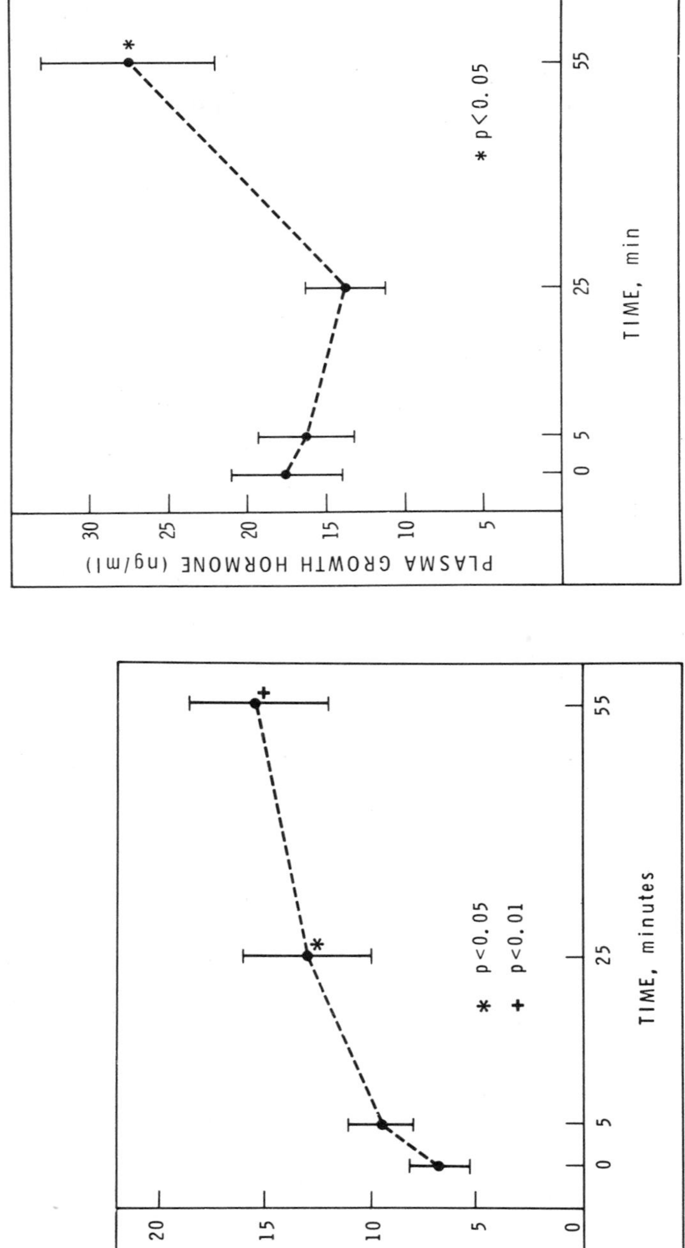

Fig.3

Fig.2

Fig.2 The effect of the first feed of E.B.M. on plasma insulin (n = 11) (± S.E.M.).

Fig.3 The effect of the first feed of E.B.M. on plasma growth hormone (n = 11) (± S.E.M.).

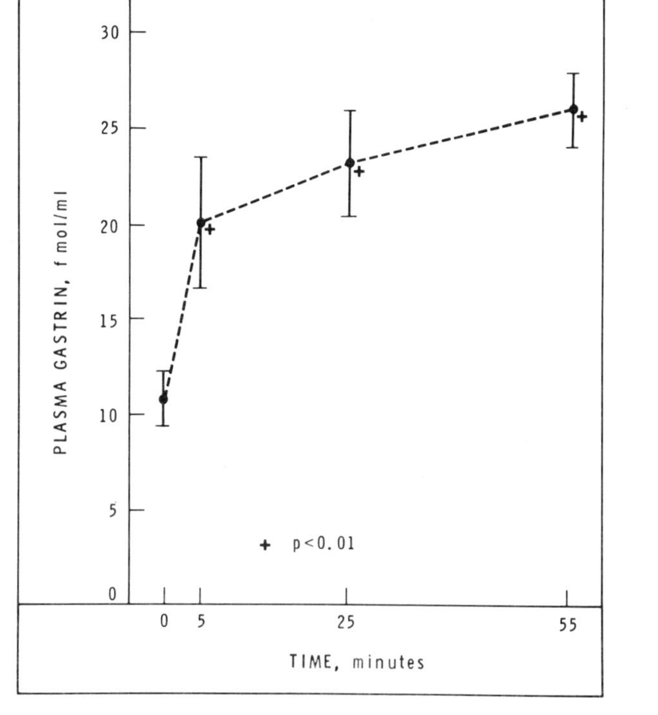

Fig.4

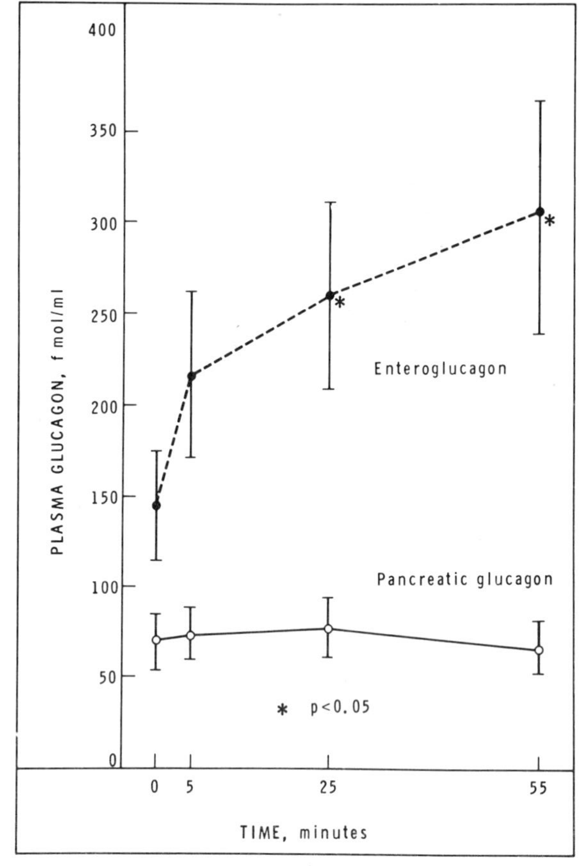

Fig.5

Fig.4 The effect of the first feed of E.B.M. on plasma gastrin (n = 9) (± S.E.M.).

Fig.5 The effect of the first feed of E.B.M. on plasma glucagon (n = 11) and plasma enteroglucagon (n = 11) (± S.E.M.).

at 55 min (Fig.2). Again, it will be of considerable interest to know how this relates to an older infant's or an adult's insulin response, but the β-cells clearly do respond to this first feed. The fact that the response was so small is probably a reflection of the small rise in blood glucose. However, even an insulin rise of 8 μU/ml would be expected to affect lipolysis in adults, and this makes the failure to change the levels of ketone bodies even more remarkable.

Figure 3 shows the effect of the feed on plasma growth hormone. The mean basal level was 17.7 ± 3.2 ng/ml, and a significant rise to 27.8 ± 5.4 ng/ml occurred 55 min after the feed. The mechanism of this increase is speculative, but it seems to coincide with the increase in glucose, and others have commented on the paradoxical increase in growth hormone after glucose in neonates (Cornblath *et al.*, 1965; Laron *et al.*, 1966). Whatever the mechanism of this stimulation, it can be seen that at least two hormones with powerful metabolic effects, i.e. insulin and growth hormone, are increased after the first feed.

The mean basal gastrin level was 10.9 fmol/ml, and within minutes of introducing the feed there was an increase, reaching a mean value of 26.1 ± 1.9 fmol/ml after 55 min (Fig.4). Of the other two gastrointestinal hormones measured, the feed caused a significant rise in plasma enteroglucagon within 25 min, reaching a mean value of 305.5 fmol/ml at 55 min (Fig.5), but no significant change occurred in the levels of Gastric Inhibitory Peptide. Mean basal GIP level was 117.7 ± 31.7 fmol/ml, and at 55 min was 154.1 ± 27.8 (p = N.S.). Further interpretation of these results is difficult since there is no information on the role of these hormones in the neonatal period, but they do indicate that the neonatal gut is capable of responding promptly to the first feed by releasing at least two gastrointestinal hormones.

The final hormone to be discussed is pancreatic glucagon. In contrast to the rise in enteroglucagon, no change was observed after the feed (Fig.5).

CONCLUSIONS

A major difficulty in interpreting our results is the fact that the infants studied were not entirely normal, in that they were all suffering from additional illness. The feed was also given by nasogastric tube, which excluded the potentially important influence of sucking (Bassett, 1974). This information may not be directly applicable to normal infants. Nevertheless, it does provide information on the effect of our standard feeding regime on these sick infants, and the following conclusions can be made.

The first feed of human breast milk given to infants approaching term causes a consistent rise in blood glucose without affecting the levels of other important intermediary metabolites. Further work is necessary to follow the pattern of metabolite changes as feeding becomes established, but the rise in glucose implies that the feed had been at least partially digested and absorbed.

The rise in glucose is accompanied by increases in the levels of insulin and growth hormone, without changing pancreatic glucagon. So at least two important 'metabolic' hormones in different endocrine systems are stimulated by the first feed. The gastro-intestinal tract appears to be primed and ready to respond at this time as shown by the increase in gastrin and enteroglucagon. The latter hormone may be of particular importance in the neonatal period in view of its postulated effect on long-term growth of absorptive intestinal mucosa (Bloom, 1974).

REFERENCES

Adam, P.A.J. (1971). *In* "Advances in Metabolic Disorders" (R. Levine and R. Luft, eds) p.183. Academic Press, London.

Albano, J.D.M., Ekins, R.P., Maritz, G. and Turner, R.C. (1972). *Acta endocr. (Copenh.)* **70**, 487.

Asplund, K. (1972). *Diabetologia* **8**, 153.

Bassett, J.M. (1974). *Australian J. Biol. Sci.* **27**, 157.

Bergmeyer, H. (1963). "Methoden der enzymatischen Analyse". Verlag Chemie, Weinheim.

Bloom, S.R. (1974). *Br. med. Bull.* **30**, 62.

Bloom, S.R. (1974). *Gut* **15**, 502.

Bradley, R.M. and Mistretta, C.M. ((1973). *Science* **179**, 1016.

Cornblath, M., Parker, M.L., Reisner, S.H., Forbes, A.E. and Daughaday, W.H. (1965). *J. clin. Endocr. Metab.* **25**, 209.

Gentz, J.C.H., Persson, B., Kellum, M., Bengtsson, G. and Thorell, J. (1971). *Life Sci.* **10**, 137.

Hey, E.N. and Katz, G. (1970). *Arch. Dis. Child.* **45**, 328.

Laron, Z., Mannheimer, A., Pertzelan, A. and Menachem, N. (1966). *Isr. J. med. Sci.* **2**, 770.

Lowy, C. and Schiff, D. (1968). *Lancet* **i**, 225.

Rogers, I.M., Davidson, D.C., Lawrence, J., Ardill, J. and Buchanan, K.D. (1974). *Arch. Dis. Child.* **49**, 796.

Rogers, I.M. Davidson, D.C., Lawrence, J. and Buchanan, K.D. (1975). *Arch. Dis. Child.* **50**, 120.

Turner, R.C., Schneeloch, B. and Paterson, P. (1971). *Acta endocr. (Copenh.)* **66**, 577.

Shelley, H.J., Basset, J.M. and Milner, R.D.G. (1975). *Br. med. Bull.* **31**, 37.

SOMATOMEDINS AND CARBOHYDRATE METABOLISM

C. La Cauza, L. Marianelli, P.A. Nicotina*, S. Seminara, R. Salti and R. Godi

Department of Pediatrics, University of Florence, Italy
**Department of Morbid Anatomy, University of Messina, Italy*

Almost all the hormones act more or less directly and ostensibly upon the carbohydrate metabolism. The role of some of them, e.g. insulin and glucagon, is of basic importance and therefore well known; the action of others, e.g. the growth hormone, is still under discussion and its mechanism hypothetical; the influence of others is still only presumable.

In our opinion, the somatomedins belong to the last category and this chapter intends to prove it.

There are various possible theories about the probable action of the somatomedins on the carbohydrate metabolism, but all of them use as their main argument the similarity of these substances to insulin and an even stronger affinity with substances which differ from the immunoreactive insulin but whose action is exactly the same.

We have known for about 15 years that the human serum exerts a biological insulin activity much superior to that of immunoreactive insulin (IRI) (Leonard *et al.*, 1962; Samaan *et al.*, 1963; Froesch *et al.*, 1963). As a matter of fact, some authors who used the glucose oxidation in the epididymal fat pads to evaluate the quantity of the biological insulin activity of the human serum through glucose proved that only 7% of this activity was due to immunoreactive insulin (Froesch *et al.*, 1963); the remaining 93% was called NSLIA (Non-Suppressible Insulin-Like Activity).

Froesch *et al.* continued their thorough research, trying to isolate the NSILA from the serum (Froesch *et al.*, 1963; Burgi *et al.*, 1966; Froesch *et al.*, 1967; Jakob *et al.*, 1968; Froesch *et al.*, 1975). In fact, they succeeded in isolating one fraction, the NSILA-S (Froesch *et al.*, 1967; Jakob *et al.*, 1968), which was shown to mimic a number of the metabolic effects of crystalline insulin (Oelz *et al.*, 1970; Hepp, 1972); however it differs from insulin in some very important characteristics. In order to explain these differences some authors supposed that the NSILA-S had a much longer half-life than that of insulin (Froesch *et al.*, 1975b).

Besides, the NSILA-S acts as a very strong growth-stimulating substance (Morell and Froesch, 1973; Zingg-and Froesch, 1973) approximately 50 times more potent than insulin (Froesch *et al.*, 1975) and its functions are nearly identical to those of somatomedins (Zingg and Froesch, 1973). Its molecular size (Froesch *et al.*, 1975c) and its amino-acid contents (Humbel *et al.*, 1971, 1972) confirm definitely its remarkable similarity to the somatomedins (Hall and Luft, 1974; Fryklund *et al.*, 1974; Hall *et al.*, 1975a; Sievertsson *et al.*, 1975) so that Van Wyck *et al.* (1973) proposed to name the NSILA-S somatomedin D.

The fact that the NSILA-S was bound to serum proteins so that in the serum of all subjects with a high amount of NSILA-S a high percentage of binding protein was also found, whereas in subjects with a low percentage of NSILA-S the amount of binding protein is also scarce, represents the latest fundamental discovery (Zapf *et al.*, 1975). These observations explain why a relatively high concentration of the NSILA-S was found in the serum of decompensated diabetics.

Foresch *et al.* (1975b) maintain that the link of the NSILA-S with the big carrier molecule makes its passage through the capillaries rather difficult. It remains to be clarified why certain tissues, such as cartilage, can extract the NSILA-S from its carrier more readily than the muscle and adipose tissues.

This binding to a serum protein is analogous to the somatomedins, as Hintz *et al.* (1974) have recently proved concerning somatomedin C.

During the last two years our knowledge of somatomedins has increased to such an extent that even a tentative synthesis of it is impossible; however, we consider it useful at least to establish certain general principles which primarily concern the assay methods.

After the isolation of the somatomedins A_1, A_2 and B (Hall, 1970, 1971, 1972; Hall *et al.*, 1975a; Sievertsson *et al.*, 1975) there were applied the radioimmunoassay with the technique of double anti-body and the radio-receptor assay (Van Wyck *et al.*, 1975; Hall *et al.*, 1975b) using specific cell membrane receptors (which differ from those used for insulin) of the human placenta as the most sensitive ones (Hintz *et al.*, 1972; Clemmons *et al.*, 1974; Marshall *et al.*, 1974).

These new assay methods for somatomedins are undoubtedly more precise and simpler than the classic biological methods but, besides the great scarcity of the necessary substances, they also present another and very serious difficulty, duly recognized by the research authors, and that is: the amounts of somatomedin obtained through these methods, although corresponding approximately to those obtained through biological methods, are generally rather higher. The most probable explanation of this discrepancy is the coexistence of inhibiting material which limits the biological action of the somatomedins.

The existence of this inhibitor has been proved by the experimental tests of Salmon (1975) and clinical ones performed by Van den Brande and Du Caju *et al.* (1973, 1974); for Van den Brande and Du Caju this has a teleological significance, since it could serve as an ideal protection to the organism in times of prolonged food deprivation, by preventing wasteful consumption of energy in the process of growth.

To conclude: until the interference of the inhibitor can be eliminated, the radioimmunoassay and radioreceptor assay as they exist now can only represent a partial aspect of the somatomedin activity, whereas the biological method furnishes its real and precise value always. Therefore, in our opinion, the biological method represents still the best research technique, particularly in the clinical field. Indeed, in our past research we applied the Hall method with the chicken embryo cartilage specific for somatomedin A.

Always using the same technique, we have begun a series of clinical and experimental research of the somatomedin activity behaviour in the pathology of carbohydrate metabolism. In this chapter we shall present the results of our clinical tests, performed in children with diabetes and glycogenosis, as well as those of our first experimental research.

The somatomedin activity in diabetics has seldom been studied. The few tests, performed exclusively on adults, go back to the period 1963-64 in which the determination of the sulphation factor was used to value indirectly the growth hormone. Jensen *et al.* (1963) using two groups of diabetics obtained the following results: in the non-obese diabetics (22 subjects, of whom one only 17 years old) the quantity of 0.97 U; in the obese (17 cases, the youngest 47 years old) the amount of 1.10 U. The difference did not change greatly for the non-obese diabetics, even after a carbohydrate restriction; whereas in the obese this restriction resulted in an 18% diminution of the sulphation factor, a difference hardly significant statistically.

More interesting and complete is the work of Yde, published in 1964. In 60 diabetic adults he found an average amount of 0.78 of sulphation factor, as compared with 0.96 in 12 control subjects. The diminution of the sulphation factor in the diabetics was statistically significant; besides, in the non-obese diabetics there existed a negative relationship between the serum sulphation factor and the serum glucose, which was absent in the obese ones. In later research (1969) Yde has confirmed this diminution of the sulphation factor in 52 newly-diagnosed and untreated diabetics.

Finally, in 1974 Van den Brande and Du Caju in their papers on somatomedin activity in certain endocrinological disorders report finding in 6 cases of untreated juvenile diabetics amounts of somatomedin within the low normal range; these results are very similar to those of Yde.

Even if we have unbeknown omitted some research, we can still undoubtedly conclude that the study of the somatomedin activity in diabetes, particularly the childhood one, is to say the least still incomplete, and therefore needs more thorough and methodical research.

We do not know of any study concerning the somatomedin activity in glycogenosis.

MATERIALS AND METHODS

The clinical tests were made on the following four groups:

1) Sixteen diabetics, aged 5 to 13; 10 of them males and 6 females, with a well-balanced metabolism, with a slight glycosuria and no acetonuria, hospitalized for the periodical control tests; their illness had been diagnosed at least 2 and at most 8 years before ("old" diabetes mellitus).

2) Four diabetics aged 6 to 10, 2 males and 2 females; their illness was at the

beginning of its evident symptomatology and their balance still unstable with considerable glycosuria and periodical acetonuria, but no chetoacidosis, the diagnosis having been made less than 3 months before ("initial" diabetes mellitus).

3) A control group of 6 patients aged 6-12, 3 males and 3 females, free from any endocrinal or metabolic illness, hospitalized with slight respiratory disease.

4) Two patients suffering from glycogenosis Type I, brothers, aged 10 years 9 months and 14 years 7 months respectively.

In all the cases blood was taken in the morning on an empty stomach in basic conditions. Afterwards the first 3 groups each received a rapid endovenous injection of ready insulin (Actrapid) in a quantity of 0.1 U/kg of real weight; the two patients of the fourth group received an injection of 0.5 g of monochlorhydrate arginine per kg of real weight.

Blood was then repeatedly taken after 30, 60, 90 and 120 min; the last sample was taken 6—8 h after the initial one, about 5 h after a meal. All the blood samples were centrifuged immediately, the glycemia measured with glucosiooxydase technique and the serum preserved at 20°C temperature.

In the serum taken in basic conditions, i.e. before the administration of insulin and arginine, the somatomedin was evaluated by Hall's method (1970), the insulin by radioimmunoassay of Herbert *et al.* (1965) and the somatothropic hormone by the method of Schalch and Parker (1964) and Morgan (1966). In the serum taken after 30, 60, 90 and 120 min the somatothropic hormone was measured together with the glycemia; finally the serum taken after 6-8 h served only to evaluate the somatomedin A.

The experimental tests were made on 72 male rats at prepuberty age and of average weight of 62.34 ± 4.98 housed and nourished in the traditional manner, their drink containing 30% of glucose; they were divided into 2 groups of 32 animals each. The first group served as control; the second was subjected to a treatment consisting of administration by gastric tube of a dose of 950 mg/kg of body weight of diazo-oxide dissolved in a 5% suspension of mucilage of gum arabic twice a day.

On alternate days, together with the second dose of diazo-oxide they were given 16 mg/kg of trichlormethyazide for the double purpose of weakening the retention of water caused by diazo-oxide and of strengthening its hyperglycemizing effect.

The first day three animals out of each group had been bled to death in order to measure the basic amount of glycemia at the start as well as at the stadium of metaphysis development.

On the eighth day, 4 h after the last administration of diazo-oxide, 6 animals out of each group were killed in order to compare the amount of glycemia in the blood of the treated animals with that of the control group.

The same tests were repeated on the 15th, 40th and 60th day, also extracting the proximal extremity of the tibia in order to study the epiphyseal cartilage.

The epiphyso-diaphysis segments of the tibias were preserved in 10% neutral formaldehyde, decalcified with a 10% solution of ethylene-diamino-tetracetic acid and enclosed in paraffin. Six-micron thick sections of them were colored with emallume-eosin and treated with Mowy's istochemical method, specific for acid mucopolysaccharides of the ground substance. The micrometric measurements of condrocyte strata were made with a calibrated lens. The results were compiled into arithmetic averages and their relative deviations as well as the relative statistical evaluation.

Table I.

Cases			Age Years	Age Months	Weight (percentiles)	Height (percentiles)	Period of Illness Years	Period of Illness Months
Group 1st								
1.	B.A.	♂	5		25°	50°–75°	2	
2.	C.E.	♀	5	6	25°	25°–50°	1	9
3.	O.F.	♀	6		25°–50°	25°	4	
4.	S.F.	♂	7		50°–75°	25°–50°	1	
5.	O.F.	♂	7	4	25°–50°	25°	1	8
6.	A.F.	♀	7	6	25°–50°	25°	3	4
7.	F.M.	♂	8		25°	50°	3	2
8.	A.C.	♂	8	2	50°	25°–50°	3	4
9.	C.F.	♂	8	6	25°–50°	25°	4	6
10.	C.A.	♂	9		50°–75°	50°–75°	5	6
11.	B.F.	♀	9	6	25°	10°–25°	4	
12.	L.M.	♂	10		25°–50°	25°–50°	3	4
13.	M.E.	♀	11	2	50°	25°–50°	3	8
14.	F.M.	♂	12		50°	50°–75°	5	2
15.	D.B.	♀	12	6	50°–75°	25°–50°	8	6
16.	P.B.	♂	13		25°–50°	25°–50°	4	
Average			y. 8	m. 9	–	–	y. 3	m. 7
Group 2nd								
1.	B.A.	♀	5	8	10°	50°	0	2
2.	A.M.	♂	6	6	10°–25°	50°	0	3
3.	S.F.	♂	7		50°	25°–50°	0	4
4.	B.E.	♀	10		25°–50°	50°	0	1
Average			y. 7	m. 3	–	–	y.	m. 2
Group 3rd								
1.	B.M.	♂	6	4	50°–75°	75°–90°	–	
2.	G.L.	♂	7	2	75°	75°	–	
3.	M.B.	♀	8		25°–50°	50°	–	
4.	S.R.	♂	9	6	50°–75°	75°	–	
5.	V.G.	♀	10	4	90°	75°–90°	–	
6.	L.G.	♀	12		75°	25°–50°	–	
Average			y. 8	m. 10	–	–	–	
Group 4th								
1.	F.M.	♂	10	9	3°	3°	6	
2.	F.F.	♂	14	7	3°	3°	13	

Clinical and auxological case history: Group 1st – "Old" diabetics; Group 2nd – "Initial" diabetics; Group 3rd – Controls. Group 4th – Glicogenosis patients Type I.

Table II.

Cases	S m A (basic)	S m A (after insulin)	Δ	Peak level HGH after insulin
Group 1st				
1. B.A. ♂	1.44	1.57	0.13	10.60
2. C.E. ♀	0.84	0.91	0.07	9.25
3. O.F. ♀	0.56	1.35	0.79	14.80
4. S.F. ♂	0.75	1.02	0.27	18.60
5. O.F. ♂	1.23	1.71	0.48	20.45
6. A.F. ♀	0.88	0.98	0.10	13.40
7. F.M. ♂	0.63	1.60	0.97	18.30
8. A.C. ♂	1.02	1.42	0.40	21.85
9. C.F. ♂	0.87	0.90	0.03	16.75
10. C.A. ♂	0.76	0.93	0.17	21.75
11. B.F. ♀	1.11	1.64	0.53	12.60
12. L.M. ♂	0.77	1.25	0.48	9.15
13. M.E. ♀	0.79	1.25	0.46	22.75
14. F.M. ♂	0.98	1.20	0.22	10.45
15. D.B. ♀	1.30	1.44	0.14	9.05
16. P.B. ♂	0.96	1.80	0.84	17.50
Average ± DS	0.93 ± 0.24	1.31 ± 0.30	0.38 ± 0.29	15.45 ± 4.92
Group 2nd				
1. B.A. ♀	0.36	0.87	0.51	18.70
2. A.M. ♂	0.50	0.73	0.23	10.20
3. S.F. ♂	0.34	0.86	0.52	12.90
4. B.E. ♀	0.52	0.75	0.23	15.20
Average ± DS	0.43 ± 0.09	0.80 ± 0.07	0.37 ± 0.16	14.25 ± 3.60
Group 3rd				
1. B.M. ♂	0.58	0.95	0.37	27.35
2. G.L. ♂	0.61	1.29	0.68	14.80
3. M.B. ♀	0.95	1.04	0.09	25.10
4. S.R. ♂	1.21	1.37	0.16	11.15
5. V.G. ♀	1.17	1.21	0.04	23.70
6. L.G. ♀	0.83	0.88	0.05	13.40
Average ± DS	0.89 ± 0.27	1.12 ± 0.20	0.23 ± 0.25	19.25 ± 6.90

RESULTS

Table I shows the main clinical and auxological characteristics of all the patients: age and sex, weight and height in percentiles, and the duration of the disease.

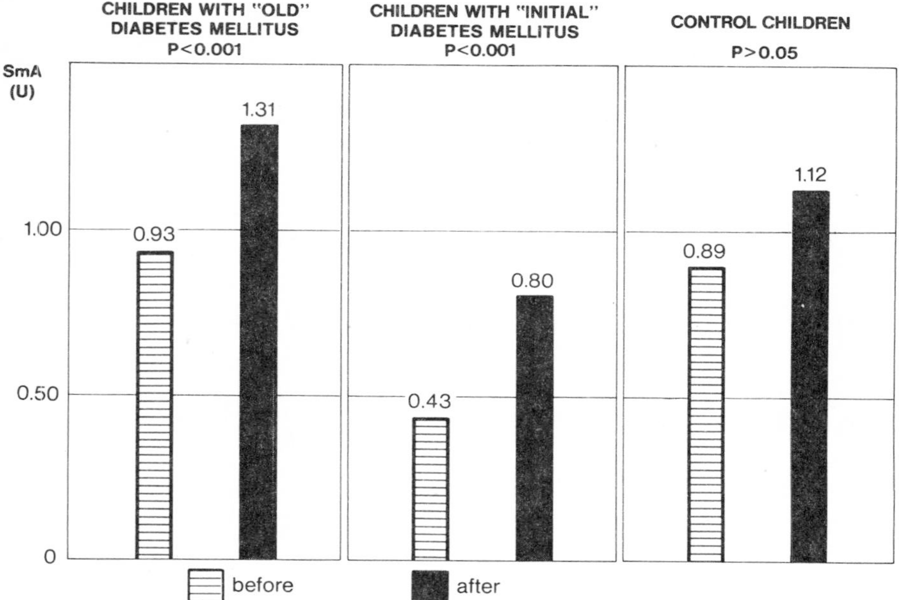

Fig. 1 The averages of SmA before and after insulin load in diabetic children and group of control.

It is evident that the diabetics do not show any significant defects of growth, either in weight or in height; only recent diabetics show a considerable weight deficiency, as demonstrated by various authors (Sterky, 1963; White and Graham, 1971; Marianelli *et al.*, 1975).

The two cases of glycogenosis described by Bartolozzi *et al.* (1975) suffer from a pronounced growth deficiency with all the characteristic symptoms of dismetabolic dwarfism.

Table II shows the amount of somatomedin A in basic conditions and after 6–8 h of insulin load, as well as the peak values of HGH during the insulin test in the two diabetic groups and in the control group with the relative averages.

In the "old" diabetics (Group 1st) in basic conditions (i.e. before the administration of insulin) the somatomedin activity remains within the normal; in the "initial" diabetics (Group 2nd) it is considerably lower than the normal average for the given age. In both groups after the insulin test we have found a significant increase of somatomedin A with an increase value Δ of 0.38 and 0.37 respectively.

In the diabetics the highest values of HGH after the insulin load were always superior to 8 nanograms, the average almost the same in both groups and almost identical with that of the control group.

Figure 1 represents comparison of the average values of the somatomedin A in the diabetics and in the controls.

Table III shows the amounts of glucosemia and insulinemia in basic conditions and the lowest value of the glucosemia after the insulin load in the diabetics and in the controls, including the relative averages. It also shows the total daily dose of insulin usually administered to the diabetics.

Table III.

Cases	Blood glucose (mg/100ml)	Serum insulin (u/ml)	Blood glucose decreased after insulin	Total insulin dose in 24 h
Group 1st				
1. B.A. ♂	170	55	120	12 U
2. C.E. ♀	180	47	98	12 "
3. O.F. ♀	130	30	67	18 "
4. S.F. ♂	200	35	105	16 "
5. O.F. ♂	306	25	210	20 "
6. A.F. ♀	120	24	50	20 "
7. F.M. ♂	240	19	115	26 "
8. A.C. ♂	140	34	67	22 "
9. C.F. ♂	302	55	48	24 "
10. C.A. ♂	100	52	46	27 "
11. B.F. ♀	110	46	55	22 "
12. L.M. ♂	210	51	106	16"
13. M.E. ♀	160	42	65	16 "
14. F.M. ♂	185	29	93	22 "
15. D.B. ♀	380	40	260	32 "
16. P.B. ♂	238	28	113	48 "
Average ± DS	198 ± 79	38 ± 12	100 ± 59	22.06
Group 2nd				
1. B.A. ♀	299	42	124	18 U
2. A.M. ♂	225	33	135	16 "
3. S.F. ♂	315	64	180	20 "
4. B.E. ♀	210	5	167	20 "
Average ± DS	262 ± 52	36 ± 24	151 ± 24	18.9
Group 3rd				
1. B.M. ♂	92	178	53	—
2. G.L. ♂	96	128	55	—
3. M.B. ♀	77	117	48	—
4. S.R. ♂	81	144	50	—
5. V.G. ♀	95	94	52	—
6. L.G. ♀	76	155	47	—
Average ± DS	86 ± 9	136 ± 29	51 ± 3	—

The variability of the hyperglycemia with the values a little higher in the "initial" diabetics is clearly visible, as well as its persistent and mostly considerable diminution after the insulin load, the low values of insulinemia and the relative variability of the 24-h insulin dose (Chiumello *et al.*, 1968).

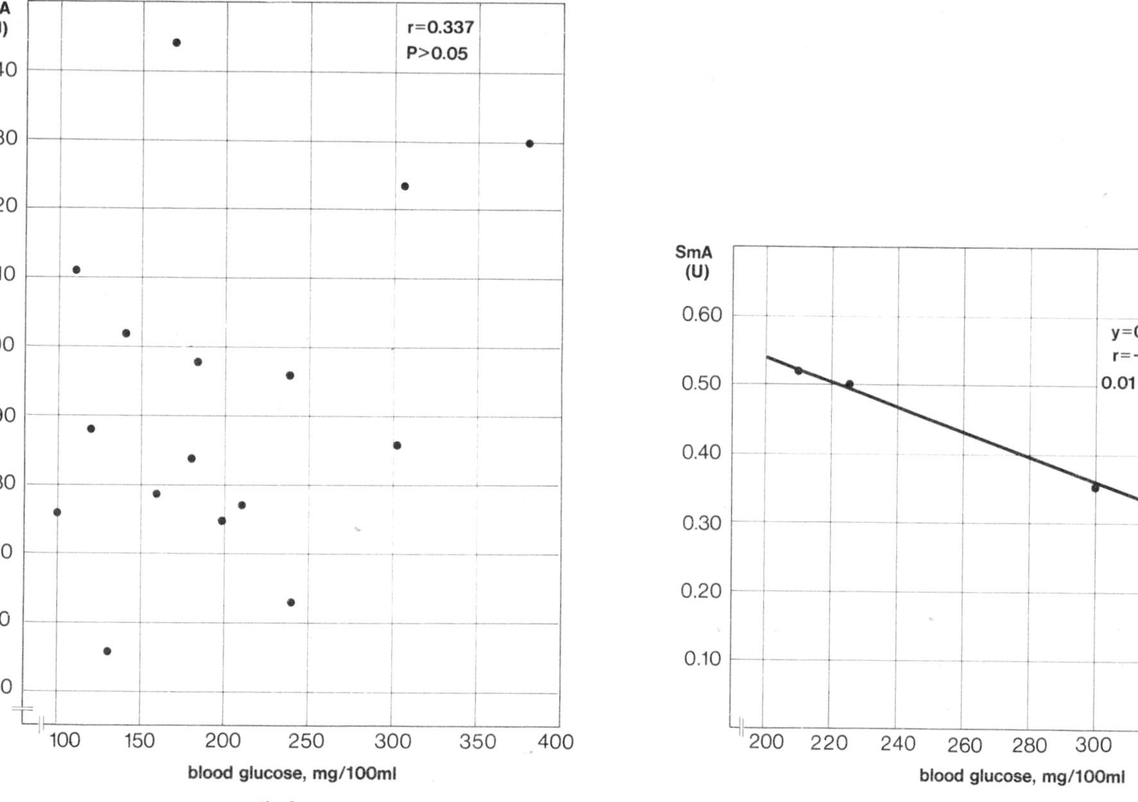

Fig. 2

Fig. 3

Fig. 2 The relationship between basal blood glucose and SmA levels in children with "old" diabetes mellitus.

Fig. 3 The relationship between basal blood glucose and SmA levels in children with "initial" diabetes mellitus.

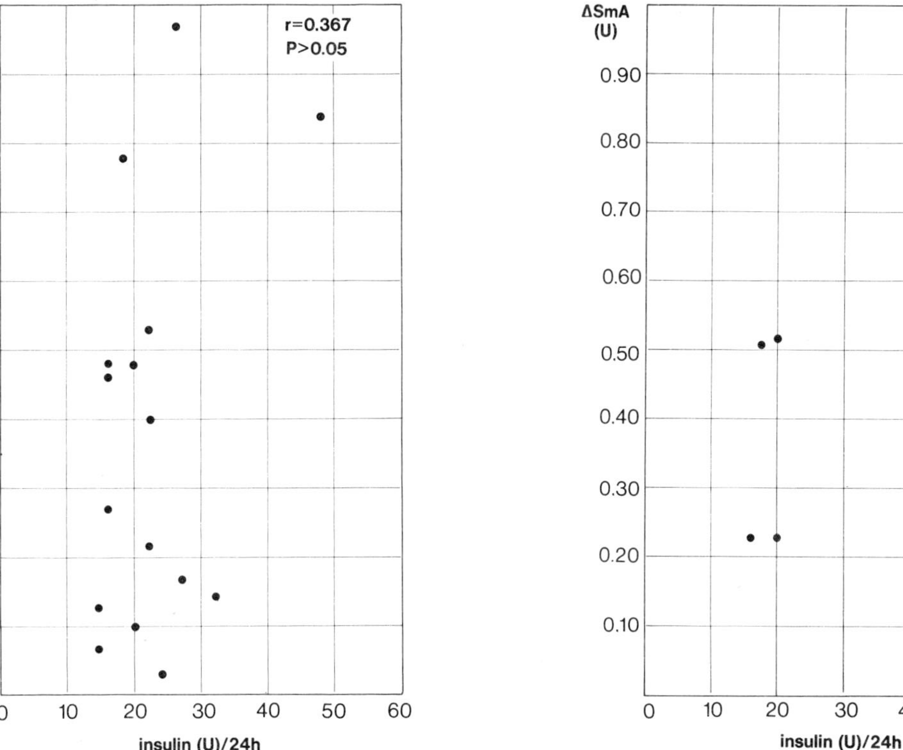

Fig.4 The relationship between SmA increase after insulin load and the total insulin dose used in daily treatment of children with "old" diabetes mellitus.

Fig.5 The relationship between SmA increase after insulin load and total insulin dose used in daily treatment of children with "initial" diabetes mellitus.

We have looked for the possible relationship between the hyperglycemia and somatomedin A in basic conditions.

In the "old" diabetics there is no interrelation, as shown in Fig.1; in the initial diabetics there exists a very considerable negative interrelation (Fig.3).

There is no relationship whatsoever between the total dose of insulin (24 h) and the basic value of somatomedin in "old" diabetics (Fig.4) as well as in the "initial" ones (Fig.5).

Table IV.

Cases		SmA Basal	SmA after arginine	Δ	Peak HGH after arginine	Blood glucose	Serum insulin
1.	F.M.	0.48	0.64	0.16	3.70	0.50	1.6
2.	F.F.	0.29	0.38	0.09	13.90	0.61	2.7

Table IV shows the levels of various parameters in the 2 cases of glycogenosis Type I. The somatomedin activity is very low and after the arginine test increases only slightly, reaching the Δ of 0.16 and 0.09 respectively.

The HGH peak has been under 4 nanograms and normal respectively.

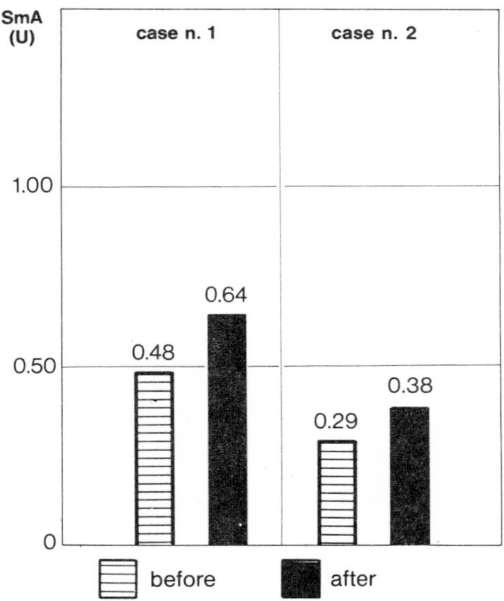

Fig.6 **SmA concentrations before and after arginine load in two cases of glycogenosis Type I.**

Figure 6 shows the scheme and comparison of the somatomedin A values; Fig.7 shows those of glucosemia and insulinemia as compared with the normal averages (Berson and Yalow, 1966; Grant, 1967). Figure 8 demonstrates the evident hypoglycemia as well as insulinemia (Havel *et al.*, 1969; Havel, 1972).

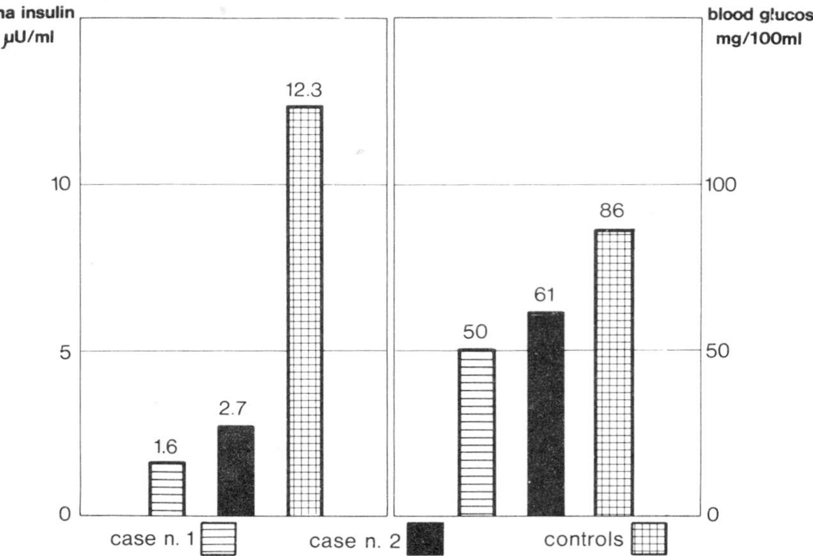

Fig. 7 **Plasma insulin and blood glucose concentrations in two cases of glycogenosis Type I.**

Concerning the experimental research on rats, the treated animals reach the state of hyperglycemia gradually, until on the 8th day the average percentages are 171.83 ± 83 ± 10.08 mg and on the 15th day 245.83 ± 20.59 mg.

The difference between these values and those of the control animals is already great on the 8th day and increases even more on the 15th day (Table V).

Table V. **Blood glucose average + SD of control and diabetic rats after 1, 8 and 15 days of treatment.**

Days	Control Rats (µ)	Diabetic Rats (µ)	Changes	t	P
1st	78 ± 8.52	—	—	—	—
8th	85 ± 9.35	171.83 ± 10.08	+ 102.15	15.47	< 0.01
15th	89.50 ± 7.79	245.83 ± 20.59	+ 174.67	19.05	< 0.01

HISTOLOGICAL RESULTS

The thickness of the cartilage strata of the diabetic rats varies considerably from that of the controls. The greatest thickness of the 15th day test was followed in later tests by a relative deficit increasing in time (Table VI).

In the control tests the epiphyseal cartilage presents, in a small enlargement, an orderly and regular cytoarchitectural disposition with a proliferating cells/vaculoating cells relationship of almost 2.

The cellular thickness, which at first seems very high, tends to decrease progressively, thus favoring the development of the preossal trabecula. The ground substance appears homogeneous and is intensively alcian-positive (+++).

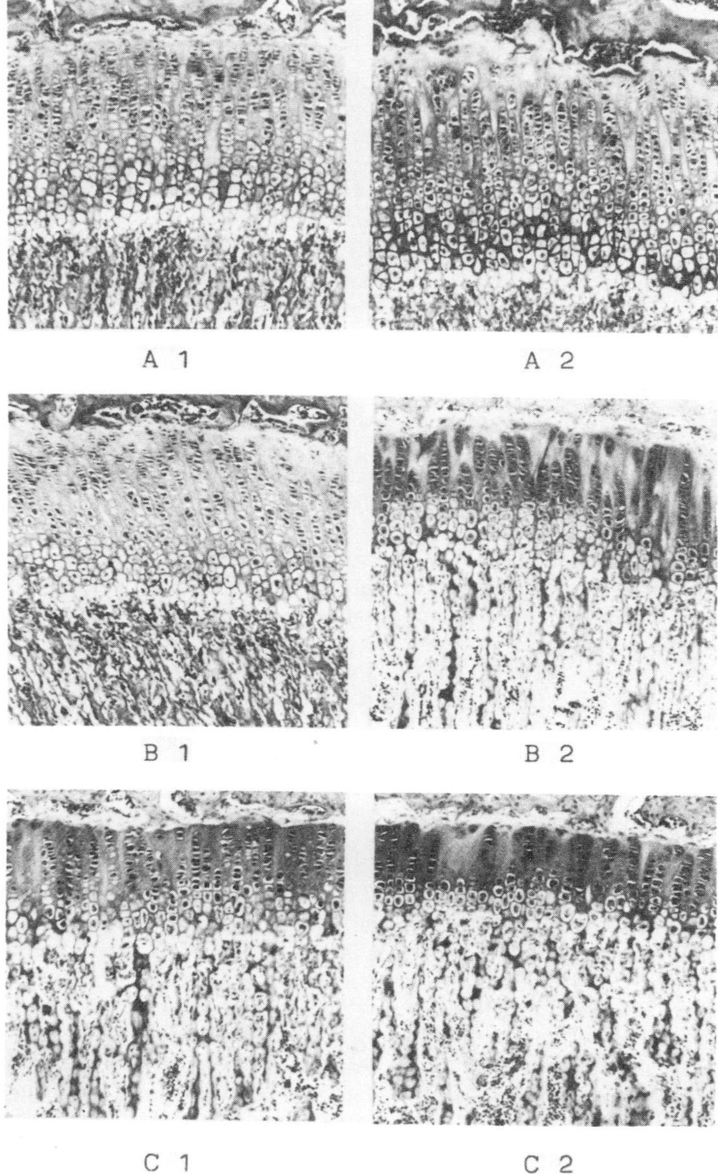

Fig. 8 **Epiphyseal cartilage of control (A1, B1, C1) and diabetic rats (A2, B2, C2) after 15, 40 and 60 days of treatment.**

The histological aspects of the preparations after a 15-day diabetogenic treatment present a normal cell structure of the epiphyseal cartilage, but also show the following alterations:

1) the proliferating cells/vacuolating cells relationship of 3;
2) a considerable increase of proliferating condrocytes;
3) a modest dishomogeneity of the ground substance;

Table VI. Epiphyseal cartilage thickness of control and diabetic rats, after 15, 40 and 60 days of treatment.

Days	Control Rats (μ)	Diabetic Rats (μ)	Changes	t	P
15th	353.84 ± 24.67	390.38 ± 32.73	+ 9.36	3.24	< 0.01
40th	268.75 ± 35.53	244.03 ± 28.62	– 16.64	3.54	< 0.01
60th	209.03 ± 15.82	149.17 ± 18.87	– 28.63	8.76	< 0.01

4) a higher percentage of transitional elements;
5) a lower amount of vaculoating condrocytes;
6) relative shortness of the preossal trabecula.

The last tests made after a 40- and 60-day treatment confirm a marked progressive decrease of the amount of condrocytes together with an increased dishomogeneity of the ground substance, which here and there seems lacunose and scarcely alcian positive (+).

The long-term results can be reduced to the following data:

1) diffused condrocyte rarefaction with sectional, almost total disappearance of proliferating cells;

2) reduced and incomplete transformation into vacuolating cartilage;

3) a visible decrease of mucopolysaccharide acids in the ground substance;

4) underdevelopment of partial disappearance of the vascular-stromal matrix in the preossal trabecula.

DISCUSSION

Our clinical research proved that in the "old" diabetics the basic SmA values correspond to the normal age averages, whereas in the "initial" diabetics they are considerably lower. Only in the last category we have found a negative relationship between hyperglycemia and SmA.

Even considering the well-known differences between childhood, juvenile and adult diabetes, it is rather suggestive that Yde (1964) found a significant decrease of the sulphate factor in the adult "initial" diabetic and a negative relationship between the hyperglycemia and the sulphation factor only in the non-obese diabetics.

However, the most important result of our research seems to be the fact that a modest insulin dose, representing a small part of the total dose necessary for 24 h could increase considerably the somatomedin activity in a state of chronic hypoinsulinism characteristic for childhood diabetes, both the "old" and the "initial". The question is whether this increase is the consequence of an indirect mechanism, i.e. the decrease of the glycemia with the resulting emission of GH into the blood stream.

We consider such hypothesis hardly probable, since in the childhood diabetes the GH concentrations do not seem to be higher (Parker *et al.*, 1968; Backer *et al.*, 1969; Chiumello *et al.*, 1971), except in the chetoacidosis phase; whereas in juvenile diabetes the data vary but the GH concentration tends to increase (Sabeh *et al.*, 1969; Johansen and Hausen, 1969, 1971; Hausen, 1970, Hausen and Johansen, 1970; Yde, 1970; Sonlesen *et al.*, 1972).

Di Natale *et al.* (1973) confirms the normality of the GH increase to pharmacological stimuli in diabetic children and finds that in these patients the peak value of GH concentration usually present in the first hours of sleep is lower than in normal children. In this our research we too have found the peak GH values normal or at the most less high than those of the controls. Therefore, in our opinion, the GH increase in the diabetic child, as reaction to the stimulus of the relative decrease of the glycemia caused by insulin, does not seem so great as to explain the SmA increase.

Diagnostically extremely useful if the somatomedin induction test in cases of dwarfism caused by global antehypophysis deficit or by isolated GH deficit, in which the somatomedin levels are considerably lower. According to Daughaday *et al.* (1969) when performing this induction test in cases of dwarfism caused by global antehypophysis deficit or by isolated GH deficit (in which the somatomedin levels are considerably lower), it is necessary to administer intramuscularly at least 5 mg of exogenous HGH daily for several days; whereas Hall (1971) considers 2 mg administered intravenously entirely and wholly sufficient. Both quantities are considerably higher than the endovenous ones passing into the blood stream under the stimulus of pharmaceutics.

A supposed variation of the circadian rhythm of somatomedin activity could represent another objection to our theory. The publications concerning the subject are very few.

Daughaday *et al.* (1959) found stable sulphation factor values during the whole 24-h period.

Van den Brande *et al.* (1975) found the amount of somatomedin in children aged 9-12 higher in the afternoon than in the morning. They admit a negative relationship between somatomedin and cortisol but, since they made a correction according to the cortisolemia values, the difference between the morning and the afternoon values was not significant statistically.

Recently Giordano *et al.* (1976) discovered that somatomedin levels are higher during the night and the first hours of the morning and that the increase of somatomedin activity follows the secretion afflux of HGH and prolactin, which might presuppose a temporary interrelation of the two processes.

To conclude: the data are discordant and too scarce to permit a definite decision. The importance of both objections may be further contested on the ground that our control group, subjected to the same insulin load as the diabetics, did not show any significant increase of somatomedin activity.

Another characteristic emerges from our study of the two cases of glycogenosis Type I: the somatomedin activity was extremely low and showed only a small increase after the arginine load. Without touching on the complicated enzymatic and metabolic problems, we would like to point out that recent science tends to lend primary importance to chronic hypoglycemia as helping to better knowledge of both the pathogenesis and the therapy of glycogenosis Type I (Greene *et al.*, 1976).

Favourable results have been obtained by a porta-cava anastomosis (Starzl *et al.*, 1973), by total parenteral nutrition (Folkman *et al.*, 1973) and, more recently, by a continuous intragastric nutrition during the night performed with a small nasal-gastric tube applied in the evening, through which was introduced a continuous infusion of 1/3 of the caloric need in the form of glucose and other monosaccarides. Green *et al.* (1976) obtained with this treatment a pronounced clinical improvement with reduction of the hepatomegalia and even a satisfactory growth increase. Our two cases, who had hardly profited from a more frequent daily alimentation, have recently begun this new type of dietetic treatment. Therefore we shall be able to observe at first hand not only the possible results but also the behaviour of metabolic and, above all, endocrinal parameters. In fact, Greene *et al.* (1976) have noticed after a certain period of treatment not only a clinical improvement but also a decrease of the initial high percentage of glucagonemia and somatot ropinemia as well as an increase of insulinemia.

Concerning GH, we would like to point out that the British authors studied and evaluated in two of their three cases only the basic value which, by itself, does not sufficiently prove the increased production of the hormone. In our two cases the basic levels were normal, the peak value absent in one case and normal in the other. Apart from the discordance of these results, the attention at least as far as growth is concerned should be centered mainly on somatomedin activity.

Our discovery of the low somatomedin concentrations sufficiently explains the dwarfism of our patients. Besides, we think that the well-known peripheral disease of the liver and the kidney, organs specifically involved in glycogenosis Type I, furnishes the more probable explanation of the somatomedin deficit since these two organs are considered to be the main somatomedin producers.

The possible involvement of other hormones, above all as probable stimulants of somatomedin activity (e.g. GH and insulin), represents a still unsolved problem and calls for a more extensive and thorough endocrinological research, particularly where glycogenosis is concerned.

Although our experimental research has so far been limited to the morphological study, it has already clearly demonstrated that a specific injury to the pancreas β cells causes a definite damage of the condro-osteogenetic activity of the epiphyseal cartilage which consists in a progressive reduction of newly-formed bone trabuculae; for a time this is compensated by a greater proliferation of cartilage cells which, however, peters out very soon.

We believe that the sum of our research demonstrates more and more clearly the still unpublished and partially-hypothetical theory of a direct influence of insulin on the somatomedin activity. We are trying, particularly through experiments, to prove definitely this theory of ours, but we think that this chapter already presents many positive elements.

Daughaday (1975) has recently formulated a hypothesis that insulin primarily regulates and prepares the substrate necessary for the production of somatomedin, while GH exercises the ultimate control of the biosynthesis, activating the formation of specific enzymes.

We conclude this chapter with still another consideration: that every hormone or family of hormones performs, besides its primary function which often decides its taxonomy, other functions, more or less known, but just as important. Therefore we are convinced that the somatomedins, besides their function of growth mediators, play an important although a still not fully-appreciated role in the control of carbohydrate metabolism.

REFERENCES

Backer, L., Root, A.W., Haque, N. and Kaye, R. (1969). *Metabolism* **18**, 110.

Bartolozzi, G., Bernini, G., Marianelli, L. and Nassi, P. (1975). *Min. Ped.* **27**, 1229.

Berson, S.A. and Yalow, R.S. (1966). *Am. J. Med.* **40**, 676.

Bürgi, H., Müller, W.A., Humbel, R.E., Labhart, A. and Froesch, E.R. (1966). *Biochim. biophys. Acta* **121**, 349.

Chiumello, G., Del Guercio, M.J. and Bidone, G. (1968). *Diabetes* **17**, 133.

Chiumello, G., Del Guercio, M.J., Carnelutti, M., Devetta, M. and Rossi, L. (1971). *J. Pediat.* **79**, 768.

Clemmons, D.R., Hintz, R.L., Underwood, L.E. and Van Wyk, J.J. (1974). *Isr. J. med. Sci.* **10**, 1254.

Creutzfeldt, W., Creutzfeldt, C., Frerichs, H., Perings, E. and Sickinger, K. (1969). *Horm. Metab. Res.* **1**, 53.

Daughaday, W.H., Salmon, W.D., Jr. and Alexander, F. (1959). *J. clin. Endocr. Metab.* **19**, 743.

Daughaday, W.H., Laron, Z., Pertzelan, A. and Heins, J.N. (1969). *Tr. A. Am. Physicians* **82**, 129.

Daughaday, W.H. (1975). *Adv. Metab. Disord.* **8**, 159.

Di Natale, B., Devetta, M., Rossi, L., Garlaschi, C., Caccamo, A., Del Guercio, M.J. and Chiumello, G. (1973). *Helv. Paediat. Acta* **28**, 591.

Du Caju, M.V.L. and Van den Brande, J.L. (1973). *Acta Paediat. Scand.* **62**, 83.

Folkman, J., Philippart, A., Tze, W.J. and Grigler, J. (1972). *Surgery* 72, 306.

Frerichs, H., Arnold, R., Creutzfeldt, C., Track, N.,and Creutzfeldt, W. (1972). *Proc. Int. Symp. on Hypoglycaemia and Diazoxide*, Padova (Cedam, ed), p.133.

Fryklund, L., Uthne, K. and Sievertsson, H. (1974a). *Biochem. biophys. Res. Commun.* **61**, 950.

Fryklund, L., Uthne, K., Sievertsson, H. and Westermark, B. (1974b). *Biochem. biophys. Res. Commun.* **61**, 957.

Froesch, E.R., Bürgi, H., Ramseier, E.B., Bally, P. and Labhart, A. (1963). *J. clin. Invest.* **42**, 1816.

Froesch, E.R., Bürgi, H., Muller, W.A., Humbel, R.E., Jacob, A. and Labhart, A. (1967). *Rec. Progr. Horm. Res.* **23**, 565.

Froesch, E.R., Schlumpf, U., Heimann, R., Zapf, J., Humbel, R.E. and Ritschard, J. (1975a). *Adv. Metab. Disord.* **8**, 203.

Froesch, E.R., Zapf, J., Meuli, C., Mäder, M., Waldvogel, M., Kaufmann, U. and Morell, B. (1975b). *Adv. Metab. Disord.* **8**, 211.

Froesch, E.R., Schlumpf, U., Heimann, R., Eigenmann, E. and Zapf, J. (1975c). *Adv. Metab. Disord.* **8**, 237.

Giordano, G., Foppiani, E., Perroni, D. and Minuto, F. (1976). *Atti XVI Congr. Soc. Ital. Endocr.*, Serono Symposium, p.175.

Grant, D.B. (1967). *Arch. Dis. Childh.* **42**, 375.

Grant, D.B., Hambley, J., Becker, D. and Pimstone, B.L. (1973). *Arch. Dis. Childh.* **48**, 596.

Greene, H.L., Slonim, A.E., O'Neill, J.A., Jr. and Burr, I.M. (1976). *New Engl. J. Med.* **294**, 423.

Hall, K. (1970). *Acta endocr. (Copenh.)* **63**, 338.

Hall, K. (1971). *Acta endocr. (Copenh.)* **66**, 491.

Hall, K. and Uthne, K. (1971). *Acta Med. Scand.* **190**, 137.

Hall, K. (1972). *Acta endocr. (Copenh.)* **Suppl. 163**, 1.

Hall, K. and Olin, P. (1972). *Acta endocr. (Copenh.)* **69**, 417.

Hall, K. and Luft, R. (1972). *Adv. Metab. Disord.* **7**, 1.

Hall, K., Takano, K., Fryklund, L. and Sievertsson, H. (1975a). *Adv. Metab. Disord.* **8**, 19.

Hall, K., Takano, K., Fryklund, L. and Sievertsson, H. (1975b). *Adv. Metab. Disord.* **8**, 61.

Hansen, A.P. (1970). *J. clin. Invest.* **49**, 1967.

Hansen, A.P. and Johansen, K. (1970). *Diabetologia* **6**, 27.

Havel, R.J., Balasse, E.O., Williams, H.E., Kane, J.P. and Segel, N. (1969). *Trans. Ass. Am. Physic.* **82**, 1969.

Havel, R.J. (1972). *New Engl. J. Med.* **287**, 1186.

Hepp, K.D. (1972). *Eur. J. Biochem.* **31**, 266.

Herbert, V., Lau, K.S., Gottlieb, C.W. and Bleicher, S.J. (1965). *J. clin. Endocrinol.* **25**, 1375.
Hintz, R.L., Clemmons, D.R., Underwood, L.E. and Van Wyk, J.J. (1972). *Proc. natn. Acad. Sci. U.S.A.* **69**, 2351.
Hintz, R.L., Orsini, E.M. and Van Camp, M.G. (1974). *Endocrinology* **94, Suppl.**, A-71.
Humbel, R.E., Bunzli, H., Mully, K., Oelz, O., Froesch, E.R. and Ritschard, W.J. (1971). *In* "Diabetes" (R.R. Rodriguez and J. Vallanee-Owen, eds) p.306. Excerpta Medica, Amsterdam.
Humbel, R.E., Bosshard, H.R. and Zahn, H. (1972). *In* "Handbook of Physiology" (D.F. Steiner and N. Freinkel, eds) **Vol.I**, p.111. Am. Physiol. Soc., Washington, D.C.
Jakob, A., Hanri, C. and Froesch, E.R. (1968). *J. clin. Invest.* **47**, 2678.
Jensen, S.E., Lundbaek, K. and Lyngsoe, J. (1963). *Acta med. scand.* **174**, 769.
Johansen, K. and Hansen, A.P. (1969). *Br. med. J.* **2**, 356-357.
Johansen, K. and Hansen, A.P. (1971). *Diabetes* **20**, 239.
Leonards, J.R., Landau, B.R. and Bartsch, G. (1962). *J. Lab. clin. Med.* **60**, 552.
Marianelli, L., Corti, R. and Bernini, G. (1975). *Min. Ped.* **27**, 1323.
Marshall, R.N., Underwood, L.E., Voina, S.J., Foushee, D.B. and Van Wyk, J.J. (1974). *J. clin. Endocr. Metab.* **39**, 283.
Morgan, C.R. (1966). *Proc. Soc. exp. Biol. Med.* **121**, 62.
Morrell, B. and Froesch, E.R. (1973). *Eur. J. clin. Invest.* **3**, 119.
Oelz, O., Jakob, A. and Froesch, E.R. (1970). *Schwiez. Med. Wochenschr.* **100**, 539.
Oelz, O., Jakob, A., Diem, S. and Froesch, E.R. (1971). *Biochim. biophys. Acta* **230**, 20.
Parker, M.L., Pildes, R.J., Knen-Lan, C., Cornblath, M. and Kipnis, D.M. (1968). *Diabetes* **17**, 27.
Sabeh, G., Mendelsohn, L.V., Corredor, D.G., Sunder, J.H., Friedman, L.M., Morgan, C.R. and Danowski, T.S. (1969). *Metabolism* **18**, 748.
Salmon, W.D, Jr. (1975). *Adv. Metab. Disord.* **8**, 183.
Samaan, N.Y., Dempster, W.J., Fraser, R. and Stillmann, D. (1963). *J. Endocrinol.* **26**, 1.
Saric, R., Moreau, F., Seguin, G., Cohen, E., Merlet, M. and Lorin, J.C. (1974). *Sem. Hôp. Paris* **50**, 1497.
Schalch, D.S. and Parker, M.L. (1964). *Nature* **203**, 1141.
Schlumpf, U., Heimann, R.P. and Froesch, E.R. (1975). *In:* Froesch, E.R., Schlumpf, U., Heimann, R., Eigenmann, E. and Zapf, J. (1975c). *Adv. Metab. Disord.* **8**, 237.
Seltzer, H.S. and Allen, E.W. (1969). *Diabetes* **18**, 19.
Sievertsson, H., Fryklund, L., Uthne, K., Hall, K. and Westermark, B. (1975). *Adv. Metab. Disord.* **8**, 47.
Sonksen, P.H., Srivastava, M.C., Tompkins, C. and Nabarro, J.D.N. (1972). *Lancet* **II**, 155.
Starzl, T.E., Putnam, C.W., Porter, K.A., Halgrimson, C.G., Corman, J., Brown, B.I., Gotlin, R.W., Rodgerson, D.O. and Greene, H.L. (1973). *Ann. Surg.* **178**, 525.
Sterky, G. (1963). *Acta Paed.* **Suppl.144.**
Van den Brande, J.L. and Du Caju, M.V.L. (1974). *In* "Advances in Human Growth Hormone Research" (S. Raiti, ed) p.98. DHEW Publ., Washington, D.C.
Van den Brande, J.L., Van Buul, S., Heinrich, U., Van Roon, F., Zurcher, T. and Van Steirtegem, A.C. (1975). *Adv. Metab. Disord.* **8**, 171.
Van Wyk, J.J., Underwood, L.E., Lister, R.C. and Marshall, R.N. (1973). *Am. J. Dis. Childh.* **126**, 705.
Van Wyk, J.J., Underwood, L.E., Baseman, J.B., Hintz, R.L., Clemmons, D.R. and Marshall, R.N. (1975). *Adv. Metab. Disord.* **8**, 127.
White, P. and Graham, C.A. (1971). *In* "Joslin's Diabetes Mellitus" , XI ed., p.339. Lea and Febiger, Philadalphia.
Wolf, F.W. and Parmeley, W.W. (1964). *Diabetes* **13**, 115.
Yalow, R.S., Hall, K. and Luft, R. (1975). *Adv. Metab. Disord.* **8**, 73.
Yde, H. (1964). *Lancet* **2**, 624.
Yde, H. (1969). *Acta endocr. (Copenh.)* **62**, 49.
Yde, H. (1970). *Acta med. scand.* **49**, 1967.
Zapf, J., Waldvogel, M. and Froesch, E.R. (1975). *Arch. Biochem. Biophys.* **168**,
Zingg, A.E. and Froesch, E.R. (1973). *Diabetologia* **9**, 472.

HYPERINSULINISM IN INFANCY: A PATHOPHYSIOLOGIC APPROACH TO DIAGNOSIS AND TREATMENT

L. Baker and C.A. Stanley

Division of Endocrinology, Department of Pediatrics
University of Pennsylvania School of Medicine and Children's Hospital of Philadelphia, USA

Over twenty years ago, McQuarrie (McQuarrie, 1954) introduced the term "idiopathic hypoglycemia of infancy" to describe a syndrome of "severe persistent hypoglycemia of unknown cause which occurs spontaneously in otherwise healthy infants". McQuarrie emphasized that idiopathic hypoglycemia of infancy should be differentiated from true hyperinsulinism. From a current point of view, idiopathic hypoglycemia of infancy is a descriptive term with no physiologic basis and it is apparent that its use as a diagnosis has obscured the true importance of hyperinsulinism in infancy. This chapter will review the Children's Hospital of Philadelphia experience over a ten-year period (1965-1975) in order to assess the relative frequency and importance of hyperinsulinism in infancy. This experience will also be used to provide recommendations regarding the steps necessary for making a specific diagnosis of hyperinsulinism, and suggestions for a rational approach to its therapy.

Hypoglycemia in the pediatric age group almost always occurs in the fasting state. A physiologic approach to hypoglycemia should therefore be based on a knowledge of the metabolic adaptation to fasting. The pinpointing of specific pathophysiologic derangements should then lead directly to more rapid diagnosis and rational therapy.

The processes involved in fuel production and utilization during fasting are shown schematically in Fig.1 (Cahill, 1970). Seven major systems involved in the maintenance of glucose homeostasis during fasting can be studied in the individual patient. These systems can be divided into three groups:

A) Those involved in glucose production:
   1. Liver glycogenolysis;

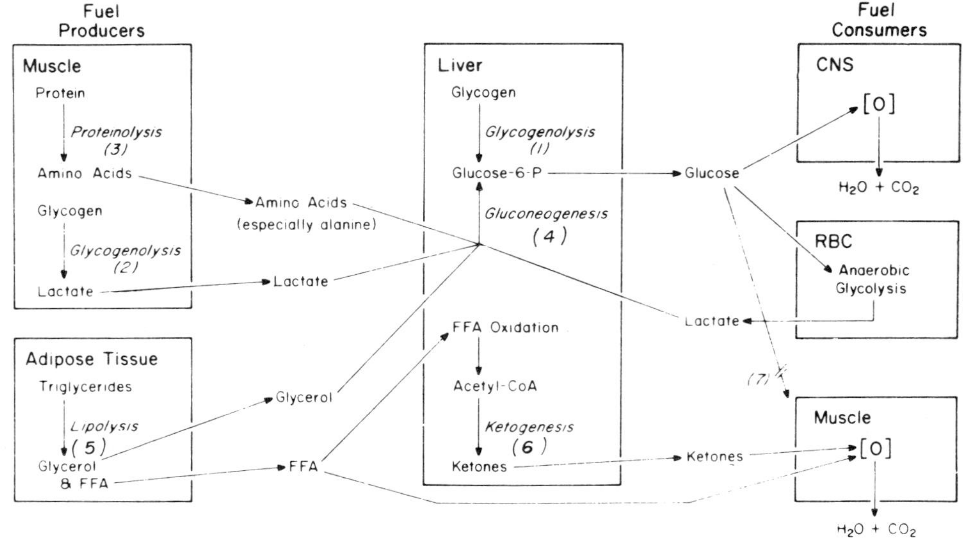

Fig. 1 Schematic representation of systems involved in fasting homeostasis. Numbers correspond to those listed in the text for the individual systems. (Adapted, with permission, from Cahill (1970).)

2. Muscle glycogenolysis;
3. Muscle protein breakdown;
4. Hepatic gluconeogenesis.

B) Those involved in the production of alternate fuels:

5. Adipose tissue lipolysis;
6. Hepatic fatty acid oxidation and ketogenesis;

C) 7. The hormonal adjustments necessary to integrate and facilitate the above.

In practical terms, this has meant the study, during fasting, of glucose, gluconeogenic substrate (lactate, pyruvate, glycerol, and alanine), capacity for gluconeogenesis (by administration of lactate, alanine or glycerol), availability of alternate metabolic fuels (free fatty acids, beta-hydroxy-butyrate, and aceto-acetate), and the hormonal milieu (insulin, growth hormone, cortisol, and glucagon). The administration of glucagon can be used to test the capacity of glycogen storage and utilization. The study of the metabolic adaptation to fasting has been used to demonstrate that a specific abnormality exists which permits the definitive diagnosis of hyperinsulinism. It has also allowed us to review the causes of hypoglycemia seen in our hospital and to place them in a classification system which eliminates the 'pseudodiagnosis' of idiopathic hypoglycemia of infancy and emphasizes the true importance of hyperinsulinism.

DIAGNOSIS

The diagnosis of hyperinsulinism is traditionally made in one of two ways: 1) the demonstration of an abnormally elevated concentration of insulin at the time of hypoglycemia; and 2) the documentation of an abnormal response to an insulin secretagogue, such as glucose, tolbutamide, leucine or glucagon. Major problems have been encountered with both approaches. An insulin level of 80 μU/ml at the time of hypoglycemia is diagnostic, but an insulin concentration of 8 μU/ml is difficult to interpret. It could be used as evidence for "relative hyperinsulinism" and "inappropriate" for a low glucose value. The problem is posed because the excessive insulin secretion of organic hyperinsulin*ism* is not always manifested by excessive concentration of circulating insulin, hyperinsulin*emia*.

The use of insulin secretagogues as diagnostic tools suffers from two major drawbacks. Both false positive and false negative responses may be seen. In addition, the extremely unstable glucose concentration in patients with hyperinsulinism often means that such provocative tests cannot be performed, since the results may be uninterpretable or one incurs the possibility of further hypoglycemic insults to the brain.

Because of these problems in diagnosis, we studied patients with hyperinsulinism to see whether a specific abnormality could be detected during fasting hypoglycemia (Stanley and Baker, 1976a). The diagnosis of hyperinsulinism in seven infants was made independently of the fasting study, based on a serum insulin of 20 μU/ml or greater at the time of spontaneous hypoglycemia, and/or a morphologic diagnosis at the time of surgery. These infants were compared to two contrast groups: an age-matched group of seven "control" infants, studied because of seizures or history suggestive of hypoglycemia, and 12 older children with ketotic hypoglycemia who were selected as "glucose-matched" controls because they demonstrated the same levels of plasma glucose at the end of fasting as did the infants with hyperinsulinism. Figure 2 presents the results of these fasting studies.

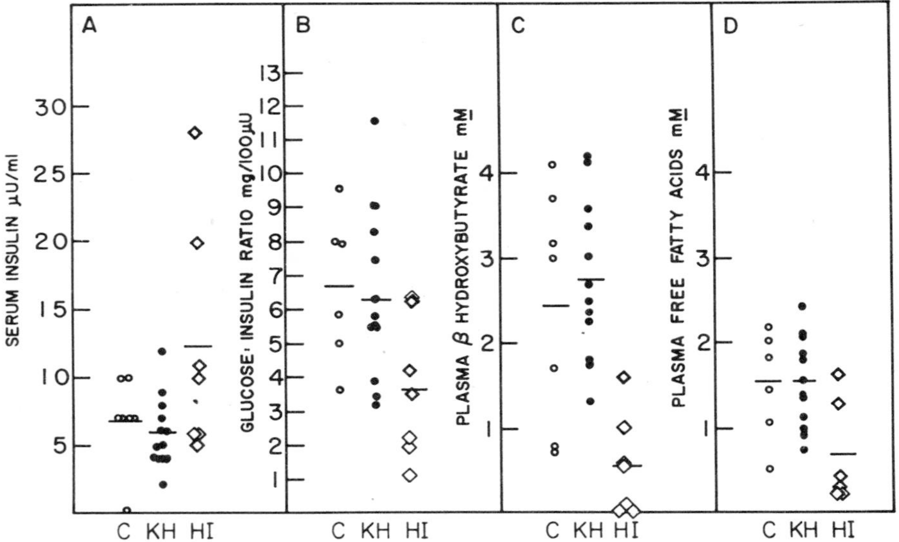

Fig. 2 Response to fasting in infants with hyperinsulinism (HI), control infants (C) and children with ketotic hypoglycemia (KH). Shown are individual values and means. A: serum insulin. B: glucose-insulin ratio. C: plasma beta-hydroxybutyrate. D: plasma free fatty acids. (From Stanley and Baker, 1976a.)

As shown in Fig.2A, three patients accounted for most of the elevation reflected in the mean insulin level found in the hyperinsulinism group. Four of the seven infants had insulin concentrations at the time of hypoglycemia which would be considered within the range of "normal" as defined by the controls and the ketotic hypoglycemic group. No further improvement in discriminating the presence of hyperinsulinism was achieved by relating the levels of glucose and insulin as a glucose-insulin ratio (Fig.2B).

The best markers for the presence of hyperinsulinism would appear to be the concentrations of free fatty acids and beta-hydroxybutyrate. Figures 2C and 2D graphically demonstrate that the overlap at the levels of beta-hydroxybutyrate and free fatty acids in the hyperinsulinism group with those in the control and ketotic hypoglycemic groups is less than that observed for levels of insulin or glucose-insulin ratios. The beta-hydroxybutyrate concentration of only one infant with hyperinsulinism fell within the range of beta-hydroxybutyrate found in infants with ketotic hypoglycemia. The fact, however, that two of the control infants demonstrated concentrations of beta-hydroxybutyrate which were in the same range as found in infants with hyperinsulinism suggests that the duration of fasting is not as critical in determining beta-hydroxybutyrate response as plasma glucose concentration. Figure 3 demonstrates the relationship between beta-hydroxybutyrate and glucose.

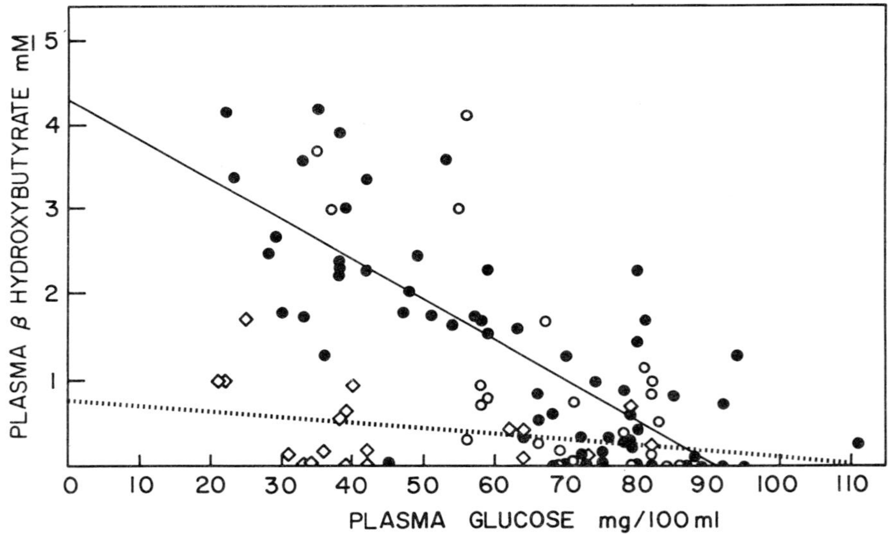

Fig.3 Relationship between plasma glucose and beta-hydroxybutyrate concentrations during fasting in infants with hyperinsulinism (◇), control infants (○), and children with ketotic hypoglycemia (•). The lines for the control and ketotic hypoglycemic groups were not significantly different; the common regression line is shown as a solid line. The dash line represents the regression line for the infants with hyperinsulinism. (From Stanley and Baker, 1976a.)

Both the control and ketotic hypoglycemic groups show a significant inverse relationship between levels of beta-hydroxybutyrate and glucose. The regression lines for the two groups are not significantly different from each other in slope or in position, so that they may be combined to form a single line. In contrast to this significant relationship, the infants with hyperinsulinism show no increase in the plasma levels of beta-hydroxybutyrate with decreasing plasma concentrations of glucose. The slope of the regression line for this group is not significantly different from zero, but is significantly different from the slope of the line for the combined control and ketotic hypoglycemic group.

Infants with hyperinsulinism thus have low concentrations of beta-hydroxybutyrate at the time of hypoglycemia. This is perhaps not surprising, since insulin suppresses ketogenesis by at least two mechanisms. It decreases the supply of free fatty acid precursors for hepatic ketone body synthesis by inhibiting adipose tissue lipolysis. In addition, insulin may have a direct effect on the liver which prevents fatty acids from being transported into mitochondria for further oxidation and ketogenesis (McGarry *et al.*, 1975).

By looking at the relationship between plasma glucose and beta-hydroxybutyrate, one can calculate the concentration of beta-hydroxybutyrate which would be considered appropriate at the time of hypoglycemia. For a plasma glucose concentration below 40 mg/100 ml, the expected value for beta-hydroxybutyrate is 2.9 mM, with a lower limit of normal (mean minus two standard deviations) of 1.1 mM. The same technique can be used to calculate "appropriate" levels for insulin at the time of hypoglycemia. The mean expected level of serum insulin for a plasma glucose below 40 mg/100 ml is 6.3 μU/ml, with an expected upper limit of normal (mean plus two standard deviations) of 12.1 μU/ml. Thus, the diagnosis of hyperinsulinism can be made on the finding, at the time of hypoglycemia, of a beta-hydroxybutyrate concentration below 1.1 mM, and/or an insulin concentration of greater than 12.1 μU/ml.

FREQUENCY AND IMPORTANCE

Using this approach to the specific diagnosis of hyperinsulinism, we have reviewed (Stanley and Baker, 1976b) the 98 cases of severe hypoglycemia presenting in infants and children at the Children's Hospital of Philadelphia in the ten-year period 1965-1975 (Table I). This does not include newborns with transient hypoglycemia, or those who were infants of diabetic mothers. Also excluded were patients in whom hypoglycemia was a relatively minor part of the presentation, as in galactosemia and hypothyroidism, or those in whom hypoglycemia was only elicited after prolonged provocative testing, as in some patients with growth hormone deficiency. In agreement with other series, ketotic hypoglycemia was found to be the most common form of hypoglycemia. Hyperinsulinism, however, was the second most common form of hypoglycemia. Of particular interest was the fact that 55% of the infants under one year of age with hypoglycemia (26 of 47) had hyperinsulinism. Hyperinsulinism was by far the most common cause of hypoglycemia in the infant under one year of age. Many patients previously diagnosed as idiopathic hypoglycemia of infancy (including such subgroups as infant giants and leucine-sensitive) had hyperinsulinism.

The importance of hyperinsulinism is not only its relative frequency, but also its role as a significant cause of brain damage in infancy. Not only is the brain deprived of glucose as a primary fuel but also the effects of hyperinsulinism are such that alternate fuels (particularly beta-hydroxybutyrate and lactate) will not be available. Thus the central nervous system of the infant with hyperinsulinism

Table I. Causes of hypoglycemia in infants and children at the Children's Hospital of Philadelphia, 1965-1975.

		All ages		Onset < 1 year	
		No.	%	No.	%
I.	Hyperinsulinism	29	30	26	55
	(with hypopituitarism)	(2)		(1)	
II.	Hypopituitarism	5	5	5	11
III.	Ketotic Hypoglycemia	50	51	5	11
IV.	Hepatic Enzyme Deficiencies:	12	12	11	23
	a. Glucose-6-phosphatase	(7)		(7)	
	b. Amylo-1,6-glucosidase	(3)		(3)	
	c. Fructose-1,6-diphosphatase	(1)		(1)	
	d. Defective ketogenesis	(1)			
V.	Classification uncertain	2	2	–	–
	Total	98		47	

is left with no fuels available to sustain normal metabolism. McQuarrie's original report emphasized the permanent brain damage seen in these children. Further corroboration of this view came from other series: 50% of infants who developed persistent symptomatic hypoglycemia before the age of six months were found to have neurologic sequelae; in another series, significant mental subnormality was present in 75% of the children with onset of hypoglycemia under age six months.

Fourteen of the 22 living infants with hyperinsulinism in the current series are now considered to be of normal intelligence and to have no significant neurologic residua. The eight children placed in the moderately or severely retarded groups are of interest. In five of these infants there was an inordinate delay between the onset of symptoms and referral. The diagnosis of hyperinsulinism was rapidly made and effective therapy instituted. The brain damage incurred by these infants could have been prevented and 19 of the 22 infants would have been spared neurologic damage. This success rate (86%) would be far better than previously seen. In the three other infants, major difficulties in the control of hypoglycemia presumably led to brain damage. The recognition of the true importance of hyperinsulinism will hopefully lead to greater awareness in the medical community and thus to early diagnosis.

THERAPY

Therapy in infants with hyperinsulinism is directed toward the prevention of brain damage by controlling blood glucose. The methods of treatment may be classified into three groups: 1) Those which suppress insulin secretion (diazoxide, epinephrine, diphenylhydantoin, low protein diet and somatostatin); 2) Those which antagonize the effects of insulin on tissues (glucocorticoids, epinephrine and glucagon); and 3) Those which destroy islet cells (surgery and streptozotocin). In practical terms, there are at present only two choices: diazoxide and pancreatic surgery. Neither is uniformly effective in controlling hyperinsulinism. Thus there is the question as to which is the treatment of choice in any given patient with hyperinsulinism.

The surgical approach to the treatment of hyperinsulinism involves exploration of the pancreas and removal of any identifiable islet adenoma. If none can be found, a subtotal pancreatectomy (± 80%) is performed, in the hope that any adenoma present will be included, or, in the event the lesion is diffuse, that sufficient tissue will be removed to control hypoglycemia. The efficacy of subtotal pancreatectomy therefore depends on the location of the lesion and whether it is localized or diffuse. An examination of the pathologic lesions found in patients with hyperinsulinism might therefore be helpful in deciding whether surgery is likely to be effective.

Table II. **Pathologic lesions found in infants and children with hyperinsulinism at the Children's Hospital of Philadelphia.**

	1965-1975		1950-1975	
age at onset	< 1 year	> 1 year	< 1 year	> 1 year
Localized lesions				
a. Islet adenoma	3	2	3	2
b. Adenomatosis of uncinate process	2	—	2	—
Diffuse lesions				
a. Nesidioblastosis	4	—	12	—
b. Beta-cell adenomatosis	1	—	1	—
c. Islet hyperplasia	—	1	2	1
Total	10	3	20	3

Table II shows the lesions found in surgical or post-mortem specimens of the pancreas in patients with hyperinsulinism at the Children's Hospital of Philadelphia from 1965-1975. The pathologic experience from 1950 to 1975 is also shown, which includes those covered in a previous report (Yakovac *et al.*, 1971). The variety of lesions found included typical islet cell adenomas, islet cell hyperplasia, beta call adenomatosis and nesidioblastosis.

The relative frequency of the pathologic lesions responsible for the hyperinsulinism appears to be related to the age of onset of the disease. Hyperinsulinism in adults is due to islet cell adenomas in 80-90% of the cases. Hyperinsulinism in infants, on the other hand, is more often associated with diffuse lesions. When the age of onset of hyperinsulinism was under one year, five out of the ten cases from 1965-1975 and 15 out of the 20 cases from 1950-1975, had diffuse lesions. In children who developed hyperinsulinism after one year of age, two of the three had adenomas. This distribution of pathologic lesions according to age has obvious therapeutic implications with respect to surgery: in the infants under one year of age, only three out of the 20 had lesions which were potentially curable by surgery.

Diazoxide was used in all 29 patients with hyperinsulinism (Table I) treated at the Children's Hospital of Philadelphia from 1965-1975. The sequence and outcome of treatment used (diazoxide or subtotal pancreatectomy) are shown

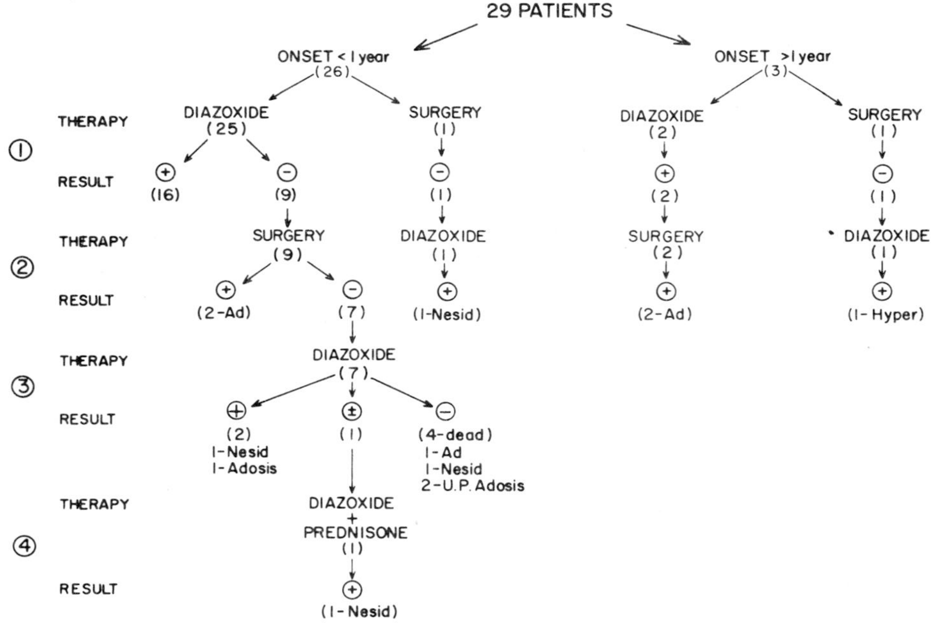

Fig.4 Therapeutic steps and response to treatment in 29 patients with hyperinsulinism at the Children's Hospital of Philadelphia, 1965 to 1975. Surgery indicates 60-80% subtotal pancreatectomy except in one case in an infant less than one year of age where an islet cell adenoma was locally resected. The response to therapy is indicated as ⊕ (good control of hypoglycemia), ⊖ (poor control), and (±) (partial improvement). The number of patients at each stage is given in parentheses. The lesion found at surgery or autopsy in 13 patients is indicated at the end of the treatment sequence: Ad (islet cell adenoma), Adosis (diffuse beta cell adenomatosis), U.P. Adosis (beta cell adenomatosis of the uncinate process), Nesid (diffuse nesidioblastosis), Hyper (islet cell hyperplasia).

schematically in Fig.4. Good control is defined as plasma glucose values above 40 mg/100 ml around the clock with spacing of meals appropriate for age. Diazoxide gave good control of hypoglycemia in 18 of 27 (67%) previously unoperated patients of all ages and in 16 of 25 (64%) of those less than one year of age. Three other infants were controlled with diazoxide following subtotal pancreatectomy. Overall, therefore, diazoxide gave good control of hypoglycemia in 23 of 29 (77%) patients less than one year of age. Nine patients who were initially started on diazoxide went to surgery because of poor control of the hypoglycemia. Three of these had nesidioblastosis, one had diffuse adenomatosis, two had adenomatosis localized to the uncinate process of the head of the pancreas, and three had single islet cell adenomas. There was no correlation between the type of lesion present and the response to diazoxide. On the other hand, in the infants less than one year of age, there appeared to be a relationship between onset of symptoms and response to diazoxide. This is graphically seen in Fig.5: only two of nine infants with onset of hypoglycemia during the first month of life responded to diazoxide, while diazoxide was effective in 14 of 16 infants with onset of hypoglycemia after the first month.

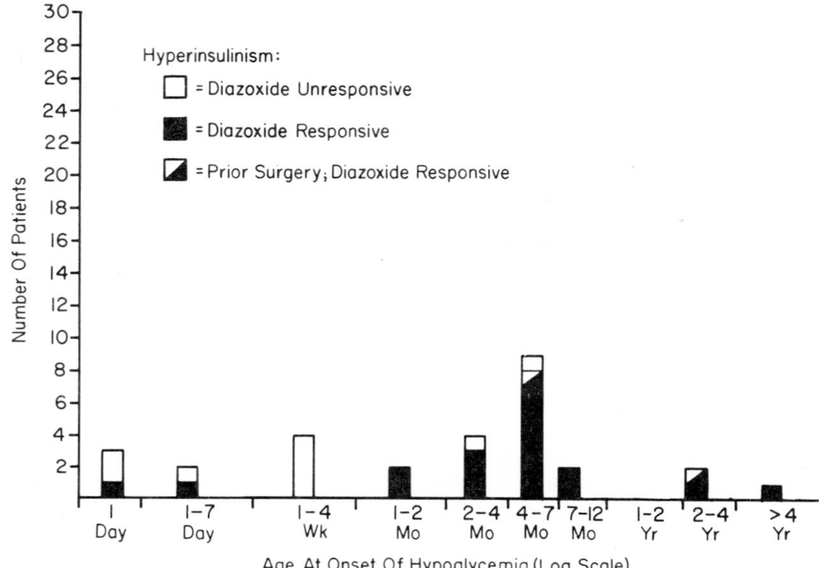

Fig.5 Age of onset of symptomatic hypoglycemia and the response to diazoxide in the 29 patients with hyperinsulinism seen at the Children's Hospital of Philadelphia, 1965-1975. The time scale is logarithmic.

From 1965-1975, subtotal pancreatectomy was used in our series only in those infants with hyperinsulinism under one year of age who failed to respond to diazoxide. Since these patients had the most severe disease, including the infants with onset under one month of age, the surgical results to be described probably underestimate the effectiveness of surgery in patients with diffuse disease. Thirteen of the patients with hyperinsulinism in the series from 1965-1975 had operations. Of these, seven had localized lesions. In one of the seven, an adenoma was identified and locally resected. In the others, subtotal pancreatectomy was done. In the four cases where the localized lesion was removed in the operative specimen, surgery was curative. In the three other cases where the lesion was not removed by subtotal pancreatectomy, the patients ultimately died with intractable hypoglycemia.

Six of the 13 patients had diffuse lesions. Subtotal pancreatectomy alone failed to control hypoglycemia. Surgery could be considered beneficial, however, in that five of the six patients could be controlled with diazoxide following the surgery. The sixth patient died despite all therapeutic endeavours.

In the pre-diazoxide era, subtotal pancreatectomy was an effective form of therapy in approximately 60-80% (Hamilton *et al.*, 1967; Pagliara *et al.*, 1973) of patients. Diazoxide appears to have approximately the same effectiveness in patients with hyperinsulinism. We have tried to answer the question of surgery versus diazoxide by weighing the efficacy and risks of long-term diazoxide therapy, the risks of surgery and the risks of overlooking a surgically curable lesion. The ten-year experience with diazoxide in the present series of the Children's Hospital of Philadelphia indicates that it is a safe drug with relatively minor side effects and no serious long-term effects. The risks of subtotal pancreatectomy are also low in the hands of an experienced pediatric surgeon, but it is a major procedure with some morbidity. It might best be avoided if surgery is not likely to cure the hyperinsulinism. A focal lesion is likely in a child who develops hyperinsulinism after the age of one year. Therefore, even though the child may respond to diazoxide, surgery should be chosen with the expectation that it will be curative. On the other hand, in the infants with onset less than one year of age only three of 20 had resectable lesions in the 1950-1975 series. This suggests that infants with hyperinsulinism with onset under one year of age are unlikely to have surgically correctable lesions. Therefore, it is our recommendation that surgery is not indicated in the infant with hyperinsulinism before one year of age who responds to diazoxide with satisfactory control of the hypoglycemia. Clearly, failure to respond to diazoxide in a patient with hyperinsulinism is an indication for surgery at any age. This recommendation differs from that proposed by Pagliara *et al.* (Pagliara *et al.*, 1973) who have stated "that any child past the neonatal period with hypoglycemia and proved hyperinsulinemia is a candiate for pancreatic exploration".

As can be seen in Fig.4, four of the infants with hyperinsulinism at the Children's Hospital of Philadelphia could not be controlled by subtotal pancreatectomy in conjunction with diazoxide and other drugs. In all of these, intractable hypoglycemia was a primary cause of death. Total pancreatectomy is probably the only choice available for such a patient at this time. Harken and co-workers (Harken *et al.*, 1971) have described five infants who were cured by "total" pancreatectomy after subtotal pancreatectomy and medical therapy failed to control the unremitting hypoglycemia. Their surgery left remnants of pancreatic tissue around the duodenum and common bile duct. Four of their five cases required insulin therapy. Four of the five infants were retarded as a result of the long delay before the hypoglycemia could be controlled.

In the series reported above, and in the present series from the Children's Hospital of Philadelphia, it has been the infants who present in the first weeks of life who have been the most difficult to manage. If mental retardation is to be prevented, these patients must be recognized early, diagnosed promptly and treated vigorously. When diazoxide, steroids, and intravenous glucose fail to control the hypoglycemia in such an infant, it is our current recommendation, as the first surgical procedure, to remove as much of the pancreas as possible if a discrete lesion is not found.

SUMMARY AND RECOMMENDATIONS FOR DIAGNOSIS AND THERAPY

Hyperinsulinism is the most common cause of recurring hypoglycemia in the first year of life. If not recognized early and treated effectively, hypoglycemia due to hyperinsulinism will produce severe brain damage. In the first year of life, hyperinsulinism is most often associated with diffuse pancreatic lesions such as nesidioblastosis. Localized lesions such as islet cell adenomas may occur at any age, but are more likely to be found in the patient developing hyperinsulinism after the first year. That the hyperinsulinism may be congenital in certain infants is indicated by the larger birth weight of these infants. Infants who are particularly large at birth and who develop symptoms in the

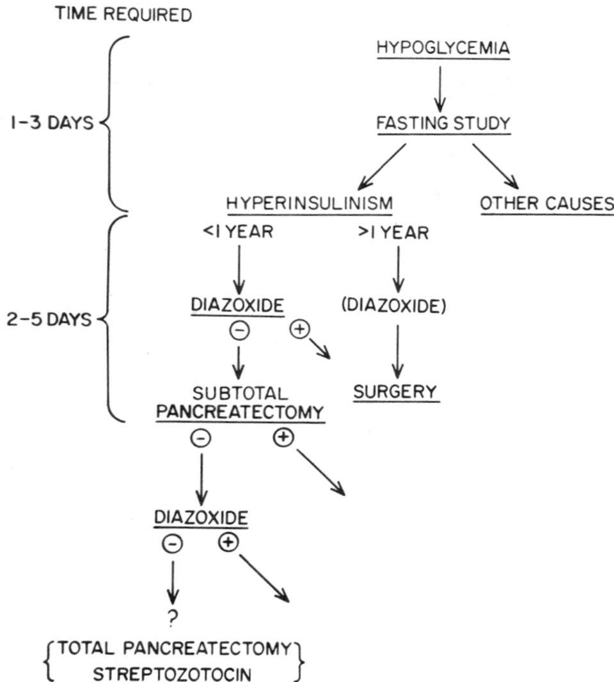

Fig.6 Suggested outline of logical sequence for the diagnosis and treatment of hypoglycemia due to hyperinsulinism. Good control of hypoglycemia is indicated by ⊕ ; inadequate control by ⊖ .

first month of life are likely to have the most severe disease and to be the most difficult to treat.

To control hypoglycemia and to prevent brain damage, a specific diagnosis of hyperinsulinism must be made rapidly and appropriate therapy to decrease insulin secretion must be instituted. Figure 6 illustrates our current recommendation for the sequence of steps for the diagnosis and treatment of hyperinsulinism. The diagnosis is made by examining the response to fasting. If, at the time of hypoglycemia, the plasma insulin concentration is elevated (greater than 12 μU/ml), and the beta-hydroxybutyrate is low (less than 1.1 mM), the diagnosis is established. If the beta-hydroxybutyrate is low, but the insulin level is not diagnostically elevated, the exclusion of hypopituitarism essentially establishes the diagnosis of hyperinsulinism. With this approach, the diagnosis of hyperinsulinism should be firmly established within one to three days after presentation.

The treatment sequence is determined by the age at which hyperinsulinism becomes manifest. In children older than one year, an adenoma should be suspected, and surgery is the treatment of choice. Diazoxide may be used both as a diagnostic test and as therapy while awaiting surgery. In infants less than one year of age, the lesion is unlikely to be surgically resectable, and diazoxide is the treatment of choice. If diazoxide is not effective, surgical exploration and subtotal pancreatectomy should be performed. The therapeutic trial of diazoxide will require only two to four days. The time required from recognition of hypoglycemia through diagnosis to a decision about surgery need not exceed one week.

Some infants may continue to have hypoglycemia following subtotal pancreatectomy. Diazoxide may be effective at this point if the lesion is diffuse, and sufficient tissue has been removed to ameliorate the disorder. If diazoxide is not effective, specific recommendations about further steps are difficult. These patients are likely to be infants with severe diffuse disease presenting in the first month of life or those with localized lesions located in the head of the pancreas. Glucocorticoids are usually without effect in this group, and total pancreatectomy may be the only choice.

If the infant with hyperinsulinism responds well to diazoxide this therapy should be continued. It is our current practice to maintain therapeutic levels of diazoxide until the age of four or five. In many of these infants, remission of the disease does occur and it will be possible to discontinue all treatment (Stanley and Baker, 1976b).

It has been the purpose of this presentation to place hyperinsulinism in its proper context. It is the most frequent cause of hypoglycemia in the young infant, with serious potential for brain damage. The recognition of the importance of hyperinsulinism should aid in earlier detection. It has also been the purpose of this presentation to make recommendations for a logical sequence which will allow for rapid diagnosis and vigorous therapy. The combination of earlier detection and more effective treatment should result in a brighter outlook for these infants.

ACKNOWLEDGEMENTS

This work was supported in part by Clinical Research Center Grant No. RR–00240 and USPHS Grant No.AM–13518.

REFERENCES

Cahill, G.F. (1970). *New Engl. J. Med.* **282**, 668.
Hamilton, J.P., Baker, L., Kaye, R. and Koop, C.E. (1967). *Pediatrics* **39**, 49.
Harken, A.H., Filler, R.M., Avruskin, T.W. and Crigler, J.F., Jr. (1971). *J. Ped. Surg.* **6**, 284.
McGarry, J.D., Wright, P.H. and Foster, D.W. (1975). *J. clin. Invest.* **55**, 1202.
McQuarrie, I. (1954). *Am. J. Dis. Childh.* **87**, 399.
Pagliara, A.S., Karl, I.E., Haymond, M. and Kipnis, D.M. (1973). *J. Pediatr.* **Part II 82**, 558.
Stanley, C.A. and Baker, L. (1976a). *Pediatrics* **57**, 702.
Stanley, C.A. and Baker, L. (1976b). *Adv. in Pediatr. (in press).*
Yakovac, W.C., Baker, L. and Hummeler, K. (1971). *J. Pediatric.* **79**, 226.

THE LATE EFFECTS OF HYPOGLYCEMIA

M. Cornblath

Department of Pediatrics, University of Maryland School of Medicine Baltimore, USA

The prognosis and late sequela of hypoglycemia depend upon multiple factors including the age at onset, the etiology, the persistence and the effective treatment of the hypoglycemia. Most important, the diagnosis of hypoglycemia must be based on reliable accurate glucose determinations (Cornblath *et al.*, 1966; Ek and Daae, 1967) and clinical criteria that clearly establish that the low blood glucose was the etiological event producing the symptoms at the time of diagnosis (Raivio and Hallman, 1968; Fluge, 1974; Cornblath *et al.*, 1966). A complete and prompt response to parenteral glucose further supports the importance of the low blood glucose as being responsible for the clinical manifestations (Shelly and Neligan, 1966; Cornblath and Schwartz, 1976). Once these basic criteria have been satisfied, it is then necessary to consider the age of onset (Haworth and Coodin, 1960; Ulstrom, 1962; Cornblath and Schwartz, 1976) and the multiple possible etiologies that can result in low blood glucose and neuroglucopenia. Events associated with or resulting in hypoglycemia must also be evaluated in assessing the outcome, especially in the neonate. The purpose of this paper is to define the criteria for the diagnosis of hypoglycemia, its frequency and manifestations in the neonate, infant, and child, as well as its late effects on growth, development, and metabolic function.

I. DEFINITION OF HYPOGLYCEMIA

Significant hypoglycemia is defined as a concentration of glucose or true sugar in whole blood below 40 mg/100 ml (<45 mg/100 ml in serum or plasma) in the infant or child, with or without clinical manifestations (Hartmann and Jaudon, 1937; Cornblath and Schwartz, 1976). In the full-sized newborn, values of blood glucose lower than 30 mg/100 ml (<35 mg/100 ml serum) during the first 72 hours of age and less than 40 mg/100 ml (<45 mg/100 ml serum) thereafter are considered abnormally low (Cornblath *et al.*, 1961; Cornblath and Reisner, 1965). In preterm or low birth-weight infants, values in whole blood less than 20 mg/100 ml (<25 mg/100 ml serum) are significant (Baens *et al.*, 1963).

The hypoglycemia may be symptomatic and associated with one or more of the following clinical manifestations: listlessness, apathy, irritability, pallor, sweating, weakness, hunger, headache, visual disturbances, mental confusion, coma, convulsions or repetitive bizarre behavior (Hartmann and Jaudon, 1937; McQuarrie, 1954; Conn and Seltzer, 1955). In the neonate, symptomatic hypoglycemia is characterized by episodes of "jitteriness", tremors, cyanosis, apnea, tachypnea, exaggerated Moro reflex (Raivio and Hallman, 1968), limpness, feeding difficulty, high-pitched cry and convulsions. Campbell *et al.* (1967) report "troublesome vomiting" as almost invariable. The clinical manifestations should subside within minutes or hours in response to adequate treatment with intravenous glucose if hypoglycemia, alone, is responsible. For reasons still unknown, some infants with hypoglycemia are rarely symptomatic, e.g., infants of diabetic mothers and older infants with Type I Glycogen Storage Disease. Recent studies in animals and in man indicate that alternate substrates, e.g., lactate, glycerol and ketones, may support brain metabolism during hypoglycemia especially in the neonatal period (Tildon *et al.*, 1975).

II. FREQUENCY OF HYPOGLYCEMIA

The incidence of hypoglycemia syndromes in infancy is virtually unknown. The frequency in the neonate depends upon the criteria for diagnosis, the population surveyed as well as the methods for blood collection and glucose analysis. In a three-year experience (1971-73), utilizing the clinical classification of early transitional (Category I), secondary (Category II), classical symptomatic (Category III) and severe, recurrent or persistent (Category IV), Gutberlet and Cornblath (1976), reported a frequency of 4.4 per 1000 total live births and 15.5 per 1000 low birth-weight infants in an inborn population. The frequency of hypoglycemia was 5.1% among 257 outborn infants transferred to this intensive care nursery during this same time period. These data are similar to those reported by other investigators for similar patients (Creery, 1966; Campbell *et al.*, 1967; Raivio and Hallman, 1968; Fluge, 1974; Haymond *et al.*, 1974).

In the older infant and child, the prevalence of hypoglycemia depends upon the referral pattern of the center reporting, the interests of the consultants and the awareness of the primary physicians. In reports from Sweden (Broberger and Zetterström, 1961), from Minneapolis (Sauls and Ulstrom, 1966; Sauls, 1974), and from Bern, Switzerland (Zuppinger, 1975), the frequency of hypoglycemia was approximately 2 to 3 per 1000 hospital admissions, significantly less than that of neonatal hypoglycemia.

III. PROGNOSIS OF HYPOGLYCEMIA

If untreated, severe and prolonged, hypoglycemia can result in death at any age. In the neonate the prognosis depends upon the severity, duration, presence of symptoms, associated pathology, and etiology as well as prompt recognition and adequate therapy (Pildes *et al.*, 1974; Cornblath and Schwartz, 1976; Gutberlet and Cornblath, 1976; Fluge, 1975; Fluge *et al.*, 1975; Koivisto *et al.*, 1974; Griffiths and Bryant, 1971; Griffiths and Laurence, 1974; Raivio and Hallman, 1968; Creery, 1966). In order to evaluate the late effects of neonatal hypoglycemia, it is critical to have a prospective study that includes a group of normoglycemic infants matched for gestational age and size, perinatal care, complications and family socioeconomic status. Furthermore, a follow-up of at least seven to nine years is necessary. Unfortunately, this is not available to date.

In assessing the late effects of any episode of hypoglycemia, a comprehensive definition of outcome is necessary and should include the following: 1) metabolic, 2) neurological and 3) growth parameters. Metabolic consequences must include consideration of the recurrence of the hypoglycemia as well as subsequent endocrine or metabolic dysfunctions or abnormalities (Fluge *et al.*, 1975). The degree of neurological handicap must include, in addition to the neurological status, developmental achievements as well as functional capacities including speech, vision, abstract thinking and concepts (Pildes *et al.*, 1975). Growth must include the growth rate, height and weight.

A. Neonatal Hypoglycemia

The definition of neonatal hypoglycemia has been expanded to include four clinical categories, each with its own frequency, severity, and prognosis (Gutberlet and Cornblath, 1976). These include:

Category I or early transitional hypoglycemia, the most common, appears to represent an abnormal response to the physiologic adjustments at birth.

Category II or secondary hypoglycemia represents underlying pathology or iatrogenic events that are associated with stress or abnormal metabolism resulting in low glucose values.

Category III or "classical" transient hypoglycemia is an extension of intrauterine disturbances that mav affect growth, endocrine interactions and perhaps gluconeogenesis for short periods of extrauterine life and rarely may recur later as ketotic hypoglycemia.

Category IV or severe, protracted or recurrent hypoglycemia is rare, usually related to a specific etiology, and is of diverse origin, but life-threatening.

Each will be briefly described and the data related to long-term prognosis summarized.

1. Early transitional hypoglycemia (Category I) occurs at or shortly after birth in infants who may be large, appropriate, and less often, small for gestational age. Included in this heterogeneous group are those infants reported by Griffiths (1968), Lubchenco and Bard (1971), and de Leeuw and de Vries (1976), as well as many in the asymptomatic groups of Creery (1966), Haworth and Vidyasagar (1971), Koivisto *et al.* (1972), Kogut (1974), Lacourt (1974), Pildes *et al.* (1974), Fluge (1975), and Gutberlet and Cornblath (1976). Asymptomatic erythroblastotic infants and infants of diabetic mothers are also placed in this group. There appears to be a positive correlation with preterm birth, complicated labor and delivery, perinatal stress or asphyxia and intrauterine malnutrition. Delayed or insufficient feedings have been implicated as well. The hypoglycemia occurs early (<12 hours of age), is asymptomatic (>80%), responds readily to oral feeds, to glucagon or to small amounts of intravenously administered glucose, and is non-recurrent.

The prognosis for this group appears to be good and is more dependent upon the associated abnormality, i.e. perinatal asphyxia, than on the low blood glucose

Table I. Differential diagnosis in newborns with episodes of apnea, cyanosis, "jitteriness', limpness, twitching, high-pitched cry, difficulty in feeding, coma and convulsions.

Clinical Entity	Secondary Hypoglycemia (Category II)
CENTRAL NERVOUS SYSTEM	
Congenital defects	+*
Congenital infections (e.g., toxoplasmosis, cytomegalic inclusion disease)	±
Acquired infections (e.g., meningitis)	±
Subdural hematoma	+
Hemorrhage	+
Kernicterus	+
SEPSIS	
Bacterial	+
Viral (rubella)	0
HEART DISEASE	
Congenital hypoplastic left heart syndrome	+
Arrhythmia	0
ASPHYXIA, ANOXIA	++ Preterminal
Perinatal	+
Meconium aspiration	±
Hyaline membrane disease	±
IATROGENIC	
Cold injury	+
Drugs to mother	
Narcotic withdrawal	±
Sulfonylureas	+
Propylthiouracil	+
Abrupt cessation of hypertonic glucose	+++
Salicylate poisoning	+
Postoperatively in neonate	++
ENDOCRINE DEFICIENCY	
Adrenal hemorrhage	±
Hypothyroid	±
MULTIPLE CONGENITAL ANOMALIES TRISOMY 18	
METABOLIC ABERRATIONS	
Pyridoxine dependency	0
Hypocalcemia	+ (10%)
Hyponatremia	0
Hypernatremia	0
Hypomagnesemia	?

* 0 = No hypoglycemia. ± to +++ = frequency and severity of hypoglycemia.

(Griffiths and Laurence, 1974). In survivors, Haworth and McRae (1967), Gentz *et al.* (1969), Koivisto *et al.* (1972), Pildes *et al.* (1974), Fluge *et al.* (1975), and Fluge (1975), report a favorable outcome with normal growth, neurological development and absence of metabolic or intellectual abnormalities. In fact, infants with difficulties at follow-up, often, had prolonged hypoglycemia (Fluge, 1974) or other associated abnormalities.

2. Secondary hypoglycemia (Category II) is precipitated by or closely associated with a variety of acute perinatal stresses. These include central nervous system abnormalities, sepsis, heart disease, asphyxia, anoxia, iatrogenic events, i.e., hypoglycemic drugs to mother, cold injury, endocrine deficiency, multiple congenital anomalies, or metabolic aberrations (see Table I and Cornblath and Schwartz, 1976, pp.163-167). This combination of events is important for two reasons: (1) a significant low blood glucose should not eliminate the consideration of other pathologic states and (2) a portion of the symptomatology and residual damage in these multiple entities may be due to the hypoglycemia. An estimate of the relative frequency of secondary hypoglycemia calculated from a total of 447 hypoglycemic infants reported by Koivisto *et al.* (1972), Fluge (1974), and Gutberlet and Cornblath (1976) revealed that 238 or 53.2% were considered to have "secondary hypoglycemia".

Neonatal mortality, due to the underlying abnormality, is significantly greater in this group than in Categories I or III (Fluge, 1975, Gutberlet and Cornblath, 1976). However, in the only known follow-up study to date, these infants seem to have little sequelae related to their hypoglycemia, but more as a consequence of the associated pathologic events (Table II). Since secondary hypoglycemia is relatively common, a prospective study with normoglycemic controls is critical to assess the late effects of the low blood glucose. Of note, two infants with hypoglycemia and central nervous system pathology developed transient diabetes mellitus following therapy with parenteral glucose and steroids (Chance and Bowers, 1966; Gentz and Cornblath, 1969), and one of the eight infants with secondary hypoglycemia had an abnormal glucose tolerance test at follow-up (Fluge *et al.*, 1975) (Table II).

3. Classical transient neonatal hypoglycemia (Category III) occurs predominantly in infants with intrauterine under-nutrition (small for gestational age or SGA). There is an increased incidence of toxemia of pregnancy and twinning. Males predominate and polycythemia, hypocalcemia and cardiomegaly may be present. The hypoglycemia is usually severe, symptomatic, recurs and requires relatively large amounts of parenteral glucose (8-10 mg/kg/min) and steroids for control (for review see Cornblath and Schwartz, 1976, pp.167-175).

If untreated, infants with Category III hypoglycemia can die (Anderson *et al.*, 1967; Banker, 1967). Furthermore, these infants are frequently of low birthweight and SGA which may be associated with all of the associated complications noted above as well as pre- and perinatal problems that may result in mental subnormality, abnormal neurologic behavior and seizures unrelated to hypoglycemia (Steward and Reynolds, 1974; Lubchenco *et al.*, 1974). Thus, to evaluate the specific long-term effects of neonatal hypoglycemia, it is critical to have a prospective study with matched normoglycemic controls at similar risk in order to balance those abnormalities unrelated to hypoglycemia and to obviate the influence of changing nursery routines.

Pildes *et al.* (1974) reported the results of a prospective controlled study of 39 hypoglycemic and 41 matched controls followed for five to seven years. This report has been critically analyzed by Haworth (1974) who correctly indicated its limitations: the original selection of infants occurred before the implications

Table II. Follow-up of neonate hypoglycemia at mean age of 3½ years (Fluge, 1975; Fluge *et al.*, 1975).

CLASSIFICATION OF HYPOGLYCEMIA AS NEONATE		No.	METABOLIC Diabetic Glucose Tol. Test	Cortisol after Insulin	Recurrent Hypoglycemia
ASYMPTOMATIC	(13)*	7	1/7	+	1/8?
SYMPTOMATIC	(11)*	9	1/8	–	
Convulsions	(7)*	6			2
Non-Convulsions	(4)*	3			
SECONDARY	(43)*	21	1/8	–	0
Convulsions	(9)*	4			
Non-Convulsions	(34)*	27			

		No.	NEUROLOGICAL Normal	M.R. +	Spastic	Later Convulsions
ASYMPTOMATIC	(13)*	7	5	1	0	0
SYMPTOMATIC	(11)*	9				
Convulsions	(7)*	6	1	2	2	3
Non-Convulsions	(4)*	3		1	2	1
SECONDARY	(43)*	21				
Convulsions	(9)*	4				
Non-Convulsions	(34)*	17				

		No.	DEVELOPMENTAL	?	MBD	Psycho-Motor Retard.	Delayed Speech
ASYMPTOMATIC	(13)*	7	6		1		
SYMPTOMATIC	(11)*	9	4	2	2	(1)**	
Convulsions	(7)*	6					
Non-Convulsions	(4)*	3					
SECONDARY	(43)*	21	16	1	1	1	2 (1)**
Convulsions	(9)*	4					
Non-Convulsions	(34)*	17					

* Original number of infants: 19 died in neonatal period; 1 died later in infancy; 9 lost to follow-up; 1 Down's Syndrome excluded. + Mental Retardation. ** Severe mental retardation.

of the concept of SGA was fully appreciated and infants were not matched for head circumference. However, the importance of a normoglycemic control group is clearly established.

At birth, more hypoglycemic infants were underweight (72% *v.* 29%) and underlength (42% *v.* 13%) than controls. However, although the mean weight of the hypoglycemic infants was significantly less than that of controls at one and two years of age, the differences were no longer significant after the age of two. By two years of age, the hypoglycemic group had caught up in height, which then remained similar to the height of controls. The mean head circumference of the hypoglycemics was significantly smaller than that of controls at birth and remained so at two, three and six years of age.

Mental development was correlated with symptoms as well as the neonatal course. Although the numbers in each subgroup are small, all 15 children with an I.Q. of 85 or less were symptomatic. Nine of the 14 had an onset beginning the first 24 hours of life, and the diagnosis was made promptly in 10 of them. In 11 infants, clinical manifestations were moderate to severe, and recurrences of hypoglycemia occurred in three patients. Therapy was less than adequate in five infants, consisting of nothing in one and oral glucose with or without steroids in four. Members of this group with a low I.Q. were significantly different from the remainder of the hypoglycemic neonates with respect to the complications of pregnancy, labor and delivery or the condition at birth. Although mean yearly I.Q. scores were not different between the hypoglycemic and control groups, a significantly larger number of hypoglycemic children (13 of 25) had scores below 86 than did the control (6 of 27) at five to seven years of age ($p < .05$). Furthermore, of 12 control children, six had I.Q. scores below 86 at age three to four years and showed improvement by ages five to seven as compared to only three of 17 hypoglycemic children. In contrast, I.Q. scores greater than 100 were found in nine of 25 hypoglycemics and in 10 of 27 controls.

Repeated EEGs throughout the seven years of follow-up revealed abnormal patterns in 43% of the hypoglycemic tracings and in 32% of the control tracings. Of note, two controls and three hypoglycemics had abnormal EEGs in the newborn period that reverted to normal by two to seven years of age. No specific EEG abnormality was present in the hypoglycemic children that would be diagnostic or distinguish them from other high-risk infants.

Neurologic abnormalities were predictably high in both the control and hypoglycemic groups, but were statistically significantly greater in number in the hypoglycemic infants at ages two, three, and six years. However, of 30 hypoglycemic infants examined neurologically for at least four years, only three had moderately severe neurologic handicaps (two had well-controlled nonfebrile seizures and one had a delay in motor and intellectual development) that could be attributed to neonatal hypoglycemia. Initially, the retarded infant had not been given any therapy for several days. The need for long-term follow-up was clearly demonstrated by the neurologic examinations. In eight of the hypoglycemic and in 11 of the control children, neurologic abnormalities noted during the first year of life had decreased or completely disappeared by school age. It is also clear that some neurological abnormalities can antedate the hypoglycemia (Haworth and McRae, 1965; Knobloch *et al.*, 1967; Harken *et al.*, 1971).

The presence of convulsions as a manifestation of hypoglycemia was associated with the most severe prognosis in all reports (Koivisto *et al.*, 1972; Fluge, 1975; Pildes *et al.*, 1974).

Recurrences of hypoglycemia, other than those associated with infiltration of parenteral fluids, occurred once in five infants during the first three months of life only and in two others who developed ketotic hypoglycemia at nine and 18 months of age (Pildes *et al.*, 1974). This represents a recurrence rate of significant hypoglycemia of 5% in this series as compared to reports of 7% (Haworth and Vidyasagar, 1971), 8% (Fluge *et al.*, 1975), and 12% (Creery, 1966).

The influence of socioeconomic factors on behavior, psychologic development and intellectual achievement can be profound. It is noteworthy that the socioeconomic and educational background, racial distribution, incidence of unmarried, divorced or separated mothers, as well as the frequency of unplanned or unwanted pregnancies and Warner ratings, were similar in both the hypogly-

Table III. Recurrent or persistent hypoglycemia (Category IV).

HORMONE DEFICIENCIES

Multiple Endocrine Deficiencies or Congenital
  Hypopituitarism
  Hypothalamic Hormone Deficiencies

Primary Endocrine Deficiency
  Growth Hormone: isolated
  ACTH: ACTH unresponsiveness
  Cortisol: (a) hemorrhage (b) adrenogenital syndrome
  Epinephrine (?)
  Glucagon (?)

HORMONE EXCESS – HYPERINSULINISM

EMG syndrome of Beckwith-Wiedemann
"Infant Giant"
Islet cell adenoma
Nesidioblastosis
Beta cell hyperplasia
Leucine sensitivity

HEREDITARY DEFECTS IN CARBOHYDRATE METABOLISM

Glycogen storage disease – Type I
Fructose intolerance
Galactosemia
Glycogen synthase deficiency
Fructose, 1-6 diphosphatase deficiency

HEREDITARY DEFECTS IN AMINO ACID METABOLISM

Maple syrup urine disease
Propionic acidemia
Methylmalonic acidemia
Tyrosinosis

IDIOPATHIC SPONTANEOUS HYPOGLYCEMIA

cemic and control groups in this one prospective controlled study. These similarities may be more important factors than the defect in not matching the infants for head circumference and gestational size in this study.

Metabolic studies at follow-up have been limited to those reported by Fluge *et al.* (1975) (Table II). One of eight symptomatic infants had a diabetic type glucose tolerance test as their only abnormality. Thus, much more controlled prospective data are needed before any definitive conclusions about outcome can be made.

4. Recurrent, severe hypoglycemia (Category IV) is caused by specific en-

zymatic or metabolic-endocrine abnormalities (Table III). Specific therapy is necessary in addition to large quantities of intravenously administered glucose. Early recognition, specific diagnostic determinations, the rapid application of a diagnostic-therapeutic trial (Cornblath and Schwartz, 1976, p.177), followed by specific therapy or surgery determine the prognosis related to the neonatal hypoglycemia. Each category noted in Table III has unique problems that affect the prognosis.

(a) Multiple hormone deficiencies or congenital hypopituitarism, most often associated with severe, even fatal, hypoglycemia during the first days of life appears to be the result of either hypothalamic hormone deficiencies (Lowinger *et al.*, 1975) or of primary "aplasia" (Sadeghi-Nejad and Senior, 1974) or hypoplasia (Cornblath, 1973) of the anterior pituitary gland. Of 26 patients either reported or known to the author, two-thirds have died, five on the first day of life, four during the neonatal period and five between two months and 17 years of life. Those alive ranged in age from six weeks to 18 years and several are retarded to varying degrees. A few appear normal. Both endocardial fibroelastosis and biliary cholestasis have been noted at post-mortem examinations.

Ultimate development and function, here, depends upon the other endocrine deficiencies present and the effectiveness of replacement therapy. Thus, the microphallus noted in 13 of 15 males responded to therapy with HGH or with monthly injections of testosterone enanthate.

(b) Hormone excess or hyperinsulinism.

(1) In the Exomphalose-Macroglossia-Gigantism (EMG) syndrome of Beckwith-Wiedemann, Filippi and McKusick (1970) suggest that the mental retardation noted at follow-up in this syndrome is probably due to untreated hypoglycemia and not to congenital abnormalities. Much of the neonatal mortality and subsequent morbidity, including microcephaly, have been attributed to unrecognized low blood glucose values. However, even with appropriate therapy, prognosis is guarded because of the multiple anomalies associated with the EMG syndrome.

(2) "Infant Giants" (Sauls and Ulstrom, 1966) or Foetopathia Diabetica (Hansson and Redin, 1963) represent a group of infants with gigantism and microcephaly who usually have severe intractable hypoglycemia refractory to every type of medical therapy and have required total pancreatectomy for control (Harken *et al.*, 1971). Death occurred in all nine patients reported before 1966. Survivors have been reported subsequently, but are usually moderately to severely retarded.

(3) Islet cell adenomas, a rarity prior to 1959, have been reported in 19 neonates since that time and others are known to the author. Of five patients reported between 1947 and 1967, three were diagnosed at autopsy; whereas of nine reported between 1967 and 1974, only one was diagnosed at autopsy while seven were operated between 19 days and seven and one-half months of age. Although follow-up studies of the 16 surviving infants have been relatively short, none have become diabetic and eight have moderate to severe neurologic or mental deficits, often with seizures. Eight are alive and well. The importance of early diagnosis and immediate surgery cannot be overemphasized.

(4) Nesidioblastosis is beginning to be recognized more frequently as a developmental abnormality responsible for severe hypoglycemia. Insufficient data prevent assigning any prognosis for development or subsequent metabolic

abnormalities in this fascinating group of infants.

(5) Beta cell hyperplasia and leucine sensitivity have both been included in the groups of infants reported by Haworth and Coodin (1960) with onset under six months of age and poor prognosis (Table III).

(c) Hereditary defects in carbohydrate metabolism associated with hypoglycemia include Type I glycogen storage disease, fructose intolerance, galactosemia, glycogen synthase deficiency and fructose 1-6 diphosphatase deficiency. The prognosis and late effects of the hypoglycemia are secondary to other problems in each of these entities. Thus, hypoglycemia may be fatal the first days of life in Type I Glycogen Storage disease, but soon the patient adapts to utilizing other substrates and tolerates his low blood glucose well. In fructose intolerance and galactosemia, hepatic and cerebral failure are more significant then the hypoglycemia. A specific diet without the offending monosaccharide results in normal growth and development.

(d) Hereditary defects in amino acid metabolism associated with hypoglycemia include Maple syrup urine disease, propionic acidemia, methylmalonic acidemia and tyrosinosis. Each has a guarded prognosis for normal development independent of the occurrence of hypoglycemia.

B. Hypoglycemia in Infancy and Childhood

Cerebral function and metabolism, especially during the first months of life, have not been adequately studied. The brain appears to have an increased vulnerability to hypoglycemia during the first months of life. In 58 patients with spontaneous idiopathic hypoglycemia reviewed by Haworth and Coodin (1960), onset was before six months of age in 35, and 51% had permanent neurologic sequelae. In 23 patients whose symptomatic hypoglycemia occurred after six months of age, only three (12%) later showed brain damage (Table IV). In reviewing 46 patients followed at the University of Minnesota for 11 years, Ulstrom (1962) reported similar results (see Table IV). In part, this may reflect more severe disease in the younger infant as well as difficulty in interpreting symptoms and diagnosing the hypoglycemia early in its course before the age of six months. On the other hand, although inordinate delays do occur before the diagnosis is made and therapy begun in patients over six months of age, brain damage in the older children is apparently less severe.

Hypoglycemia, depending upon its etiology, tends to be less severe and protracted in the older infant and child, but can result in personality changes, abnormal behavior, and neurologic abnormalities. Furthermore, there appears to be a rather specific age susceptibility with ketotic hypoglycemia beginning at nine to 12 months of age, peaking at 18 to 30 months and "curing" itself by age 4 to 7 years. The frequency of recognition of islet cell adenoma after the neontal period begins to increase during the decade between 5 and 15 years of life. Reactive hypoglycemia, which often follows meals and rarely predicts future diabetes mellitus, begins to appear at 8 to 10 years of age and increases through adolescence and early adulthood. The long-term effects of the latter have not been well documented. On the other hand, low blood glucose values have not been well documented in the multiple behavior, emotional and learning disorders that have been attributed to hypoglycemia. The diagnosis of significant hypoglycemia is based on critical criteria at every age and reliable laboratory studies (*supra vide*). The abuse of the diagnosis of hypoglycemia as a cause of behavior disorders is to be condemned.

Table IV. The age of onset of spontaneous symptomatic hypoglycemia and neurologic sequelae or mental subnormality.

	Age of Onset	Neurologic Sequelae Present	Absent (Per Cent)	
Haworth and Coodin (1960)	< 6 months	18	17	(49)
	> 6 months	3	20	(88)
		I.Q. < 80	> 80	
Ulstrom (1962)	< 6 months	12	3	(20)
	7 months - 1 year	2	6	(75)
	1 year - 5 months	1	18	(95)

Only the prognosis in islet cell adenoma will be discussed here because of the long delays reported between the onset of symptoms and diagnosis. In review of the literature, Cornblath and Schwartz (1976) found that whereas 36% of the children were diagnosed in less than six months, 50% required one to two years and 14% over two years and as long as ten years before the diagnosis and appropriate therapy was instituted. At follow-up of a series of such children treated surgically, one died of operative causes (Bell *et al.*, 1970), one became a permanent insulin-requiring diabetic (Francois *et al.*, 1962), one required insulin for 28 days and eight have either neurologic sequelae or major personality and behavior problems. Fourteen (56%), fortunately, are completely well.

In conclusion, studies of the outcome of patients with documented hypoglycemia are needed. These must include investigations of the hypothalamic-endocrine-metabolic factors influencing homeostasis. Fat and amino acid metabolism must be included to appreciate carbohydrate regulation. Finally, it cannot be over-emphasized that precise definitions of the initial episode of hypoglycemia are essential if one is to understand their late effects, be they on neurological, endocrine, metabolic or intellectual functions.

ACKNOWLEDGEMENTS

This work was supported in part by research grant HD 03959-08 from the National Institute of Child Health and Human Development, NIH, and by grants from the John A. Hartford Foundation and the Morris Singer Research Fund.

REFERENCES

Anderson, J.M., Milner, R.D.G. and Strich, S.J. (1967). *J. Neurol. Neurosurg.* **30**, 295.

Baens, G.S., Lundeen, E. and Cornblath, M. (1963). *Pediatrics* **31**, 580.

Banker, B.Q. (1967). *Dev. Med. Child Neurol.* **9**, 544.

Bell, W.E., Samaan, N.A. and Longnecker, D.S. (1970). *Arch. Neurol.* **23**, 330.

Broberger, O. and Zetterström, R. (1961). *J. Pediatr.* **59**, 215.

Campbell, M.A., Ferguson, I.C., Hutchison, J.H. and Kerr, M.M. (1967). *Arch. Dis. Childh.* **42**, 353.

Chance, G.W. and Bower, B.D. (1966). *Arch. Dis. Childh.* **41**, 279.

Conn, J.W. and Seltzer, H.S. (1955). *Am. J. Med.* **19**, 460.
Cornblath, M. (1973). *In* "Advances in Human Growth Hormone Research", p.809. DHEW Publication No. (NIH) 74-612.
Cornblath, M., Ganzon, A.F., Nicolopoulos, D., Baens, G.S., Hollander, R.J., Gordon, M.H. and Gordon, H.H. (1961). *Pediatrics* **27**, 378.
Cornblath, M., Joassin, G., Weisskopf, B. and Swiatek, K.R. (1966). *Pediatr. Clin. North Am.* **13**, 905.
Cornblath, M. and Reisner, S.H. (1965). *New Engl. J. Med.* **273**, 278.
Cornblath, M. and Schwartz, R. (1976). "Disorders of Carbohydrate Metabolism in Infancy", 2nd Ed. Saunders & Co., Philadelphia.
Creery, R.D.G. (1966). *Dev. Med. Child Neurol.* **8**, 746.
Ek, J. and Daae, L.N.W. (1967). *Acta Paediatr. Scand.* **56**, 461.
Filippi, G. and McKusick, V.A. (1970). *Medicine* **49**, 279.
Fluge, G. (1974). *Acta Paediatr. Scand.* **63**, 826.
Fluge, G. (1975). *Acta Paediatr. Scand.* **64**, 629.
Fluge, G., Stoa, K.F. and Aarskog, D. (1975). *Acta Paediatr. Scand.* **64**, 280.
Francois, R., Pradon, M., Sherrer, M. and Uglienco, A.R. (1962). *J. Pediatr.* **60**, 721.
Gentz, J.C.H. and Cornblath, M. (1969). *Adv. Pediatr.* **16**, 345.
Gentz, J., Persson, B. and Zetterström, R. (1969). *Acta Paediatr. Scand.* **58**, 449.
Griffiths, A.D. (1968). *Arch. Dis. Childh.* **43**, 688.
Griffiths, A.D. and Bryant, G.M. (1971). *Arch. Dis. Childh.* **46**, 819.
Griffiths, A.D. and Laurence, K.M. (1974). *Dev. Med. Child. Neurol.* **16**, 308.
Gutberlet, R.L. and Cornblath, M. (1976). *Pediatrics* **58**, 10-17.
Hansson, G. and Redin, B. (1963). *Acta Paediatr.* **52**, 145.
Harken, A.H., Filler, R.M., AvRuskin, J.W. and Crigler, J.R., Jr. (1971). *J. Pediatr. Surg.* **6**, 284.
Hartmann, A.F. and Jaudon, J.C. (1937). *J. Pediatr.* **11**, 1.
Haworth, J.C. (1974). *Pediatrics* **54**, 3-4.
Haworth, J. and Coodin, F.J. (1960). *Pediatrics* **25**, 748.
Haworth, J.C. and McRae, K.N. (1965). *Can. med. Assoc. J.* **92**, 861.
Haworth, J.C. and Vidyasagar, D. (1971). *Clin. Obstet. Gynec.* **14**, 821.
Haymond, M.W., Karl, I.E. and Pagliara, A.S. (1974). *New Engl. J. Med.* **291**, 322.
Knobloch, J., Sotos, J.F., Sherard, E.S., Jr., Hodson, W.A. and Wehe, R.A. (1967). *J. Pediatr.* **70**, 876.
Kogut, M.D. (1974). *Curr. Probl. Pediatr.* **4**, 3.
Koivisto, M., Blanco-Sequeiros, M. and Krause, U. (1972). *Dev. Med. Child Neurol.* **14**, 603.
Lacourt, G. (1974). *Medicine Sociale et Preventive* **19**, 101.
deLeeuw, R. and deVries, I. (1976). *Pediatrics* **58**, 18-22.
Lovinger, R.D., Kaplan, S.L. and Grumbach, M.M. (1975). *J. Pediatr.* **87**, 1171.
Lubchenco, L.O. and Bard, H. (1971). *Pediatrics* **47**, 831.
Lubchenco, L.O., Bard, H., Goldman, A.L., Coyer, W.E., McIntyre, C. and Smith, D.M. (1974). *Dev. Med. Child Neurol.* **16**, 421.
McQuarrie, I. (1954). *Am. J. Dis. Child.* **87**, 399.
Pildes, R.S., Cornblath, M., Warren, L., Page-El, E., deMenza, S., Merritt, D.M. and Peeva, A. (1974). *Pediatrics* **54**, 5.
Raivio, K.O. and Hallman, N. (1968). *Acta Paediatr. Scand.* **57**, 517.
Sadeghi-Nejad, A. and Senior, B. (1974). *J. Pediatr.* **84**, 749.
Sauls, H.S. (1974). *In* "Metabolic Endocrine and Genetic Disorders of Children" (V.C. Kelly, ed), p.683. Harper and Row, Pubs., Inc., New York.
Sauls, H.S., Jr. and Ulstrom, R.A. (1966). *In* "Brennemann's Practice of Pediatrics" (V.C. Kelly, ed), **Vol.I**, Chapter 6. W.F. Prior Co., Hagerstown, Maryland.
Shelly, H.J. (1964). *Br. med. J.* **I**, 273.
Steward, A.L. and Reynolds, E.O.R. (1974). *Pediatrics* **54**, 724.
Tildon, J.T., Ozand, P.T. and Cornblath, M. (1975). *In* "The Normal and Pathological Development of Metabolsim" (F.A. Hommes and C.J. Vandenberg, eds), p.143. Academic Press, New York.
Ulstrom, R.A. (1962). *In* "Erbliche Stoifwechselkrankheiten" (F. Linneweh, ed), p.225. Urban and Schwartzenberg, Berlin.
Zuppinger, K.A. (1975). *In* "Monographs in Pediatrics" (F. Falkner, N. Kretchmer and E. Rossi, eds) **Vol.4**, S. Karger, Basel.

KETOTIC HYPOGLYCEMIA

J. L. Chaussain, P. Georges, L. Calzada and J.C. Job

Laboratoire de Recherches sur la Croissance
Hôpital St-Vincent de Paul, Paris, France

Ketotic hypoglycemia is the commonest form of hypoglycemia in childhood. First recognized by Ross and Joseph in 1924, this syndrome was clearly defined by Colle and Ulstrom in 1964. The combination of seizures, hypoglycemia and acetonuria may be associated with various etiologies, such as pituitary and adrenal deficiencies and hepatic enzymatic defects. The term ketotic hypoglycemia is generally attributed only to apparently idiopathic cases. But if the cause of idiopathic ketotic hypoglycemia remains unknown, recent studies have cast some light on the mechanism of this syndrome.

CLINICAL MANIFESTATIONS

Hypoglycemic episodes occur exclusively in the morning and are often preceded by vomiting. Seizures and/or coma are the two major clinical symptoms. Episodes recur at intervals of a few months or of a year or more. In recent years, we had the opportunity to study 15 cases of ketotic hypoglycemia. Clinical data on these patients are given in Table I. The major characteristics in the history of these children correspond to those previously reported (Sauls and Ulstrom, 1965; Gabilan and Chaussain, 1968). They are: occurrence after one year of age, predominance in males and low birth weight in two thirds of the cases. The association to a cataract of the crystalline lens, also reported previously (Cornblath and Schwartz, 1966; Gabilan and Chaussain, 1969), was found in 3 children of the present group. An important factor must be added: the spontaneous disappearance of hypoglycemic crisis at 8 or 9 years of age. Neurologic damage, non-hypoglycemic seizures and mental retardation may persist as sequelae.

Table I. Clinical data in 15 children with ketotic hypoglycemia.

No.	Sex, Age (years)	Premature	Birth weight (kg)	Neonatal hypoglycemia	Age of onset (years)	Cataract
1.	M, 1.4/12	+	0.895		1.4/12	
2.	M, 1.4/12	+	1.600		1.3/12	
3.	M, 1.6/12		1.800	+	1.6/12	+
4.	M, 1.8/12	+	1.420	+	1.3/12	
5.	M, 1.11/12		4.000		1.8/12	
6.	F, 2	+	1.680		2.	+
7.	M, 3		2.900	+	1.9/12	
8.	M, 3.2/12		3.380		3.1/12	
9.	M, 3.3/12		4.000		3.3/12	
10.	M, 3.10/12	+	2.000	+	1.3/12	
11.	M, 4	+	2.000		2.5/12	
12.	M, 4		1.650	+	2.	+
13.	M, 4.3/12		3.150		4.	
14.	M, 4.5/12		3.060		2.1/12	
15.	M, 7		1.630	+	2.3/12	

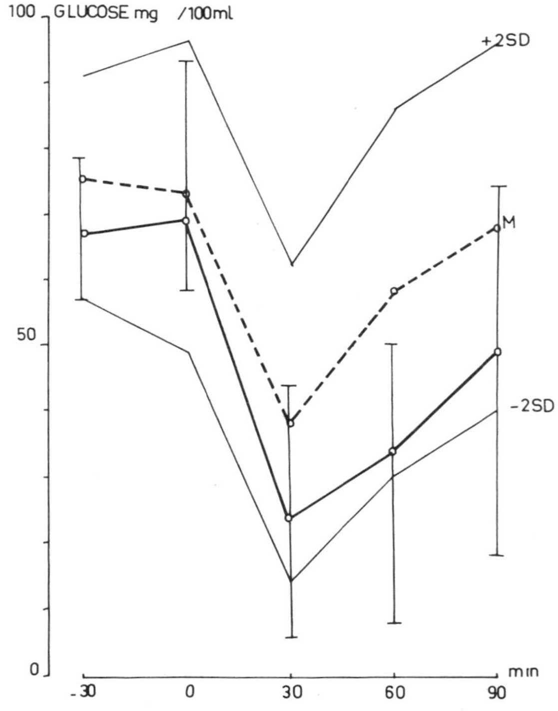

Fig. 1 Blood glucose response to insulin (0.05 u/kg) in children with ketotic hypoglycemia, by comparison with controls (M ± 2 SD, 0.1 u/kg).

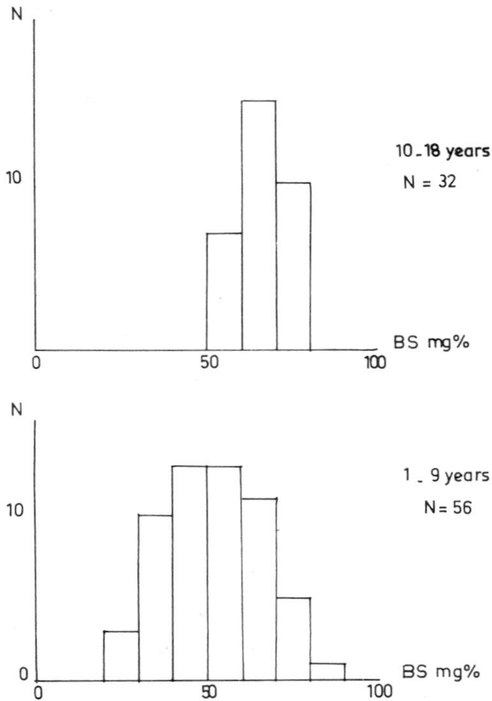

Fig.2 **Distribution of blood glucose 24 hour fasting values in normal children aged 1 to 9 years and 10 to 18 years.**

LABORATORY FINDINGS

At the time of the seizures the blood sugar is lower than 40 mg/100 ml and the research of the ketonuria is strongly positive. The glucagon injection fails to increase the blood glucose concentration.

The increased sensitivity to insulin is the only characteristic finding between the spontaneous episodes (Fig.1). Between crises the glycemic response to glucagon and the growth hormone and cortisol responses to specific stimuli are normal.

MECHANISM

If the etiology of ketotic hypoglycemia remains unknown, recent reports lead to a better understanding of the mechanism of the syndrome. Ketotic hypoglycemia may be considered as the consequence of the simultaneous occurrence of 2 out of 3 factors: nutritional disorder, age-related sensitivity to fasting, and hormonal deficiency.

The nutritional disorder is present, in most cases, in the days preceding the hypoglycemia episode. Anorexia and vomiting may be related to an intercurrent infection, especially a pharyngitis, or to various circumstances including prolonged travels by car.

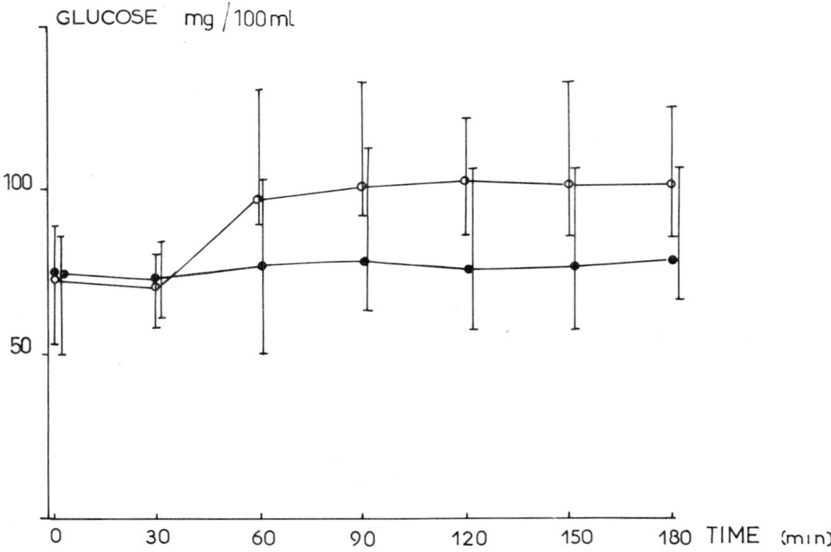

Fig.3 **Blood sugar response to 2-deoxyglucose in normal children (open circles) and in 8 children with ketotic hypoglycemia (black circles).**

The age-related sensitivity to fast has been clearly established in children with ketotic hypoglycemia (Chaussain, 1973), but systematic studies of the effects of fast in normal children (Chaussain *et al.*, 1974; Haymond *et al.*, 1974) emphasized the inability of children to sustain a normal blood sugar level, during a relatively short period of time. According to Pagliara *et al.* (1972) this sensitivity to fast may be related to a deficient gluconeogenesis, attested by low alanine levels. This phenomenon appears to be more marked in children with ketotic hypoglycemia. Similar conclusions were drawn from studies using the ketogenic low caloric diet (Colle and Ulstrom, 1964; Cornblath and Schwartz, 1966; Senior and Loridan, 1969).

The sensitivity to fast appears to be age-related. In normal young children (Fig.2) the blood sugar values after a 24 h fast are distributed according to a Gaussian curve and 22% exhibited a fasting blood sugar level in the hypoglycemic range. Above 10 years of age, fasting blood sugar values are also distributed according to a Gaussian curve, but no values in the hypoglycemic range were founded. This age-related improvement of the sensitivity to fast in children may be secondary to a better gluconeogenesis attested by fasting alanine levels increasing proportionally with age (Chaussain *et al.*, *in press*). The spontaneous disappearance with age of hypoglycemic episodes in children with ketotic hypoglycemia may be secondary to this age-related improvement of the glycemic response to fasting.

The hormonal factor is evidenced by ketotic hypoglycemic syndrome secondary to a growth hormone and/or cortisol deficiency. The practical consequence of this fact is that hypopituitarism and adrenal insufficiency must be eliminated by appropriate tests in children with ketotic hypoglycemia.

The possibility of a deficient epinephrine secretion in idiopathic ketotic hypoglycemia has been raised on indirect (Sizonenko *et al.*, 1973; Chaussain

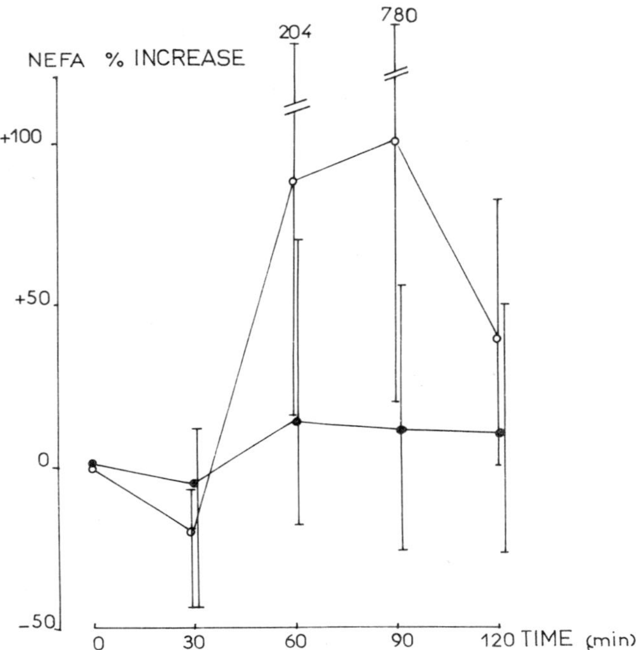

Fig.4 FFA response to 2-deoxyglucose in normal children (open circles) and in 8 children with ketotic hypoglycemia (black circles).

et al., 1973) and direct (Köffler *et al.*, 1971; Christensen, 1974) arguments. Indirect arguments are provided by studies performed with 2-deoxyglucose. The administration of this glucose analogue induces in normal subjects an intracellular glucopenia which results in epinephrine discharge with secondary increase of the biological parameters: blood sugar, serum FFA and plasma renine activity. The effects of 2-deoxyglucose (50 mg/kg I.V. in 30 min) on blood sugar and FFA in a group of 8 children with ketotic hypoglycemia are represented in Figs 3 and 4, in comparison with controls. A significant decrease of blood glucose ($p < 0.001$) and FFA ($p < 0.02$) responses is observed in children with ketotic hypoglycemia, but the study of individual patients shows that only half of them are non-responders. This variability in the response of 2-deoxyglucose in children with ketotic hypoglycemia may signify that the altered epinephrine secretion may be a secondary phenomenon, or that the syndrome is heterogeneous.

Another point which may be considered is the relative hypoinsulinism of children with ketotic hypoglycemia, attested by the sensitivity to exogenous insulin, and by the direct measurements of plasma insulin after a period of fasting (Chaussain *et al.*, 1974). The fasting increase of branched chain aminoacids in children with ketotic hypoglycemia appears to be also related to this hypoinsulinism (Chaussain *et al.*, 1974; Hambraeus *et al.*, 1972). The role played by this phenomenon in the mechanism of ketotic hypoglycemia is at present not clear. It may indicate an adaptation of pancreatic β cells to the reduced state of hepatic glucogenesis.

THERAPY

Glucose infusion is the only treatment of the acute episodes. Frequent vomiting excludes oral glucose, Glucagon injection fails to increase the blood sugar during hypoglycemic seizures of these patients.

In order to prevent recurrence, prolonged periods of fasting must be avoided and systematic nocturnal feeding must be recommended to prevent depletion of gluconeogenesis substrates. In case of repeated vomiting, glucose infusion is immediately necessary.

REFERENCES

Chaussain, J.L. (1973). *J. Pediat.* **82**, 438.

Chaussain, J.L., Georges, P., Olive, G. and Job, J.C. (1973). *Arch. Franc. Pediat.* **30**, 1081.

Chaussain, J.L., Georges, P., Olive, G. and Job, J.C. (1974). *J. Pediat.* **85**, 776.

Chaussain, J.L., Georges, P., Olive, G. and Job, J.C. *Pediat. Res. (in press).*

Christensen, N.J. (1974). *J. clin. Endocr. Metab.* **38**, 107.

Colle, E. and Ulstrom, R.A. (1964). *J. Pediat.* **64**, 632.

Cornblath, M. and Schwartz, R. (1966). "Disorders of Carbohydrate Metabolism in Infancy". W.B. Saunders Co., Philadelphia and London.

Gabilan, J.C. and Chaussain, J.L. (1968). *Rev. Pediat. (Paris)* **9**, 323.

Gabilan, J.C. and Chaussain, J.L. (1969). *Arch. Franç. Pédiat.* **26**, 633.

Hambraeus, L., Westphal, O. and Hagberg, B. (1972). *Acta Paediat. Scand.* **61**, 81.

Haymond, M.W., Karl, I.E. and Pagliara, A.S. (1974). *J. clin. Endocr. Metab.* **38**, 521.

Koffler, H., Schubert, W.K. and Hug, G. (1971). *J. Pediat.* **78**, 448.

Pagliara, A.S., Karl, I.E., De Vivo, D.C., Feigin, R.D. and Kipnis, D.M. (1972). *J. clin. Invest.* **51**, 1440.

Ross, S.G. and Josephs, H.W. (1924). *Am. J. Dis. Childh.* **28**, 447.

Sauls, H.S. and Ulstrom, R.A. (1965). *In* "Brinnemans Practice of Pediatrics" (V.C. Kelly, ed). W.F. Prior Co., Hagerstown, M.D.

Senior, B. and Loridan, L. (1969). *J. Pediat.* **74**, 529.

Sizonenko, P.C., Paunier, L., Vallotton, M.B., Cuendet, G.S., Zahnd, G. and Marliss, E.B. (1973). *Pediat. Res.* **7**, 983.

GLUCAGON, INSULIN AND GROWTH HORMONE IN NEONATAL HYPOGLYCEMIA AND HYPERGLYCEMIA DURING THE ACUTE DISEASE AND AFTER FOLLOW-UP

P. Stubbe

Department of Pediatrics, University of Goettingen, West Germany

This investigation was performed to study insulin, glucagon, growth hormone and glucose concentrations following arginine, glucose and other infusions in hypoglycemic new-born infants in order to explore a possible causative relation of these hormones to hypoglycemia.

Lack of growth hormone (GH) production has rarely been found to be responsible for neonatal hypoglycemia. Insulin concentrations were found to be higher than expected when compared with low blood glucose in cases of islet cell adenoma or nesidioblastosis. Glucagon determinations have not been performed to a great extent in hypoglycemic infants, since difficulties with the assay and small plasma increments usually available in new-borns limited the experience. So far I know of only 2 infants where absence of glucagon was claimed to be present with hypoglycemia. Another report showed the insulin-to-glucagon molar ratio to be different between appropriate for age (AGAI) and hypoglycemic small for gestational age infants (SGAI), hypoglycemic infants having a ratio of 2-3 compared to 1-2 in normoglycemic SGAI and AGAI (Falorni *et al.*, 1975).

We have studied a total of 13 hypoglycemic and one hyperglycemic infants. I would like to present two infants in detail and summarize the findings of the remaining 12. All these 12 were with one exception SGAI and pregnancy was usually complicated by toxemia. Despite early feedings, these infants developed hypoglycemia below 20 mg/100 ml between the 1st and 3rd day of life. All were showing symptoms which may have been due to hypoglycemia. I.v. glucose tolerance tests demonstrated persistent elevated kg values for months or even years. GH, insulin and glucagon determinations showed presence of all hor-

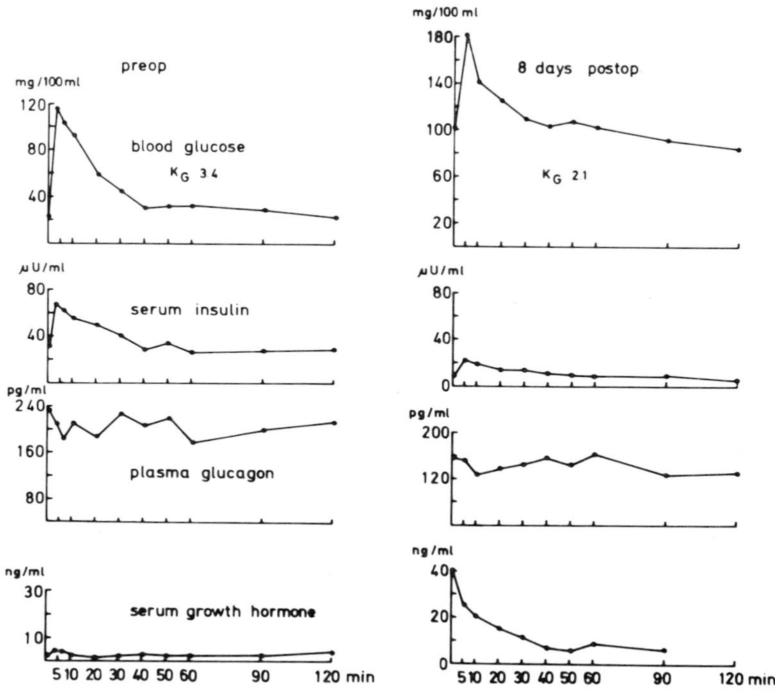

Fig. 1 Glucose, insulin, glucagon and growth hormone before and after operation following i.v. glucose tolerance test in an infant with focal adenomatosis of the pancreatic gland.

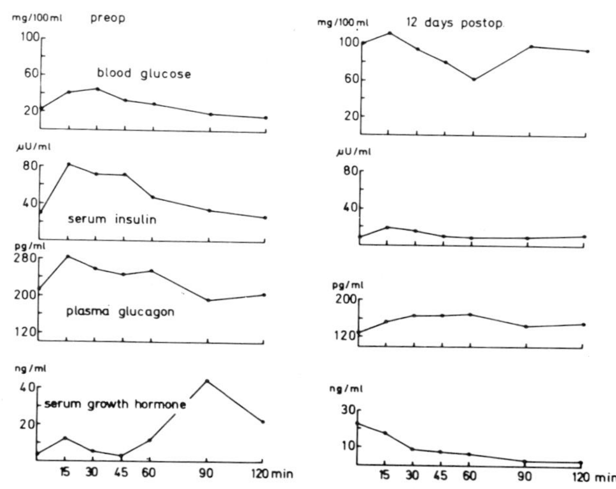

Fig. 2 Glucose, insulin, glucagon and growth hormone following i.v. arginine infusion in focal adenomatosis.

mones and secretion following i.v. glucose or arginine were considered to be normal. Of these twelve, two died, three have neurological deficits and developmental retardations, three are too young for final diagnosis and four appear to be normal.

The infants to be presented in detail are firstly a hypoglycemic infant appropriate for gestational age and secondly a small for gestational age infant with hyperglycemia caused by septicemia. The female infant with persisting hypoglycemia was investigated when she was almost 2 months of age. The birth weight was 3850 g. From the 9th day of life, low blood glucose concentrations were repeatedly observed and symptoms including seizures were recognized. When investigated at almost 2 months of age the child was on steroids and diazoxide and had signs of iatrogenic Cushing's syndrome. Figure 1 shows the i.v. glucose tolerance test before and after operation. The kg value was high before and normal after operation. The basal insulin was 32 μu/ml and high in the presence of a low blood glucose of 24 mg/100 ml. The insulin increased and returned to baseline after 60 min. The glucagon was initially depressed. The molar insulin to glucagon ratio was 3 initially and rose to 7.6 after 6 min. After operation the hormones were within normal limits, the molar ratio being 1.1 at first and 3.4 at 5 min.

Figure 2 shows the hormonal response following arginine before and after operation. Insulin and glucagon were increasing, the initial molar ratio was 3.1, and 6.4 at 15 min. Blood glucose rose continuously during the arginine infusion. When glucose later decreased to 20 mg/100 ml, GH was 44 ng/ml. After operation insulin and glucagon behaved normally. The molar ratio was 1.4 initially, and 2.7 at 15 min.

Figure 3 shows that i.v. tolbutamide was not a potent stimulus for insulin secretion before and after operation. Molar insulin/glucagon ratio was 3.7 in the beginning and 4.0 at 40 min before operation. After operation, the ratio decreased to 1.8 initially and to values lower than 1.0 during the next two hours.

Figure 4 shows the hormonal response to i.v. glucagon. Glucagon was the most powerful stimulus to insulin secretion in this infant, reaching almost 100 μu/ml at 10 min. Glucose and insulin decreased below starting levels at 90 min. At this time, growth hormone increased to 17 ng/ml. After operation the insulin and glucagon responses were normal.

Figure 5 shows the oral leucine tolerance test performed shortly before operation. Blood glucose decreased progressively to 10 mg/100 ml at 15 min. Insulin increased on the other hand progressively, reaching 72 μu/ml at 30 min shortly before the infant had a seizure and received i.v. glucagon. The injected glucagon then caused a further increase of insulin concentration in excess of 200 μu/ml. The infant was operated thereafter and a 70% removal of the pancreatic gland was performed. The electronmicroscopic and immunohistological work-up was done by Dr. Creutzfeld and Dr. Arnold from the Department of Internal Medicine. The diagnosis was focal adenomatosis, a tumor between islet cell hyperplasia and adenoma. Many B cells with typical granula formation and atypical cells identified as D_1 or F cells were found. Immunohistochemistry identified 4 pancreatic hormones: insulin, glucagon, somatostatin and pancreatic polypeptide.

The second patient I wish to consider in more detail was a SGAI who developed hyperglycemia of 950 mg/100 ml at 48 h of life while on 5% glucose because of septicemia caused by enterobacter cloacae. The blood glucose concentration responded favourably to a single injection of 1 unit regular insulin

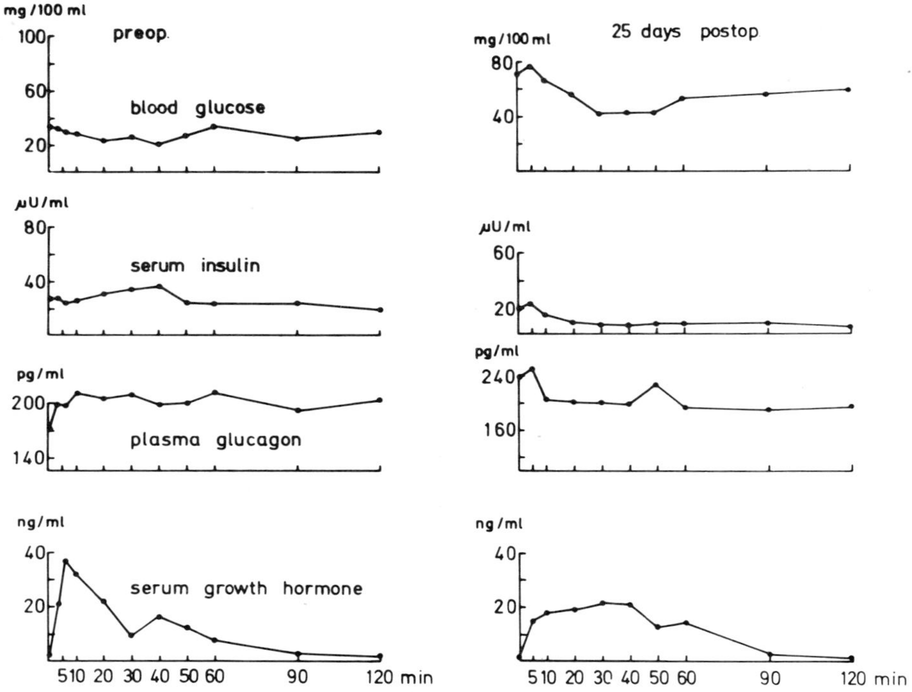

Fig. 3 Glucose, insulin, glucagon and growth hormone following i.v. tolbutamide test in focal adenomatosis.

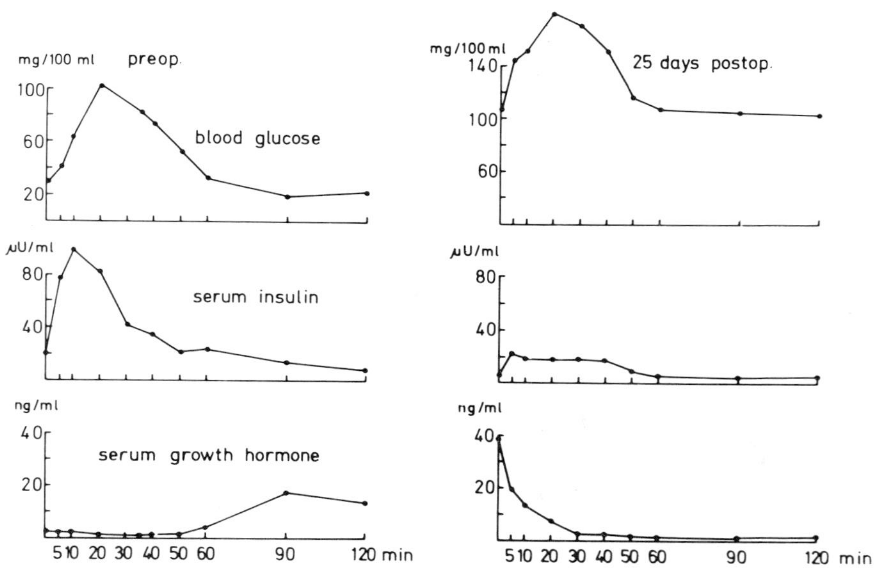

Fig. 4 Glucose, insulin and growth hormone following i.v. glucagon in focal adenomatosis.

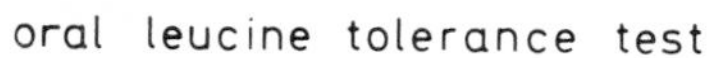

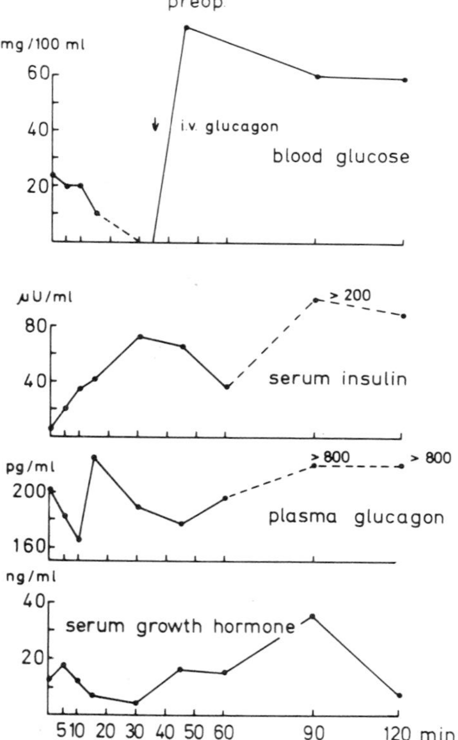

Fig.5 **Glucose, insulin, glucagon and growth hormone following oral leucine tolerance test in focal adenomatosis before operation.**

and within 24 h the glucose was normal without further insulin supplementation. At three days of age the infant required an exchange transfusion because of hyperbilirubinemia.

Figure 6 shows glucose, insulin, glucagon and growth hormone concentrations during the exchange. Glucose increased steadily, insulin remained fairly constant with 21 μu/ml at the end of the exchange procedure. Glucagon rose despite increasing blood glucose and showed a biphasic course. The molar insulin/glucagon ratio remained below 0.4; GH rose from 9 to 22 ng/ml. Compared to investigations done by Milner *et al.* (1972) during exchange transfusions in erythroblastotic infants, this infant behaved quite differently in that the insulin remained low, the molar insulin/glucagon ratio was lower and the growth hormone response to ACD blood was blunted.

I.v. glucose tolerance tests were repeated at 19 days, 2½ months and 6 months. The insulin increased and glucagon decreased within normal limits. At 6 months the kg value was 1.3. Insulin and glucagon were normal; the initial molar ratio was 2.3.

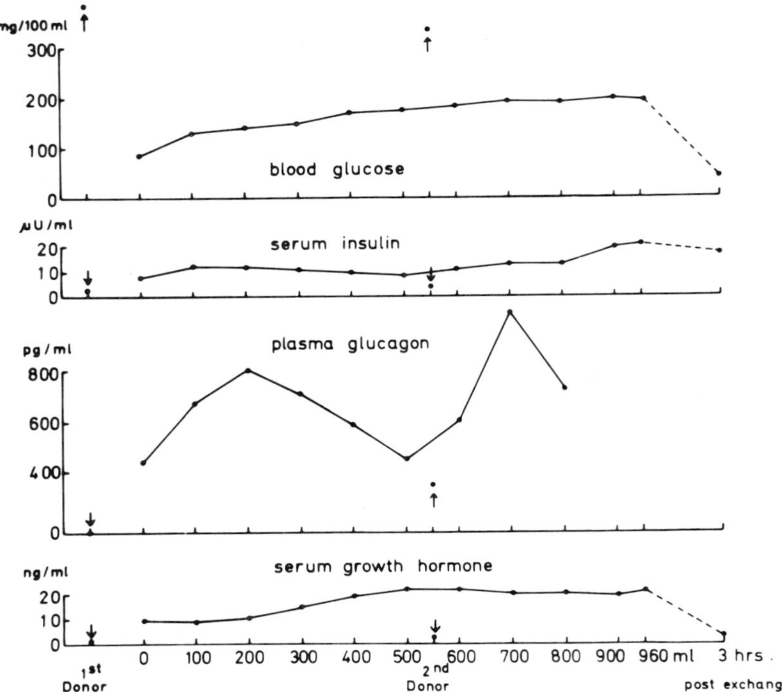

Fig.6 Glucose, insulin, glucagon and growth hormone during exchange transfusion one day after hyperglycemia in an infant with enterobacter septicemia.

In summary, we have shown persisting hyperinsulinism in a hypoglycemic infant due to focal adenomatosis. I.v. glucagon appeared to be the most potent stimulus to insulin secretion. In a temporarily hyperglycemic infant relative hyperglucagonemia appeared to be a possible explanation of the disease.

REFERENCES

Falorni, A., Massi-Benedetti, F., Gallo, S. and Rominzi, S. (1975). *Pediat. Res.* **9**, 55-60.
Milner, R.D.G., Fekete, M., Assan, R. and Hodge, J.S. (1972). *Arch. Dis. Child.* **47**, 179-185.

REMARKS ON GLUCOSE LEVELS IN THE CEREBROSPINAL FLUID IN NEW-BORNS WITH SEVERE HYPOGLYCEMIA

L. Brunelli

Department of Paediatrics, Regina Elena Hospital, Milan, Italy

During the period May 1974–May 1976, at the Regina Elena Hospital, about one hundred children, suffering from hypoglycemia in the neonatal period, were hospitalized. In the first 72 hours of life, the glycemic levels were lower than 30 mg% in the normal new-borns and lower than 20 mg% in the low-weight new-borns. Among these new-borns, we have selected 12 who suffered from a particularly evident hypoglycemia, with values lower than 15 mg%. To tell the truth, another group of 6 new-borns with glycemic values lower than 15 mg% has not been taken into consideration, in order to standardize the experimental group. In fact, the clinical picture was marked by serious cardiopathies, protracted asphyxia with difficulty of reanimation, and evident electrolytic disorders.

In the group of 12 new-borns, clinical symptoms could not always be detected which, though varying, are often present in severe hypoglycemia (Cornblath *et al.*, 1964; Dubois *et al.*, 1973; Nicolini, 1973; Flauto and Vaccari, 1973). Some of them were born immaturely, others were small for date, and some others were born normally by eutocic or instrumental delivery. In all these babies, together with glycemia, the glucose dose in the cerebrospinal fluid was also determined, almost simultaneously.

For the determination of the glucose the enzymatic method of glucosamine-oxidase was used; the deproteinization was carried out with the acetate of uranyl for the blood and with the perchloric acid 0.33 N for the cerebrospinal fluid (Werner *et al.*, 1970). The results obtained are shown in Table I.

From examination of the Table, it appears that in the babies we examined, with the exception of Case No.6, the glycorrhachia is not different from the values pointed out by Ammon and Richterich (1970) in normal new-borns. These authors, using the same method as ours, found glucose rates in the cerebrospinal fluid

Table I.

N.	Case	Sex	Weeks gestation	Delivery	Weight (grams)	Glucose mg% Blood	CSF	Age (days)	Symptomatology
1	S.T.	m	40	Eutocic Asph.	4000	5	49	3	Convulsions
2	B.L.	f	39	Eutocic	3650	13	43	3	Asymptomatic
3	T.G.	m	40	Eutocic	3150	8	53	3	Tremors
4	S.C.	m	39	Eutocic	2700	9	55	2	Asymptomatic
5	M.M.	m	40	Forceps-Asph.	3500	9	34	2	Tremors
6	F.A.	f	40	Eutocic Twin	2050	0	19	1	Asymptomatic
7	F.M.	f	40	Eutocic Twin	2350	14	48	1	Asymptomatic
8	R.L.	m	38	Eut. Plac. Insuff.	1750	1	70	1	Hypertonia
9	G.M.	m	38	Eutocic	2250	14	35	7	Asymptomatic
10	R.G.	f	38	Eutocic	2900	12	64	2	Asymptomatic
11	R.F.	f	40	Cesar. Sect.	4000	10	38	2	Asymptomatic
12	R.M.	f	36	Eutocic	2050	11	69	3	Apathy

Table II. F.A. new born, twin, 2050 grams (N.6) Asymptomatic Hypoglycemia

Day		1	2	3	4	5	6	7	8	9	10	11	12	13
Glucose infusion		—	—	—	—	—	—	—						
Glucose mg%														
Blood	0	2	2	7	2	16	7	34	30	41	53	42	39	61
CSF	19								42					

ranging from 29.8 mg% to 87.8 mg%, values similar to ours in a limited number of controls.

All this, should our data be confirmed, could let us think of a certain independence of the glucose levels in the cerebrospinal fluid as regards the hematic rates. In fact, according to the majority of modern opinions (Plum and Siesjo, 1975) the secretion of the cerebrospinal fluid is a process requiring energy, and it differs substantially from a simple plasma ultrafiltrate. In these circumstances, we can think that the cerebrospinal fluid is able to maintain a certain stability as long as possible, which is essential for the close homeostasis necessary for the function of the neuron.

The above does not exclude that the infusion of glucose in the hypoglycemia (Table No.II), especially if protracted avoiding sudden increase of the glycemia, can affect the cerebrospinal fluid levels and therefore confirm further on how the barrier blood-fluid is barely efficient in the neonatal period (Adinolfi *et al.*, 1976; Saunders *et al.*, 1976).

REFERENCES

Adinolfi, M., Beck, S.E. Haddad, S.A. and Seller, M.J. (1976). *Nature* **259**, 140-141.

Ammon, J. and Richterich, R. (1970). *Schweiz. med. Wschr.* **100**, 1317-1320.

Cornblath, M., Baens, G.S., Wybregt, S.H. and Klein, R.I. (1964). *Pediatrics* **33**, 388-402.

Dubois, O., Menne, T., Lefebvre, C. and Berquin, J. (1973). *Pédiatrie* **28**, 782-783.

Flauto, U. and Vaccari, A. (1973). *Min. Ped.* **25**, 353-359.

Nicolini, A. (1973). *Min. Ped.* **25**, 240-245.

Plum, F. and Siesjo, B.K. (1975). *Anesthesiology* **42**, 708-730.

Saunders, N.R., Dziegielewska, K.M., Malinowska, D.H., Reynolds, M.L., Reynolds, J.M. and Møllgard, K. (1976). *Nature* **262**, 156.

Werner, W., Rey, H. and Wielinger, H. (1970). *Z. analyt. Chem.* **252**, 224.

CONSTITUTIONAL DELAY OF GROWTH AND PUBERTY

A. Prader

Department of Pediatrics, University of Zürich, Kinderspital, Switzerland

Constitutional delay of growth and puberty constitutes a well-defined pattern of growth and development and is the most frequent cause of short stature in children and of the absence of expected puberty (Wilkins, 1965; Rappaport, 1968; Bierich, 1975; Prader, 1975). It carries a good prognosis and should not be regarded as a disorder, but rather as an extreme variant of normal growth and development.

Lack of puberty at an age when other children manifest sexual maturation and the associated spurt of growth and physical strength is a matter of concern for the parents and frequently the cause of unhappiness and misery for the affected individual. For psychosocial reasons, which will be discussed later, the problem usually has a stronger impact on boys than on girls.

There are many possible causes for the lack of pubertal development. If in a boy aged 16 puberty is absent and the cause for this is unknown, it is preferable to call the situation "lacking" puberty and not "delayed" or "retarded" puberty which would indicate only a temporary absence of puberty. Although a temporary absence or delay frequently occurs, there are certain causes which involve permanent hypogonadism. Differential diagnosis of constitutional delay of growth and puberty (Table I) includes endocrine disorders (hypothalamo-pituitary disorders, primary hypogonadism and primary hypothyroidism), chronic disease (examples are mucoviscidosis, renal insufficiency, poorly controlled diabetes mellitus, thalassemia, etc.) and malnutrition and deprivation. We will come back to the differential diagnosis after having discussed the various practical and theoretical aspects of constitutional delay of growth and puberty.

DEFINITION AND INCIDENCE

For the patient and his parents the definition of what constitutes a significant delay is an individual psychological problem. A boy aged 13 may be unhappy because he is retarded in comparison with his peers, whereas another boy aged 15 may

Table I. Lack of expected puberty.

1. Constitutional Delay of Growth and Puberty
2. Endocrine Disorders
   a) Hypothalamo-pituitary disorders
      – Multiple hormone deficiency
      – Isolated growth hormone deficiency
      – Isolated gonadotropin deficiency
      – Increased prolactin
   b) Primary hypogonadism
      ♀ – Turner-syndrome
      – Pure gonadal dysgenesis
      ♂ – Anorchia
      – Testicular atrophy
   c) Primary hypothyroidism
3. Chronic Diseases
4. Malnutrition, Deprivation

accept to be not yet in puberty without being disturbed.

Statistically, the normal timing of puberty is defined as the range between the mean plus and minus 2 standard deviations (SD). By definition, 2.5% mature earlier and 2.5% later. According to the Zürich longitudinal growth study (Prader, 1975), the upper age limit defined as the mean +2 SD is 15.2 years for the appearance of pubic hair in boys, 13.4 years for the beginning of breast development in girls and 15.6 years for menarche (Fig.1). It is important to realise that in 2.5% of all children puberty occurs later. Considering this, and the experience with families of patients it is clearly seen that there is no sex difference in the incidence of constitutional delay of growth and puberty. However, as already mentioned, there are psychosocial reasons which explain why many of the boys but only few of the girls ask for help.

CLINICAL ASPECTS AND NATURAL HISTORY

A typical example is a boy aged 15 or 16 who is unhappy because he is not yet in puberty. He looks younger, is rather short but in good health, and physical examination does not reveal any abnormal findings. The following questions and simple examinations are of importance in order to clarify the situation.

The *family history* will frequently reveal that one or both parents and/or some of the older siblings were also late maturers. One will ask about the age of menarche of the mother and whether the father was early or late in puberty. One will also note the height of the parents and age, height and pubertal development of the siblings. An impressive family history is given in Table II. Several adult male members of this family are slightly or considerably taller than when measured at the age of 18 as military conscripts.

The previous *growth pattern* is unfortunately not always known. A typical example is the lower growth curve in Fig.2. At birth and during the first years the growth curve lies within the normal range. Later it crosses through the percentiles

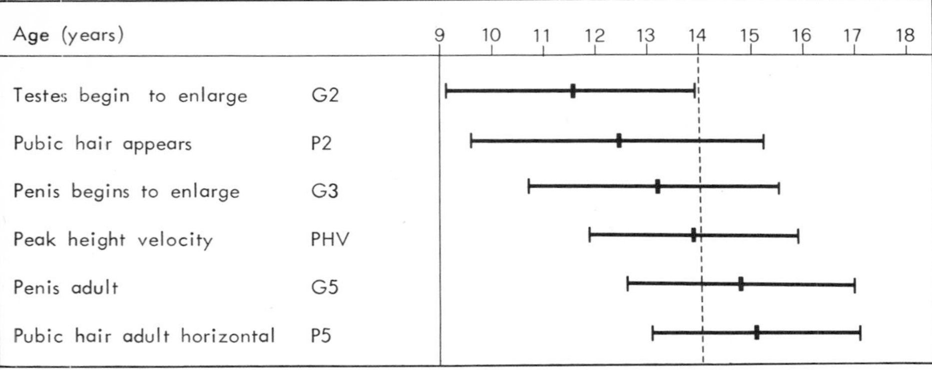

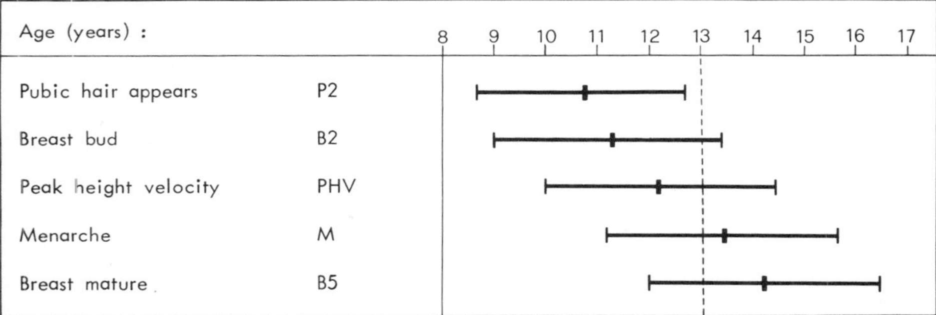

Fig. 1 Normal timing of puberty in boys (upper part) and in girls (lower part) in the Zürich longitudinal growth study.

into a lower or subnormal range; may run for a certain period along a lower percentile or below and parallel to the 3rd percentile; is far below the 3rd percentile when the other children undergo the pubertal growth spurt and finally catches up when the other children come to the end of their growth. Between the age of 6 and 12, many of these children are regarded as having simply short stature. On the same growth chart is also shown the growth of the patient's elder brother who grew much taller. However, his growth pattern is exactly the same. He was first in the upper percentiles, dropped below the 50th percentile when the majority of boys had their pubertal growth spurt and moved into the upper percentiles again when he had his delayed growth spurt and puberty. Thus, a boy with constitutional delay of growth and puberty has a normal height if he is to become a tall adult and is short if he is to become an adult of average or short stature. Many of our patients are not only delayed in puberty but also very short because of the combination of familial or constitutional short stature with constitutional delay of growth and puberty.

There are some additional growth characteristics of constitutional delay of growth and puberty: the prespurt growth velocity which is always low ("minimal height velocity" in contrast to "peak height velocity", seen at the height of the growth spurt) becomes even lower if puberty is delayed (the parents

Table II. **Constitutional delay of growth and puberty.**

	Age (years)	Height (cm)	Bone Age (years)
Patient (R. Hans)	16 3/12	140	9 10/12
	18 10/12	152	13 6/12
Father	18 6/12	158	
	28	170	
Brother R.	18 11/12	159	
	21 6/12	167	15 6/12
Brother A.	18 3/12	173	
	21	175	

and the patient will say that he has not grown at all during the last year) and the relative length of the extremities, which in normally timed puberty is always at its maximum just before and at the beginning of puberty, becomes frequently exaggeraged and impresses as "eunuchoid" proportions (Fig.3).

Since *testicular growth* precedes the appearance of the secondary sex characteristics it is important to assess testicular volume with the help of an orchidometer (Zachmann *et al.*, 1974). A volume of more than 2 ml indicates that the appearance of the secondary sex characteristics and the pubertal growth spurt may be expected within the next 1 or 2 years.

Bone age, as assessed on an X-ray film of the hand according to Greulich and Pyle, is always delayed. Compared to bone age, height and growth velocity are usually in the normal range.

Predicted adult height calculated from age, height and bone age according to Bayley and Pinneau or one of the newer methods is usually normal, or within the range to be expected from the parents' height.

Bone age also allows to predict quite well the timing of puberty and the growth spurt because puberty and the growth spurt will in general begin at the appropriate bone age. In boys the testes will increase in volume at a bone age of about 11 to 12 and pubic hair will appear at a bone age of about 13. The pubertal growth spurt will manifest itself soon afterwards, and peak height velocity will be reached at a bone age of about 14. In girls breast development and pubic hair will appear at a bone age of about 11 and menarche will occur at a bone age of 13.

The most important aspect of constitutional delay of growth and puberty is the *psychological problem.* Only those parents and those patients who suffer psychologically are brought to our attention. They seek medical advice because of their anxieties. The parents' anxieties concern mainly the future. Will their son ever become sexually mature? Will he become fertile? Will he reach adult height? In contrast to the parents the boy is mainly concerned with his present psychological problems which may be serious enough to cause depression, social withdrawal, aggression or delinquent behaviour. Being smaller, physically less mature and weaker than his peers, he is unable to compete physically, is excluded

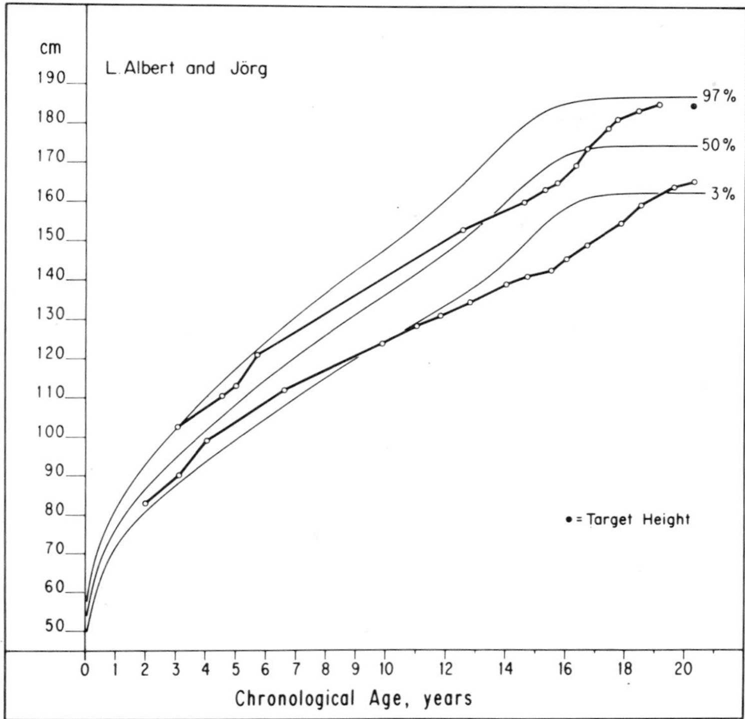

Fig. 2 **Constitutional delay of growth and puberty in two brothers.**

from adolescent activities and is frequently subjected to indignities and humiliations from his peers. It is important to discuss the situation first with the parents alone and then with the boy alone. Some of the crucial questions are: How is the patient accepted by his peers? How is his physical performance? Does he have friends of his own age? Does he use the common shower room, or is he ashamed to be seen in the nude by the others? Does he hate and avoid the shower room because he is exposed to indignities? It is this situation which may be truly terrible for such a boy. During the interview he may suddenly burst out crying and expose a state of extreme misery. The severity of the psychological reactions varies greatly, depending on the emotional stability of the patient, the social setting and the type of school he attends. Boys tend more than girls to terrorize and to exclude those who are different and weaker. This explains why most patients with constitutional delay of growth and adolescence seen in medical practice are boys.

ENDOCRINE FINDINGS

Endocrinological investigations give essentially normal results (Sizonenko, 1975). The response of plasma growth hormone to insulin and other stimulation tests is normal or low (Illig and Prader, 1970; Vanderschueren, 1976). If it is low it can be normalized by giving sex steroids during a very short period (Martin *et al.*,

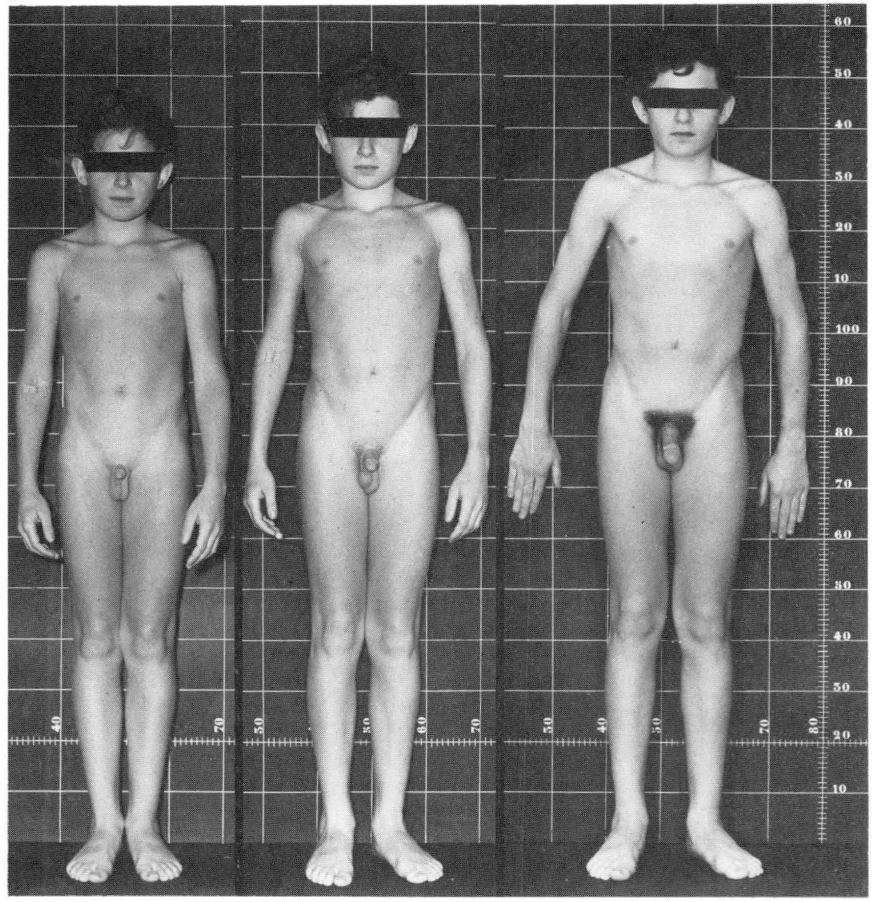

Age	**14 1/12**	**15 3/12**	**16 2/12 y.**
Height	**142,6**	**146,6**	**155,4 cm**

Fig.3 Constitutional delay of growth and puberty, demonstrating the good prognosis.

1968; Illig and Prader, 1970). In true growth hormone deficiency such treatment has no influence on the test results. The levels of the gonadotropins LH and FSH and their response to the hypothalamic LH releasing hormone are low for the chronological age of the patients, but normal for their bone age (Roth *et al.*, 1973; Illig *et al.*, 1974; Job *et al.*, 1976). The same is true for the urinary 17-ketosteroids and for testosterone and estrogens in urine and plasma. After stimulation with human chorionic gonadotropins plasma and urinary testosterone increases insufficiently for the patient's chronological age, but is normal for his bone age (Zachmann, 1972; Rudd *et al.*, 1973). These tests are rarely necessary and have certainly less importance than the family history, the physical examination and the assessment of bone age.

ETIOLOGY AND PATHOGENESIS

What is the etiology and pathogenesis of constitutional delay of growth and puberty? It is clearly a familial condition but there is no typical hereditary pattern. It is not transmitted according to the mendelian rules. This is the reason why the old and vague word "constitutional" is more appropriate than the word "hereditary". Height and growth velocity are of multifactorial etiology and independent of each other. "Multifactorial" means that they depend on multiple genetic and environmental factors. The lack of a relation between height or stature on the one hand, and growth velocity or developmental tempo on the other hand, has been clearly shown in the analysis of the data of our longitudinal growth study (Largo *et al.*, 1977) and is exemplified by the two brothers in Fig.2 whose stature is very different but whose growth and developmental tempo show an identical pattern.

It is tempting to speculate that the mechanism which leads to constitutional delay of growth and puberty is a specific temporary and mild deficiency of growth hormone (Tanner *et al.*, 1971; Joss, 1975; Trygstad and Foss, 1975; Gourmelen *et al.*, 1976) or somatomedin (Van den Brande, 1973; Hall and Filipsson, 1975). As mentioned, in some studies the growth hormone response to insulin has been low and could be normalized by giving sex steroids. However, it has been shown that the mean blood level of growth hormone during a 24-h period is normal (Blizzard *et al.*, 1974; Butenandt *et al.*, 1976). Thus it is difficult to offer an endocrine explanation. Furthermore, one should bear in mind that the retardation of growth and bone age begins at a very early age, many years before the normal age of puberty.

DIFFERENTIAL DIAGNOSIS

After the discussion of the clinical, psychological and endocrinological aspects and of the problem of etiology and pathogenesis we come back to the differential diagnosis. Most conditions listed in Table I can be excluded by thorough physical examination. It is important to know that the same growth pattern with the same retardation of bone age as in constitutional delay of growth and puberty may be seen in chronic disease (Fig.4) and in partial growth hormone deficiency, with or without gonadotropin deficiency. If the family history is typical and if the boy already has slightly enlarged testicles and a bone age of 11 or 12 years, the clinical diagnosis cannot be doubted, and there is no need to perform any endocrine tests.

If bone age is above 11 in girls and above 13 in boys in the absence of any signs of puberty, constitutional delay of growth and puberty is unlikely and one has to consider hypothalamo-pituitary or primary hypogonadism. In isolated gonadotropin deficiency and in primary hypogonadism of boys, growth is not usually retarded. In some patients with a very severe delay of growth and bone age and without puberty, a true deficiency of growth hormone with or without a deficiency of gonadotropins cannot be excluded, and it is mainly in these patients where the appropriate tests are indicated. If the response of growth hormone to insulin and other stimulation tests is insufficient it should be repeated after a short course of testosterone. If the LH and FSH response to the LH releasing hormone (LHRH) is normal for bone age, true gonadotropin deficiency is unlikely. During the 2 years preceding the appearance of the secondary sex

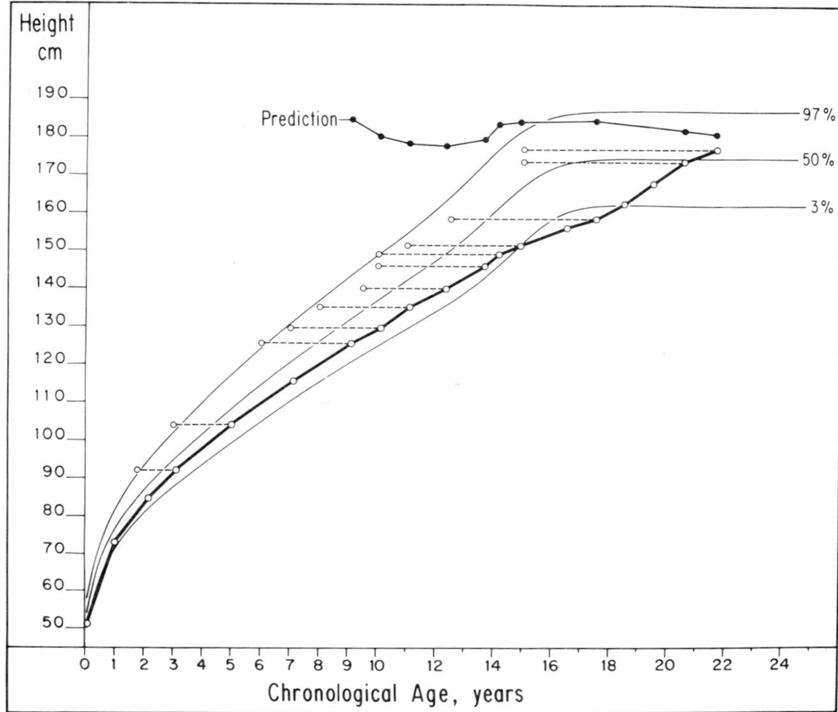

Fig.4 Delay of growth and puberty in a boy with mucoviscidosis. For most height measurements not only the chronological age, but also the retarded bone age is indicated. At the age of 22, bone age is only 15½ and adult height is not yet reached. The pattern of growth and puberty is identical with that in constitutional delay of growth and puberty.

characteristics, the LH and FSH response is usually as high as in early puberty which excludes a gonadotropin deficiency. However, sometimes the result of this test is equivocal and leaves one in doubt. A prolonged test protocol may allow a better discrimination. We need a prospective study to find out whether it is possible to differentiate long before puberty between constitutional delay of growth and puberty and true gonadotropin deficiency.

A newly-discovered endocrine disorder causing lack of puberty by suppressing the gonadotropic effect is hyperprolactinemia due to a pituitary adenoma or of idiopathic nature (König *et al.*, 1976). In typical cases, gynecomastia and galactorrhea are present, but there may be exceptions. This condition is probably extremely rare in the age group of early adolescence.

THERAPY

From a purely somatic point of view, very little needs to be said about treatment. In patients with true endocrine disorders permanent hormone replacement therapy is indicated. In constitutional delay of growth and adolescence there is no clear indication for such therapy because puberty will eventually occur spontaneously. However, one has also to consider the psychosocial situation which may present an urgent indication for at least a temporary therapy with sex hormones. Sex hormone therapy should be avoided if there is no urgent psychosocial indication because it may suppress the physiological increase of the gonadotropins and gonadal maturation, and it may slightly decrease ultimate height. However, the latter is not necessarily true (Kaplan *et al.*, 1973). The full information about the good prognosis and about the approximate time period for the expected appearance of the secondary sex characteristics and the pubertal growth spurt, together with a friendly supporting discussion will frequently be sufficient to reassure the patient and to give him the necessary patience and courage to go through the difficult waiting period before puberty sets in spontaneously. If, however, the patient's anxieties still persist and if there is a real psychosocial indication as described above, one should not hesitate to prescribe sex hormone therapy for a limited period of some months in replacement dosage. This treatment should be temporary in order to avoid the disadvantages mentioned and because puberty will continue spontaneously after a bone age of 13 in boys and 11 in girls has been reached. Such therapy quickly induces the pubertal development and the desired acceleration of growth and strength and greatly improves the patient's self confidence. In a boy, a long-acting intramuscular testosterone preparation in a dosage of 100 mg given every 3 or 4 weeks for a period of several months is recommended. This is sufficient to induce partial puberty and is less than the replacement dosage necessary for full maturation. It has been argued that human chorionic gonadotropin constitutes a more physiological therapy because of its stimulating effect on testicular maturation. It is questionable whether such treatment is really better than testosterone. It leads to unphysiologically high gonadotropin peaks and presumably suppresses the hypothalamic secretion of LH releasing hormone. From a practical point of view, testosterone therapy is much simpler and cheaper and does not prevent post-treatment spontaneous testicular maturation. In girls, where there is rarely a real psychosocial indication for treatment, a similar temporary low dosage estrogen therapy (e.g. ethinylestradiol 0.01–0.02 mg daily for 3 months) may be given. Good psychological and hormonal management of a child who is miserable and desperate because of his delay in growth and lack of puberty is one of the most rewarding experiences in adolescent medicine.

REFERENCES

Bayley, N. and Pinneau, S.R. (1952). *J. Pediat.* **40**, 423-441.

Bierich, J.R. (1975). *Mschr. Kinderheilk.* **123**, 301-306.

Blizzard, R.M., Thompson, R.G., Baghdassarian, A., Kowarski, A., Migeon, C.H. and Rodriguez, A. (1974). *In* "The Control of the Onset of Puberty" (M.M. Grumbach, G.D. Grave and F.E. Mayer, eds) pp.342-366. John Wiley & Sons, New York, London, Sydney, Toronto.

Butenandt, O., Eder, R., Wohlfarth, K., Bidlingmaier, F. and Knorr, D. (1976). *Europ. J. Pediat.* **122**, 85-92.

Greulich, W.W. and Pyle, S.I. (1959). "Radiographic Atlas of Skeletal Development of the Hand and Wrist". 2nd Ed., 256 pp. Stanford University Press, Stanford, California.

Gourmelen, M., Pham-Huu-Trung, M.T. and Girard, F. (1976). *Europ. Soc. Pediat. Endocr.*, Rotterdam.

Hall, K. and Filipsson, R. (1975). *Acta Endocr.* **78**, 239-250.

Illig, R., Pluznik, S., Werner, H. and Prader, A. (1974). *Horm. and Metab. Res.*, **Suppl.5**, 156-162.

Illig, R. and Prader, A. (1970). *J. clin. Endocr. Metab.* **30**, 615-618.
Job, J.C., Caussain, J.L., Garnier, P.E. and Toublanc, J.E. (1976). *J. Pediat.* **88**, 494-498.
Joss, E.E. (1975). *Monographs in Paediatrics* **5**.
Kaplan, J.G., Moshang, T., Jr., Bernstein, R., Parks, J.S. and Bongiovanni, A.M. (1973). *J. Pediat.* **82**, 38-44.
König, M.P., Zuppinger, K. and Leichti, B. (1976). *Europ. Soc. Pediat. Endocr.*, Rotterdam.
Largo, R.H., Stutzle, W., Gasser, Th., Huber, P.J. and Prader, A. (1977). *To be published.*
Martin, L.G., Clark, J.W. and Connor, T.B. (1968). *J. clin. Endocr. Metab.* **28**, 425-428.
Prader, A. (1975). *Mschr. Kinderheilk.* **123**, 291-296.
Rappaport, R. (1968). *Ann. Péd.* **44**, 313-320.
Roth, J.C., Grumbach, M.M. and Kaplan, S.L. (1973). *J. clin. Endocr. Metab.* **37**, 680-686.
Rudd, B.T., Rayner, P.H.W., Smith, M.R., Holder, G., Jivani, S.K.M. and Theodoridis, C.G. (1973). *Arch. Dis. Childh.* **48**, 590-595.
Sizonenko, P.C. (1975). *Clinics in Endocrinol. and Metab.* **4**, 173-206.
Tanner, J.M., Whitehouse, R.H., Hughes, P.C.R. and Vince, F.P. (1971). *Arch. Dis. Childh.* **46**, 745-782.
Trygstad, O. and Foss, I. (1975). *Internat. Symp. on Growth Hormone and Related Peptides*, Milan.
Van den Brande, J.V.L. (1973). Thesis, Rotterdam.
Vanderschueren, M. (1976). Thesis, Leuven.
Wilkins, L. (1965). "The Diagnosis and Treatment of Endocrine Disorders in Childhood and Adolescence", 3rd Ed., 619 pp. Charles C. Thomas, Publisher, Springfield, Illinois.
Zachmann, M. (1972). *Acta Endocr.* **70, Suppl.164**, 1-94.
Zachmann, M., Prader, A., Kind, H.P., Häfliger, H. and Budliger, H. (1974). *Helv. paed. Acta* **29**, 61-72.

USEFULNESS OF THE LH-RH TEST IN THE CHOICE OF THERAPY IN DELAYED PUBERTY IN BOYS

Z. Laron

Institute of Pediatric and Adolescent Endocrinology, Beilinson Medical Center Petah Tikva and Sackler School of Medicine, Tel Aviv University, Israel

Because of wide individual and often familial variability in the time of onset of puberty (Laron, 1963; Marshall *et al.*, 1970) the diagnosis of delayed puberty is often made only after the involved adolescent himself becomes aware that he is different from his peers. Until recently it was virtually impossible to predict a future delay in the onset of puberty, and the diagnostic tools available to differentiate between the various disorders which may cause a disturbance in the mechanism of puberty were limited, so that the usual approach was that of "wait and see" (Kulin *et al.*, 1974).

In boys delayed puberty may be due to a lesion anywhere along the hypothalamic-pituitary-gonadal-peripheral end-organ axis and may be congenital or acquired or transitory (Jones *et al.*, 1950; Root, 1973).

CLINICAL ASPECTS

In those cases in which there has been a prolonged intrauterine lack of gonadotrophins and/or androgens, the penis and testes will be small even in the prepubertal period (Table I), but when the intrauterine lack has been of shorter duration or of low intensity they may be of normal size. In most groups linear growth is normal in the prepubertal period but serves as one of the most sensitive indices of delayed puberty subsequently. The laboratory tests now available to investigate the integrity of the hypothalamic-pituitary-testicular axis are listed in Table II.

Unquestionably, the possibility of performing radioimmunoassays for LH, FSH (Midgley, 1966; Midgley, 1967) and testosterone (Weinstein *et al.*, 1972) and the synthesis of LH-RH (Schally *et al.*, 1971) constitute a major break-

Table I. The prepubertal development of the gonads and genitalia as related to linear growth in boys with disturbances related to the hypothalamic-pituitary-testicular axis.

Diagnosis	Linear Growth	Penis Size	Testicular Size	Ref. No.
Isol. Gonadotrophin Deficiency	N	Small	Small	(6)
Multiple Pit. Hormone Deficiency inc. Gonadotrophins ±	Ret.	Small	Small	(7)
Isolated LH or FSH Deficiency	N	Small or N	Small or N	
Const. Delayed Puberty	N	N	N	
Primary Testicular Failure (Klinefelter Syndr.	N	N		(8)
Bloom Syndr.	Ret.	or Small	Small	(9)
Other)				
End-Organ Failure (Reifenstein Syndr.)	N	Small	N	(10)

N = Normal.

Table II. Laboratory aids used to test the hypothalamic-pituitary-testicular axis.

Plasma FSH and LH
Clomiphene Test (50 mg/d – 5 days)
LH-RH Test (50 $\mu g/m^2$ i.v.) Single or Repeated
Plasma Testosterone
HCG Test (5000 U i.m.) or 1500 u i.m. × 7/2 weeks

through in this field. Measurement of the basal gonadotrophin levels is of limited value (Dickerman *et al.*, 1976; Laron *et al.*, 1974) while the determination of the night peak of LH secretion (Kulin *et al.*, 1976) is a cumbersome procedure. Furthermore, the clomiphene test is not useful until late puberty (Kulin *et al.*, 1972) and the HCG test is of only limited value in the prepubertal age group (Josefsberg *et al.*, 1976). The one-bolus LH-RH test, however, has proven to be of utmost usefulness in discriminating between a normal and subnormal axis even in prepuberty (Dickerman *et al.*, 1976; Dickerman *et al.*, 1976).

The LH and FSH response to a standard dose of LH-RH in normal boys in prepuberty and the various stages of puberty has been determined (see Figs 1 and 2). This now makes it possible to establish the diagnosis of isolated gonadotrophin deficiency due to LH-RH deficiency of a selective pituitary failure (Table

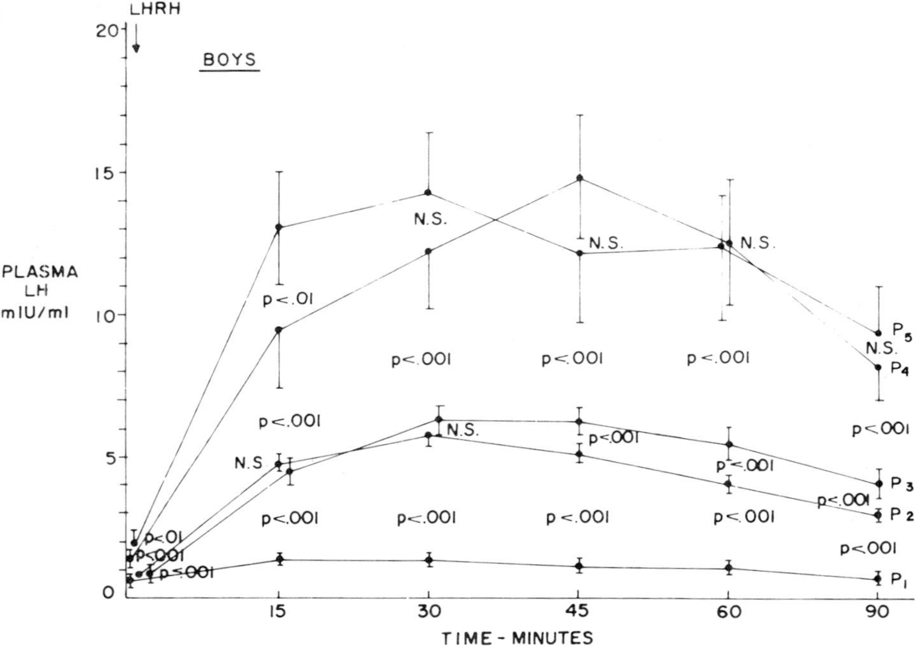

Fig.1 LH-RH test (50 $\mu g/m^2$) in different pubertal stages. Mean levels ± SD. N.S. = Not significant. Reproduced with permission of the *American Journal of Diseases of Children.*

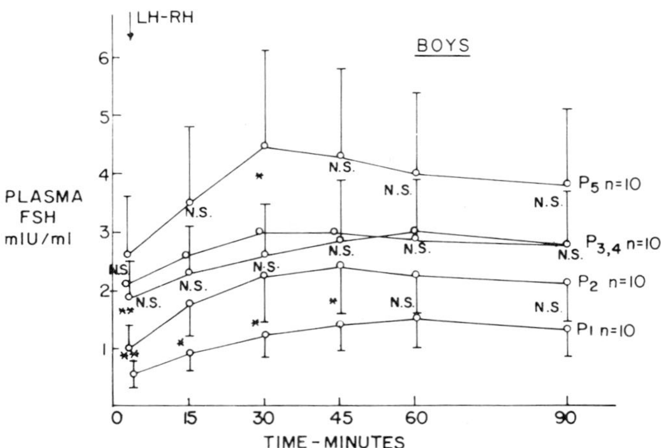

Fig.2 LH-RH test (50 $\mu g/m^2$ i.v.) in different pubertal stages (P_{1-5}). Mean ± SD. N.S. = Not significant. * P ⩽ 0.1–0.02. ** P ⩽ 0.01–0.001. (P = Significance between nearest means.) Reproduced with permission of the *American Journal of Diseases of Children.*

Table III. Isolated gonadotrophin deficiency due to LH-RH deficiency diagnosed before the age of puberty.

D.F. Kallman's Syndrome, Fam.

	C A (Yrs.)	B A (Yrs.)	Test. Vol. ml	Pubic Hair cm	Penis cm	Plasma LH mIU/ml *b* – *p*	Plasma FSH mIU/ml *b* – *p*	Testo. ng/dl
A)	8^{10}	7	0.5	0	3.3 × 0.7	0.25 – 0.4	1.2 – 2.7	20
B)	9^{6}	8	0.5	0	3.5 × 1.0	0.9 – 2.4	1.2 – 4.7	12
C)	10^{4}	8^{6}	0.5	0	4.0 × 1.0			7.4 – 95

A) LRH Test (50 μg/m²)
B) LRH Test (50 μg/m²) post 100 μg LRH/day for 5 days
C) HCG Test (1500 U × 7) on alternating days

CA = Chronological age; BA = Bone age; b = Basal; p = Peak.

Table IV. M.N. Incomplete hypogonadotrophic hypogonadism of pituitary origin LRH tests (50 μg/m²).

	C A (Yrs.)	B A (Yrs.)	Height –SD	Test. Vol. ml.	Pubic Hair cm	Penis cm	Plasma LH mIU/ml *b* – *p*	Plasma FSH mIU/ml *b* – *p*	Testo. ng/dl
A)	17^{6}	13	3	2 – 2	±	7 × 1.5	0.5 – 2.4	0.9 – 3.7	39
A)	18		3	2 – 2	±	,,	0.7 – 2.3	0.5 – 1.3	60
B)	18^{3}	14	3	2.5 – 2	±	,,	0.3 – 2.2	0.6 – 3.4	65
D)	18^{6}		3	3 – 3	±	,,	0.6 – 0.8	0.5 – 0.5	60

A) Post 100 μg LRH/day for 5 days
B) Post 100 μg LRH/day for 5 days
D) Post clomiphene citrate 50 mg/day for 2 months

CA = Chronological age; BA = Bone age.

Table V. Sequential LH-RH tests (50 μg/m² i.v.) in a pubertal male.

CA (Yrs.)	BA (Yrs.)	Height –SD	Test. Vol. ml	Pubic Hair	Penis cm	Ejac.	LH mIU/ml		FSH mIU/ml		Testo. ng/dl
							b	*p*	*b*	*p*	
11^{8}	10^{6}	2.5	2 – 2	0	5.5/1.2	–	0.3	3.1	0.6	1.1	10
13^{8}	13		3 – 3	1+	7./1.6	–	0.7	5.5	0.7	3.0	29
14^{3}	13^{6}		5 – 5	2+	9./2	–	0.5	6.8	1.0	2.8	35
15^{6}	14		8 – 8	2+	10./2.3	?	1.3	15.4	1.2	3.5	134
16^{3}	15^{6}	0.7	15 – 15	3+	11./3	+	3.4	13.2	2.0	4.8	325

CA = Chronological age; BA = Bone age.

Table VI. Patient O.Z. A 14-year-old male with constitutional delayed puberty (no pubertal signs). Effect of methandrostenolone (1.5 mg/d for 3 months) on the plasma LH and FSH response to LH-RH (50 μg/m²) and on hGH response to arginine (0.5 g/kg).

LH-RH Arginine Test, Time (min)	0′		30′		60′		90′	
	b	*a*	*b*	*a*	*b*	*a*	*b*	*a*
LH (mIU/ml)	0.4 –	0.7*	3.8 –	1.8*				
FSH (mIU/ml)	0.8 –	0.5*					1.6 –	0.5*
hGH (ng/ml)	1.3 –	2.9*	3.7 –	13*	3.9 –	17.6*	8.1 –	11.2*
hGH Sum 30′ + 60′ + 90′			15.7 –	41.8				

* Test on last day of methandrostenolone treatment. b = Before R_X; a = After R_X.

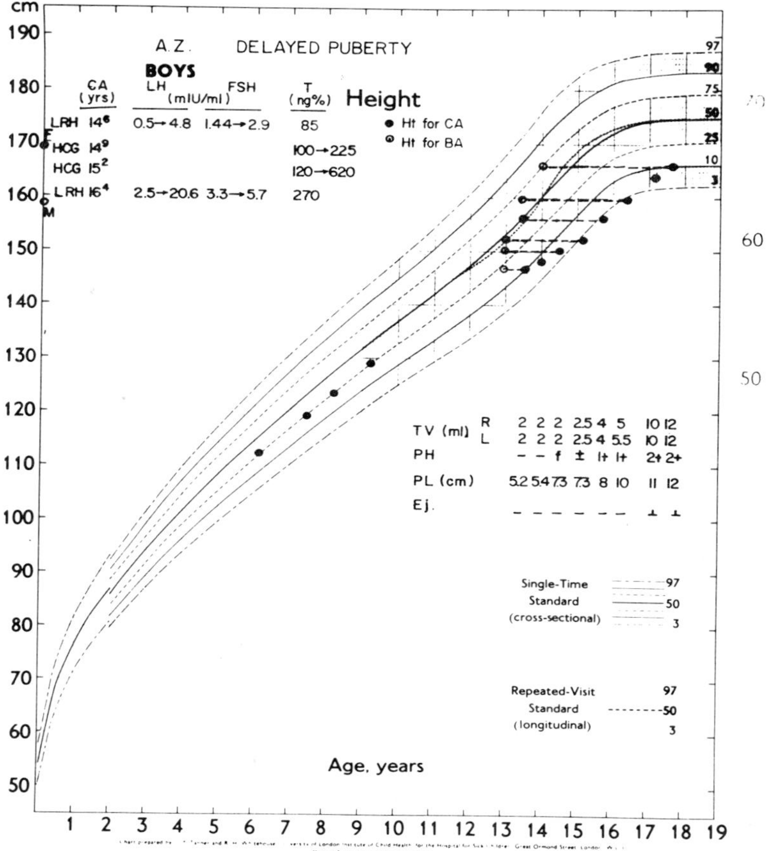

Fig.3 Linear growth, sexual development and sex hormone responses to LH-RH and HCG in a boy with constitutional delayed puberty.

III). The diagnosis is confirmed by a lack of gonadotrophin response upon repeated LH-RH stimulation (Table IV). In contrast, in cases of early primary testicular failure the gonadotrophin response to LH-RH may already be increased in prepuberty (Kauli *et al., in press*).

In normal prepubertal children there is usually a slight increase in both LH and FSH (sometimes only of LH) in response to the LH-RH test (Figs 1 and 2). Table V shows the findings at later ages in a typical subject. What happens in cases of "constitutional delayed puberty"? Figure 3 illustrates the linear growth, bone age, sexual development and sex hormone responses to LH-RH and HCG in an untreated boy. Despite a growth spurt and a testicular volume in the normal range for age, at age 17 8/12 years he is not fully virilized and his bone age corresponds to 14 years. Note that at age 14, when he showed a decrease in growth rate, there was an increasing lag in bone and sexual maturation. In treating such a boy, manifold factors must be taken into consideration, and each individual case must be carefully weighed. We find that the psychological factors (to be discussed in an

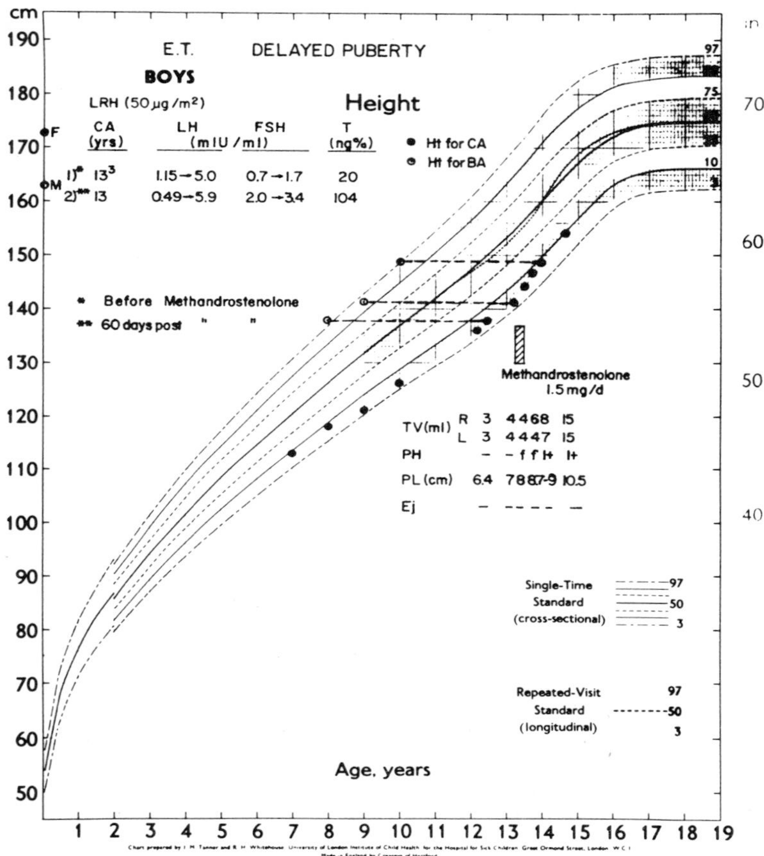

Fig.4 Linear growth, sexual development and sex hormone responses to LH-RH in a boy with constitutional delayed puberty before and after a 3 month course of methandrostenolone.

adjacent chapter) are usually the decisive ones.

There are two types of therapy employed in our Institute:

A) Initiation of puberty – to be performed only when there are no signs of puberty or only early ones.

B) Acceleration of puberty – when puberty is very slow and prolonged. Both types of treatment are usually administered for short periods, from 3 to 6 months at the most.

INITIATION OF PUBERTY

For this type of therapy we use methandrostenolone (Dianabol^{Rx} - CIBA), an anabolic steroid with low androgenic activity (Laron, 1962; Laron, 1966). Figure 4 illustrates the results of this type of intervention. It is evident that despite the short course of 1.5 mg/day for 3 months, patient E.T. had showed an immediate growth spurt. At the end of such a course in another patient (Table

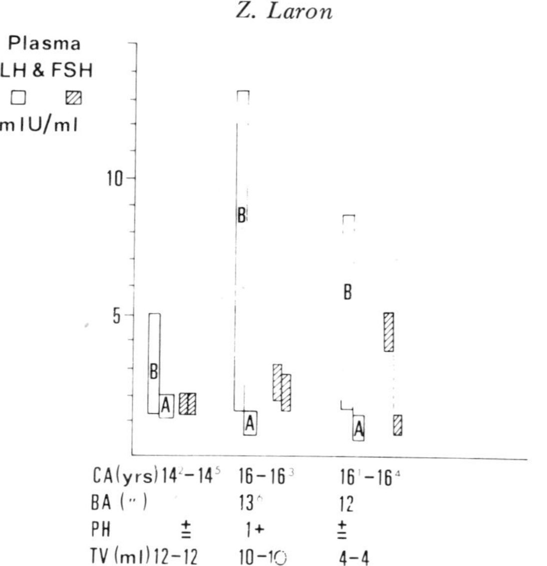

Fig.5 Suppression of gonadotrophin response to LH-RH (50 μg/m²) during treatment (1.5 mg/d — 3 months) with methandrostenolone in boys with delayed puberty.

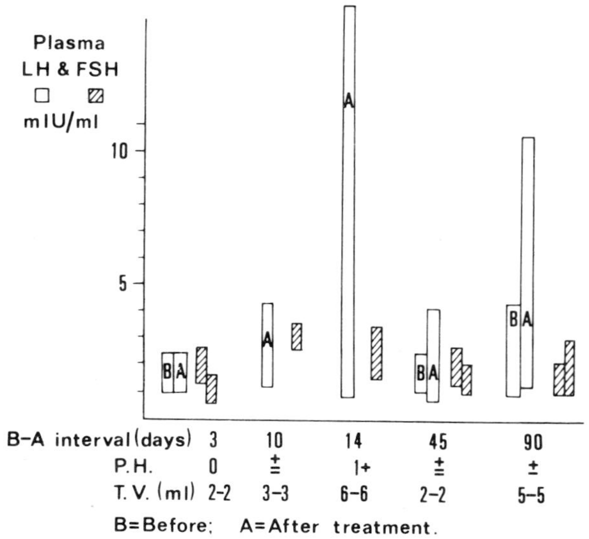

Fig.6 Recovery of gonadotrophin response to LH-RH (50 μg/m²) after methandrostenolone treatment (1.5 mg/d — 3 months), in boys with delayed puberty.

VI) we find a suppression of the LH and FSH response to LH-RH, but a rise in plasma hGH response, as we have described previously (Laron *et al.*, 1972).

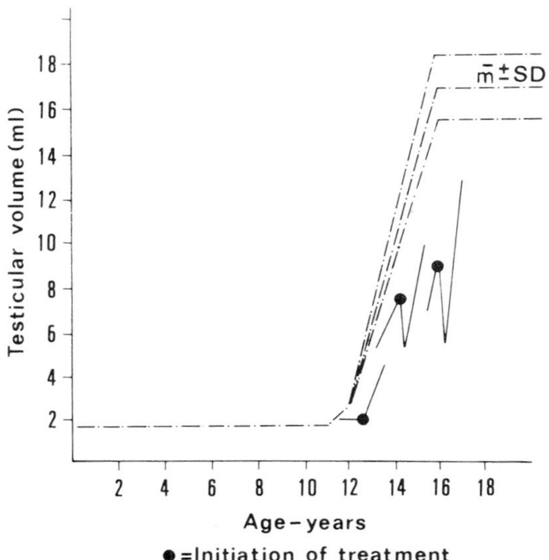

Fig. 7 Effect of methandrostenolone (1.5 mg/d — 3 months) on testicular volume in boys with delayed puberty. (Norms from Zilka and Laron, 1969).

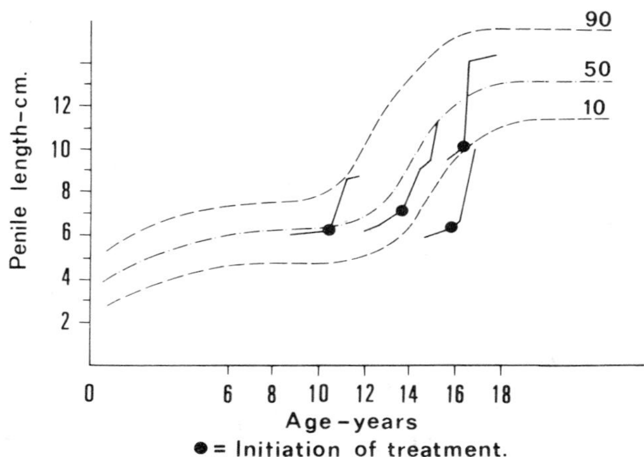

Fig. 8 Effect of methandrostenolone (1.5 mg/d — 3 months) on penile length in boys with short stature and delayed puberty.

What is the mechanism by which methandrostenolone acts on puberty? Initially, it suppresses the gonadotrophins (Fig.5), perhaps through the effect of its androgenic properties upon the pituitary LH. Later, as it is converted in the body to estrogens (Laron, 1962), it is possible that there is also a suppression of FSH and not just a central LH-RH suppression. Discontinuation of the methandrostenolone leads to a rebound phenomenon, i.e. an increase in the response of LH and to a lesser degree of FSH, as would be expected in boys (Fig.6).

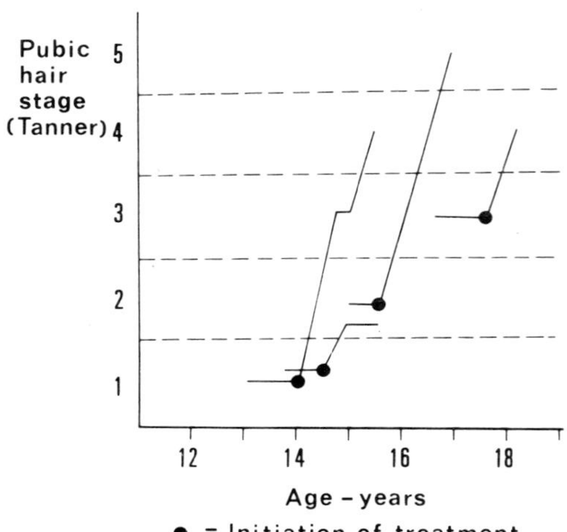

Fig.9 Effect of methandrostenolone (1.5 mg/d — 3 months) on pubic hair development in boys with delayed puberty.

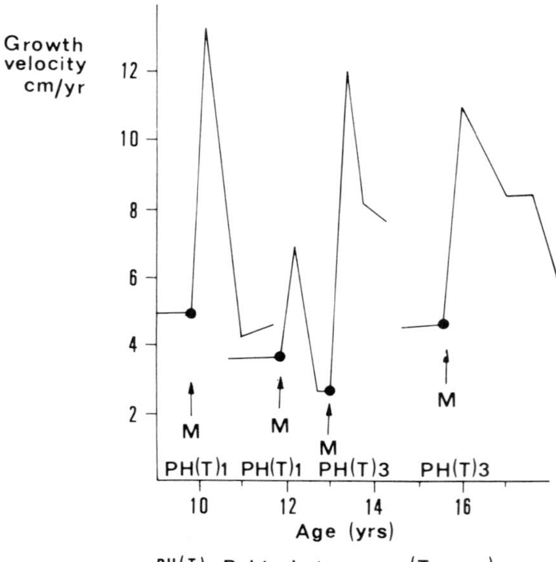

Fig.10 Effect of methandrostenolone (M) (1.5 mg/d — 3 months) on growth velocity in boys with short stature.

Clinically, a 3-months course of methandrostenolone has the following effects: after an initial decrease in size induced by the gonadotrophin suppression, the testes show a growth spurt (Fig.7), the penis rapidly enlarges (Fig.8) and the abundance of pubic hair increases (Fig.9). Growth velocity (Fig.10) rises steeply

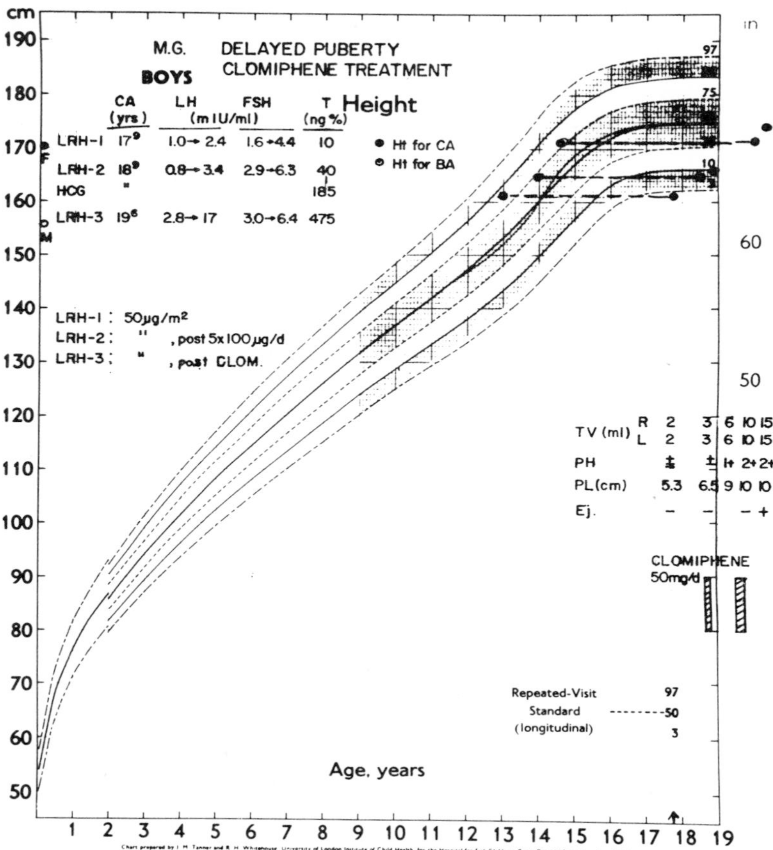

Fig.11 Linear growth, sexual development and sex hormone response to LH-RH in a boy with constitutional delayed puberty before and after clomiphene therapy (50 mg/d).

and then falls, in younger children to pretreatment values and in older ones to intermediate values.

In conclusion, with this type of therapy, for which other androgens could certainly be used, the induction of puberty is probably caused by a rebound rise of the gonadotrophins following their suppression (Table VII). It is possible that a threshold-sensitivity may also play a role in the results attained. The boost in growth which is partly induced by an increase in hGH secretion is psychologically very beneficial to these boys, especially to those in whom there is pronounced shortness in stature.

ACCELERATION OF PUBERTY

Some boys mature very slowly, as exemplified by M.G. (Fig.11), who at age 17 9/12 years was short (161 cm) and had a bone age of 13 years, with the only

Table VII. **Hypothesis of methandrostenolone effect on the induction of puberty in delayed puberty.**

	Before	During	After	
	Methandrostenolone Administration			
hGH	Low	High	Normal	
GnRH	Low	Lower	High)	Rebound Phenomenon
LH	Low	Lower	High)	
FSH	Low	Lower	High)	

sexual sign being the presence of pubic fuzz. An LH-RH test showed that there is no lack of gonadotrophins, which increase upon repeated stimulation. Two courses of clomiphene therapy (50 mg/day) given for 2 and 3 months respectively, accelerated sexual development.

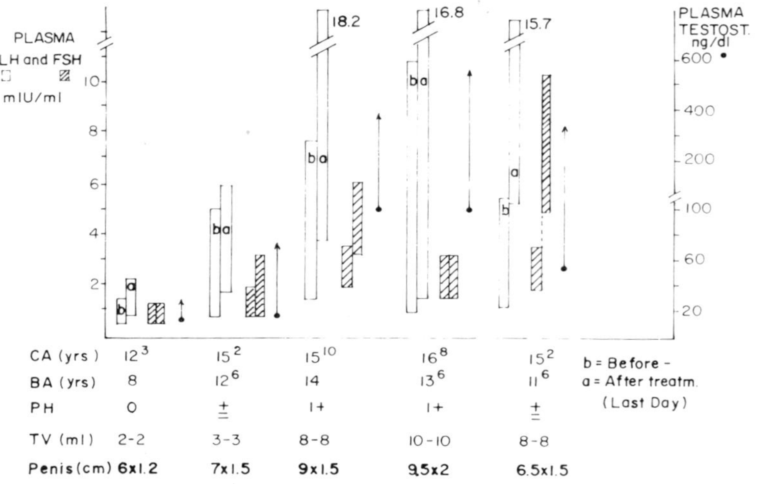

Fig.12 **Effect of clomiphene citrate (50 mg/d — 2 months) on plasma testosterone level and the gonadotrophin response to LH-RH (50 μg/m²) in boys with delayed puberty.**

How does clomiphene act? Measuring LH and FSH response to LH-RH before and after 2 months of administration (Fig.12), we found that clomiphene increased the responses of both LH and FSH. In young and immature boys, as in a patient aged 12 3/12 years with no sexual characteristics, there was no response. There was also no response in patients with hypogonadotrophic hypogonadism — thus this may constitute an additional tool for differential diagnosis. Table VIII lists the various mechanisms presumed to play a role in accelerating puberty when clomiphene is administered.

In conclusion it is of utmost importance that delayed puberty be diagnosed at an early age, so as to determine which patients may respond to appropriate therapy. In this we are aided by the LH-RH test, which now allows us to make the differential diagnosis between primary, secondary and tertiary gonadal failure.

Table VIII. Hypothesis of clomiphene effect on the acceleration of puberty.

Increases GnRH Release by Acting as a Positive Estrogen Feed Back
Directly Increases LH and FSH Output
Raises the TeBG and the True Testosterone Level
Exerts a Weak Estrogen Effect

GnRH = LH + RH + (FSH–RH?)
TeBG = Testosterone Binding Globulin

ACKNOWLEDGEMENT

The authors are indebted to Dr. J. Mulder of Ferring AG, Malmö, Sweden for the generous supply of LH-RH and to Mrs. Ruth Fradkin for her assistance in the preparation of the manuscript.

REFERENCES

Dickerman, Z., Prager-Lewin, R. and Laron, Z. (1976). *Am. J. Dis. Child.* **130**, 634.
Dickerman, Z., Prager-Lewin, R. and Laron, Z. (1976). *Fertil. Steril.* **27**, 162.
Dickerman, Z., Landmann, J., Prager-Lewin, R. and Laron, Z. *Isr. J. med. Sci. (in press).*
Flatau, E., Josefsberg, Z., Prager-Lewin, R., Markman-Halabe, E., Kaufman, H. and Laron, Z. (1975). *Helv. Paediat. Acta* **30**, 377.
Jones, M.C. and Bayley, N. (1950). *J. Educ. Psychol.* **41**, 129-148.
Josefsberg, Z., Markman-Halabe, E., Magazanik, A., Kaufman, H. and Laron, Z. (1976). *Isr. J. med. Sci.* **12**, 139.
Kauli, R., Prager-Lewin, R., Kaufman, H. and Laron, Z. *Clin. Endocrinol. (in press).*
Kulin, H.E. and Reiter, E.O. (1974). *In* "The Control of the Onset of Puberty" (M.M. Grumbach, G.D. Grave and F.E. Meyer, eds) pp.238-257. John Wiley & Sons, New York, London.
Kulin, H.E., Grumbach, M.M. and Kaplan, S.L. (1972). *Pediat. Res.* **6**, 162.
Kulin, H.E., Moore, R.G., Jr. and Santner, S.J. (1976). *J. clin. Endocr. Metab.* **42**, 770.
Laron, Z. (1962). *In* "Protein Metabolism" (F. Gross, ed) p.398. Springer-Verlag, Berlin-Göttingen-Heidelberg.
Laron, Z. (1962). *J. clin. Endocr. Metab.* **22**, 450.
Laron, Z. (1963). *Acta Paediat.* **52**, 133.
Laron, Z. (1966). *In* "Somatic Growth of the Child" (J.J. Van der Werff ten Bosch and A. Haak, eds) p.281. H.E. Stenfert Kroese N.V., Leiden.
Laron, Z. and Hochman, I.H. (1971). *J. clin. Endocr. Metab.* **32**, 671.
Laron, Z. and Kaushanski, A. (1975). *Pediat. Res.* **9**, 671.
Laron, Z. and Sarel, R. (1970). *Acta endocr. (Copenh.)* **63**, 625.
Laron, Z., Hochman, H. and Keret, R. (1972). *Clin. Endocrinol.* **1**, 91.
Laron, Z., Elion, D., Hochman, H., Scharf, A. and Franchimont, P. (1974). *Harefauah* **87**, 11.
Marshall, W.A. and Turner, J.M. (1970). *Arch. Dis. Childh.* **45**, 13.
Midgley, A.R. (1966). *Endocrinology* **79**, 10.
Midgley, A.R. (1967). *J. clin. Endor. Metab.* **27**, 295.
Root, A.W. (1973). *J. Pediat.* **83**, 187.
Schally, A.V., Arimura, A., Kostin, A.J., Matsuo, H., Baba, Y., Redding, T.W., Nair, R.M. and Debeljuk, L. *Science* **173**, 1036.
Weinstein, A., Lindner, J.R., Friedlander, A. and Bauminger, S. (1972). *Steroids* **20**, 789.
Zilka, E. and Laron, Z. (1969). *Harefuah* **77**, 511.

PSYCHOLOGICAL ASPECTS OF DELAYED PUBERTY IN BOYS

A. Galatzer, V. Kaufman and Z. Laron

Institute of Pediatric and Adolescent Endocrinology, Beilinson Medical Center Petah Tikva and Sackler School of Medicine, Tel Aviv University, Israel

The psychological problems present in boys with delayed puberty may be of "primary" origin, due to a concomitant central nervous and hypothalamic disturbance, or of "secondary" origin, due to the retardation in sexual development and/or short stature.

A study was therefore carried out to determine the effect of treatment with methandrostenolone (Dianabol^{Rx} - CIBA), administered at a dose of 0.03–0.05 mg/kg/day for a period of 3 months, upon 15 boys selected at random from among a large group of children with constitutional delayed puberty who are under the observation of our Institute. These boys ranged in age from 12 8/12 to 21 years. For control purposes, they were individually matched according to age, socio-economic class and intelligence with a group of normal children (it is of note that the latter were sexually more advanced than the 15 patients). The 15 patients underwent a psychological evaluation before the institution of treatment and 3 months after its discontinuation (6 months after the initial interview). Before therapy was started the subjects were interviewed regarding their feelings towards their body image and their social relationships, and were also given a battery of psychological tests, including the Tennessee Self Concept Scale (Fitts, 1965), Body Focus Questionnaire (Fisher, 1964) and Draw a Person Test (Fisher, 1959).

RESULTS

The results of the Self-Concept and Self-Acceptance tests were found to be better in the controls than in the experimental group of boys with delayed puberty when the latter were tested before institution of treatment. The boys with delayed puberty had a lower self-concept together with a large amount of conflict between several areas of self-description, especially in the physical and social areas.

There were evident feelings of inferiority in the boys with delayed puberty. Their level of psychological harmony was lower than in the controls, there was less self-actualization and a larger amount of conflicts and defence mechanisms related to their physical and social self-perception. They demonstrated an overall psychological discomfort and a lack of general integration of their personality.

In daily life, these feelings caused them to lead a life apart from their age mates. They were often not accepted by their age peers and many reported being ashamed to join friends in sports or outings at which they would have had to expose themselves to the other boys. The relationship with the opposite sex was very poor – none of the older boys had a steady girl friend and the interest of these children in sex seemed to be considerably lower than that of the control group.

At the time of the second psychological evaluation, 6 months after the initial evaluation and 3 months after discontinuation of methandrostenolone, a moderate improvement in growth rate and sexual development was apparent in all the patients. Thirteen of the boys sensed the change in growth and 11 reported increased virilization. Psychologically the principal change for the better was seen in an improved harmony and emotional stability. The physical self-concept was still lower than that of the control group. These findings indicate that a further normalization in sexual development and/or growth may be needed before the boys with delayed puberty manifest marked psychological improvement. It is also possible that the process of adjustment to the physical changes of the body requires additional time.

DISCUSSION

The results of the tests performed in the pre-treatment phase of this study corroborates those obtained by others in studies of delayed puberty. The feelings of inferiority and rejection and the low self-image have also been reported by Bayley (1965), Mussen and Jones (1957) and Jones and Bayley (1950). There is every likelihood that these feelings, born and nurtured during adolescence, may be carried through adulthood, thus affecting his mental health (Money and Alexander, 1967). If hormonal treatment, even though of short duration, is sufficient to induce a change in the emotional status of the boy with delayed puberty, then its importance becomes self-evident.

Our findings and those reported in the literature, stress the importance of psychological evaluation and counselling of boys with delayed puberty, as well as of well-timed treatment when indicated. Psychological counselling, with or without medication, can be of help to these boys during this difficult period of life and may also assist them to reach adulthood in a well-adjusted emotional state.

ACKNOWLEDGEMENT

The authors are indebted to Mrs. Ruth Fradkin for her assistance in the preparation of the manuscript.

REFERENCES

Bayley, N. (1965). *Merrill-Palmer Quarterly*, **II, 183**, 2-8.
Fisher, S. (1959). *J. Consult. Psychol.* **23**, 54-59.
Fisher, S. (1964). *Psychological Monographs* **78**, 1-22.
Fitts, W.H. (1965). "Tennessee Self Concept Scale Manual". Department of Mental Health, Nashville, Tenn.
Jones, M.C. and Bayley, N. (1950). *J. Educ. Psychol.* **41**, 8-15.
Money, J. and Alexander, D. (1967). *J. Sex Res.* **3**, 31-47.
Mussen, P.H. and Jones, M.C. (1957). *Child Develop.* **28**, 243-256.

PLASMA STEROID LEVELS IN PREPUBERTAL AND PUBERTAL GIRLS AND IN CASES OF DELAYED PUBERTY

C. Pintor, A.R. Genazzani, F. Facchinetti, S. Romagnino, R. Corda and P. Fioretti

First Department of Pediatrics, Obstetrics, University of Cagliari
Department of Obstetrics, University of Siena, Italy

INTRODUCTION

One of the major topics in endocrinology which has been developed in the last few years is the study of reproductive function and, in particular, the analysis of the relationships between the different hormones involved in the hypothalamus-pituitary-gonadal axis in humans.

In this field, one of the major areas which has to be clarified from many aspects, is the physiology of the onset of reproductive function, i.e. puberty. Recent studies have clearly indicated the important role of adrenal androgens in the beginning and maintenance of sexual maturation in both sexes. However, the real importance of this adrenal activation which has been named adrenarche (Albright, 1947) in the development of the secondary sexual characteristics and in the establishment of new feed-back levels in the hypothalamus between sexual steroids and gonadotropins, has not been completely clarified.

In prepubertal girls, Sizonenko (1974), Hopper and Yen (1975), Sizonenko and Paunier (1975) and Ducharme *et al.* (1976) found that dehydroepiandrosterone (DHA) plasma levels increased slightly from 6-8 years of age, until the first stage of puberty (Tanner, 1962). The same authors, and also Korth-Schutz *et al.* (1976) report further, progressive rises, reaching the highest concentrations at the fourth-fifth stage of puberty (P_{4-5}).

As far as dehydroepiandrosterone-sulphate (DHA-S) is concerned, no data are reported in literature regarding subjects less than 8 years of age. Hopper and Yen (1975) report values around 0.5 μg/ml in girls; these values do not vary between 8 and 12 years. The authors report a subsequent rise in DHA-S, which continues up to the adult age group.

As far as other adrenal steroids are concerned, no data are available regarding plasma levels in the prepubertal or pubertal age groups, of pregnenolone (Δ_5-P) and its sulphate (Δ_5-P-S) or 17-hydroxy derivative (17OH-Δ_5-P).

Ducharme *et al.* (1976) have recently reported that cortisol does not vary in the plasma of prepubertal or pubertal subjects of either sex.

Of the other steroids of both adrenal and gonadal origin, after a progressive decrease after the first two months of life (Winter *et al.*, 1976) androstenedione (A) does not seem to show any particular variations in girls up to 8 years. Then the A values increase progressively in relation both to the chronological age (Ducharme *et al.*, 1976) and to the stage of puberty (Korth-Schutz *et al.*, 1976).

Testosterone (T) values have been reported to be significantly higher in peripheral than in cord blood at birth (Forest and Cathiard, 1975); these values decrease progressively in females during the first week of life (Forest *et al.*, 1974, 1975; Winter *et al.*, 1976) and remain unmodified during the prepubertal period (Gupta, 1974; Forest *et al.*, 1974; Gupta *et al.*, 1975; Sizonenko and Paunier, 1975; Ducharme *et al.*, 1976; Korth-Schutz *et al.*, 1976). At puberty, a significant and progressive rise has been demonstrated by Sizonenko and Paunier (1975), Ducharme *et al.* (1976) and Korth-Schutz *et al.* (1976) occurring between P_1 and P_3.

No data are available regarding dihydrotestosterone (DHT) plasma levels in prepubertal life; at P_1 stage, plasma levels have been reported to be close to 50 pg/ml, by Gupta *et al.* (1975) and Korth-Schutz *et al.* (1976), and slightly lower levels have been reported by Ducharme *et al.* (1976). A progressive rise has been described by the same authors, until adult age.

As far as estrogens are concerned, estrone (E_1) levels in prepubertal girls from 6 to 8 years are constant around 30 pg/ml (Ducharme *et al.*, 1976). A progressive increase to the adult values has been described by Angsusingha *et al.* (1974), Gupta *et al.* (1975) and Ducharme *et al.* (1976), with some disagreement, however, in the absolute concentrations. A similar pattern, with constant plasma levels in the prepubertal phase and a progressive increase during sexual maturation, has been described in the case of estradiol (E_2) by Jenner *et al.* (1972), Angsusingha *et al.* (1974), Gupta *et al.* (1975) and Ducharme *et al.* (1976); Kantero *et al.* (1975) have described the same situation regarding total urinary estrogen excretion.

No data are available on progesterone (P) and 17 hydroxyprogesterone (17-P) plasma levels in prepubertal and pubertal girls. In a limited study of the first two years of life, Winter *et al.* (1976) indicate the existence of a progressive decrease in plasma 17-P; this decrease was significantly more marked in females than in males, where the 17-P plasma levels showed a behaviour pattern similar to that of T.

Before concluding this short analysis of the literature on the steroid levels in prepubertal and pubertal girls, some mention should be made of the proteic hormones involved in pubertal maturation: adrenocorticotrophic hormone (ACTH), follicle-stimulating hormone (FSH), luteinizing hormone (LH) and prolactin (Prl).

No data are available on the ACTH plasma levels, although important modifications have been found during the menstrual cycle (Genazzani *et al.*, 1975), in relation to the adrenal androgen variations throughout the cycle (Genazzani,

1975). In prepubertal girls, constantly low levels of both FSH and LH have been described by Sizonenko *et al.* (1970) and Sizonenko and Paunier (1975).

During sexual maturation, a progressive rise in FSH, first described by Sizonenko *et al.* (1970), has been confirmed by Jenner *et al.* (1972), Angsusingha *et al.* (1974) and Sizonenko and Paunier (1975). On the other hand, the LH values always remain around the P_1 values (Sizonenko *et al.*, 1970; Jenner *et al.*, 1972; Sizonenko, 1974; Angsusingha *et al.*, 1974; Kantero *et al.*, 1975; Sizonenko and Paunier, 1975).

It is of interest to note, moreover, that significant rises in LH and FSH plasma levels have been described in pubertal males and females during slęep (Boyar *et al.*, 1972, 1973). This phenomenon is particularly evident in mid-puberty, decreasing in late puberty and is absent in adult life (Boyar *et al.*, 1973; Kapen *et al.*, 1974). Furthermore, in males the LH variations during sleep were correlated to simultaneous variations in plasma testosterone (Parker *et al.*, 1975).

The last proteic hormone to be involved in puberty, at least in rodents, is prolactin (Dohler and Wuttke, 1974). No changes have been found in prepubertal girls, in plasma prolactin levels (Ehara *et al.*, 1975; Aubert *et al.*, 1976), but rises are found at the end of puberty (Ehara *et al.*, 1975; Aubert *et al.*, 1976), related to the simultaneous increases in plasma E_2 levels (Del Pozo *et al.*, 1976; Robyn *et al.*, 1976).

The present research has been carried out with the aim of studying the behaviour pattern of some plasma steroids and to clarify the role of the adrenal gland, during the prepubertal period, i.e. from the first to the ninth year of age, and in the first stage of puberty according to Tanner (1962).

A group of patients with delayed onset of puberty was also investigated in detail, and compared with a small group of pubertal girls, and also with our previous results (Genazzani *et al.*, 1976) obtained in adult women during different phases of the menstrual cycle, in order to facilitate a clearer evaluation of the mechanism involved in this pathological condition of sexual maturation.

A. *Patients*

1. *Prepubertal girls*

This group included 32 girls from 1 to 9 years of age, who had been admitted to the Department of Pediatrics, University of Cagliari, because of minor, non-endocrinological complaints.

2. *Pubertal girls*

This group included 11 girls between 10 and 13 years of age, at different stages of sexual maturation according to Tanner (1962); subdivided, there were 5 cases at stage P_1, 2 cases at stage P_2, 3 cases at P_3 and 1 at stage $P_{4\text{-}5}$. These girls, who had been admitted to the Department of Pediatrics with complaints other than gonadal or adrenal disturbances, were found to be endocrinologically normal.

3. *Delayed puberty*

This group included 10 patients admitted to the Department of Obstetrics and Gynecology, University of Cagliari, with primary or secondary amenorrhea; clinical, biochemical and endocrinological examinations confirmed the diagnosis of delayed puberty.

As reported in Table I, each case was examined according to Tanner's criteria (1962): development of the breasts, genitalia and pubic hair was scored. On the basis of these evaluations, the various cases ranged from stages P_2 to P_4, while the chronological ages ranged from 16 to 25 years. Four cases (D.F.M., M.O., P.M.C.

Table I. **Delayed puberty: clinical data, basal plasma levels of LH, FSH, Prl, GH, TSH, Tiroxine and Cortisol and maximal gonadotropic response to LH-RH stimulation.**

N.		Name	Age	Pub. Stage B.	P.H.	G.	Amenorrhea	FSH (mU/ml) Basal	LH-RH*	LH (mU/ml) Basal	LH-RH*	Prl ng/ml	GH ng/ml	TSH μU/ml	T_4 ng/ml	Cortisol ng/ml
1.		R.L.	17	2	2	2	Primary	3.6	7.1	1.8	6.7	9	1.2	1.8	68	110
2.		A.C.	18	2	2	2	Secondary	2.9	9.2	2.8	29	10	1.4	1.4	57	70
3		B.M.	20	2	3	2	Primary	4.1	12.6	3.1	67	6.7	1.6	1.5	57	150
4		P.L.	19	2	3	2	Primary	1.0	4.6	2.8	3.4	2.1	1.3	0.7	56	110
5		S.A.	25	3	3	2	Primary	11.0	23.5	5.0	25	6.0	1.7	1.2	63	120
6	a	D.F.M.	20	3	3	2	Secondary	8.8	21.4	11.5	36	6.6	2.0	2.1	70	85
	b	"	21	4	4	2	"	3.6	18.2	8.7	42	2.0	1.8	1.6	76	105
7	a	M.O.	16	2	3	3	Primary	6.3	10	3.2	7	12.5	1.6	2.4	75	120
	b	"	17	3	3	3	"	7.2	10.5	5.5	12.5	14.5	1.2	2.2	82	135
	c	"	18	3	4	3	"	8.2	11.8	5	17	13.6	1.4	2.1	70	115
8	a	P.M.C.	18	2	3	3	Secondary	10.8	33	9.4	14	7.6	2.3	1.8	71	90
	b	"	19	3	3	3	"	6.7	18	12	55	6.5	2.0	1.7	66	85
9	a	M.A.	17	3	3	3	"	4.8	35	2.9	30	3.2	3.5	1.0	48	80
	b	"	18	4	4	3	"	5.1	24	6.0	42	4.0	1.7	1.2	54	120
	c	"	18½	4	4	3	"	6.5	27	6.5	51	6.1	2.4	1.3	61	95
10		F.G.	21	4	4	4	Primary	7.7	19	2.6	20	4.1	2.1	3.8	62	130

* Highest plasma levels after 50 μg of LH-RH e.v.

and M.A.) were followed up to 1-2 years to check the progress of sexual maturation. Six subjects were cases of primary amenorrhea; the remaining 4 patients had a history of a single episode of spontaneous vaginal bleeding, referred to as menarche, but never followed by further episodes. The basal levels of the following pituitary hormones were controlled in each patient: LH, FSH, Prl, Growth Hormone (GH) and Thyro-stimulating hormone (TSH), and the pituitary response to 50 μg of i.v. Luteinizing Hormone-Releasing Hormone (LH-RH) (Relisorm L, Serono, Rome, Italy) was also studied. The basal plasma levels of Thyroxine (T_4) and Cortisol were also measured. The single values reported in Table I, indicate that amenorrhea and delayed puberty were not linked with a primary pathological condition of the pituitary's non-gonadotropic activities, or of a primary disease of the thyroid or adrenal glands. The FSH basal values were lower than expected (Genazzani *et al.*, 1976) for the chronological age in cases 1-2-3-4; the FSH response to LH-RH stimulation was also diminished in these cases, and in case 7. The LH plasma resting levels were also lower than normal (Genazzani *et al.*, 1976) in cases 1-2-3-4, and in the first samples taken from cases 7 and 9; a reduced LH response to LH-RH was found in cases 1 and 4, and at the first examination in cases 7 and 8. It is interesting to point out the progressively improving response to LH-RH seen in the cases followed up for one or more years.

4. Samples

Blood samples for steroid analysis were taken, in all cases, after informed consent of the parents, or of the patients themselves if already adult. Blood samples were taken from the cubital vein at 8-9 a.m. after overnight fasting and bed rest. The heparinized blood was immediately centrifuged at 4°C and the plasma frozen in different vials and stored at −20°C until the time of assay. No sample was defrozen more than once.

B. Materials and Methods

1. Solvents, standard steroid hormones, tritiated steroids

All solvents were of analytical grade, and were purchased either from Carlo Erba S.p.A. (Milan, Italy) or from Merck AG (Darmstadt, Germany). Chromatographically pure standard steroid hormones were obtained from Vister (Italy), with the exception of Pregnenolone, which came from Ikapharm (Sweden).

Tritiated molecules were obtained from NEN (England).

2. *Column chromatography*

After 1:10 ether extraction of the plasma samples, two kinds of celite-ethylene glycol chromatographic columns were set up, according to Abraham (1973), modified by Magrini *et al.* (1973) and subsequently by Facchinetti *et al.* (1976). The first kind of column was used to separate P, A, T and E_2, whilst the second served to separate Δ_5-P, DHT, DHA and 17-P.

A 25% aliquot of each chromatographic fraction was used to evaluate the recovery of tritiated hormones (3,000 cpm) added to the plasma prior to extraction. The recovery (in %) of each tritiated hormone is reported in Table II.

Table II.

Steroid		Antiserum	Recovery (%) M ± Sem	Water Blank (pg)	Std. Curve Range (pg)
Progesterone	(P)	Biodata	68.4 ± 1.8	6	16 – 500
Androstenedione	(A)	Endocr. Sci.	51.5 ± 1.9	5.5	9 – 300
Testosterone	(T)	C.I.S.	58.6 ± 2.2	6.5	12.5 – 400
Estradiol	(E_2)	Biodata	71.9 ± 2.3	7	12.5 – 400
Dihydrotestosterone	(DHT)	Endocr. Sci.	63.0 ± 1.7	8.5	12.5 – 400
Pregnenolone	(Δ_5P)	Dr. Abraham	72.4 ± 1.7	7	16 – 500
Dehydroepiandrost.	(DHA)	Biodata	38.7 ± 2.7	14	31 – 1000
07OHProgesterone	(17P)	Biodata	56.2 ± 1.7	13.5	16 – 500
Cortisol		C.I.S.	94.2 ± 0.4	–	250 – 8000
Dehydroepiandrost. Sulphate	(DHA-S)	Dr. Serio	100	–	100 – 1600

3. *Radioimmunoassays*

The following proteic hormones were measured directly in the plasma: FSH and LH, with C.I.S. kits (Saluggia, Italy); TSH, Prl and Thyroxine by Biodata Kits (Milan, Italy). DHA-S was measured directly in the plasma, according to Cattaneo *et al.* (1975). Cortisol was measured by a solid-phase method using C.I.S. kits (Saluggia, Italy), after washing the plasma in petroleum ether (1:10) and extraction with methylene chloride, as proposed by Melis *et al.* (1976). The RIA's of the chromatographic fractions were made using the antisera reported in Table II. The assays were characterized by an overnight incubation, and a dextran-coated charcoal separation.

4. *Statistical analysis*

The statistical analysis of the results was made according to Student's "t" test, using a Hewlett-Packard 9810 desk computer.

RESULTS

A. *Prepubertal Girls*

The results have been divided into different groups according to the chronological age (1 to 4 years, 5-6 years and 7-9 years), and are shown in Tables III–V and in Figs 1–5.

1. *Gonadotropins and prolactin*

LH plasma levels were found to be similar in all three groups of prepubertal girls (Tables III, IV and V); no significant difference was found (Fig.1). On the

Table III. Prepubertal girls of 1–4 years: LH, FSH, Prl and steroids plasma levels.

Name	Chron. Age	LH mU/ml	FSH mU/ml	Prl ng/ml	Cortisol ng/ml	DHA-S ng/ml	DHA pg/ml	Δ_5-P pg/ml	P pg/ml	17-P pg/ml	A pg/ml	T pg/ml	DHT pg/ml	E_2 pg/ml
F.S.	17 m	2.9	1.6	2.3		15.5	384	151	73	351	307	55	26.7	17
P.E.	17 m		2.4	4.4	110	11	135	277	32	367	312	51	29	18
D.L.	2 yrs	3.5	3.5	4.6	140	27	375	152	54	135	120		13	63
A.R.	2 yrs	2.0	1.1			17				365	181		18.8	19
M.G.	2½ yrs	4.5	1.75		140	28.5	395	135	142			47	24	19
F.M.	3 yrs	3.2	1.0		170		245	346	65	195	101	139	12.8	68
D.B.	3 yrs	3.0	1.75	6.7		28.5	435	131		271		90	27	
O.M.	4 yrs		1.0	8.7	160	15	409	314	57	341			17	48
P.S.	4 yrs	3.2	1.75			25	640		35		155	53	23.2	21
S.S.	4 yrs	4.2	2.1	13.8	80	60	477	207		414	272		21	27.5
Mean		3.31	1.79	6.75	133	25.2	388.3	214.1	65.4	304.8	206.8	72.5	21.2	33.4
± Sem		0.27	0.23	1.8	15	5.1	49.8	32.7	15.0	36.4	36.3	16.1	1.9	7.3
N		8	10	6	6	9	9	8	7	8	7	6	10	9

Table IV. Prepubertal girls of 5–6 years: LH, FSH, Prl and steroid plasma levels.

Name	Chron. Age	LH mU/ml	FSH mU/ml	Prl ng/ml	Cortisol ng/ml	DHA-S ng/ml	DHA pg/ml	Δ_5-P pg/ml	P pg/ml	17-P pg/ml	A pg/ml	T pg/ml	DHT pg/ml	E_2 pg/ml
A.M.	5 yrs	2.6	2.5			17	392	721		299	308			
S.F.	5 yrs			10.6		35	272	709		490	347			52
M.G.	5 yrs	5.7	3.5	8.7		42.5	342	480	155	274		126	17	68
B.S.	5 yrs	5.2	2	5		37.5	293	582	194	304	212	146	28	
S.M.T.	5 yrs	2.2	2	10.8	60	180	858		162	102	114	83	26	58
D.K.	5 yrs	3.2	2.4	5	105	180	904		163	360	239	56	56	63
P.O.	5 yrs				80	130			215	154	205	84		
C.G.	6 yrs			3.8			684	830	41	380	397	101		84
L.M.A.	6 yrs	3.2	2.4		140		780	753		227		180	14	
P.A.	6 yrs			6.9	200	175	364	229	67	452			33	65.5
P.M.	6 yrs	3.1	5.9	12.5		20	923	429	120	501	206		26	
S.M.	6 yrs			4.6	120		545		180					
N.P.	6 yrs	3.1	5		130	105	939		202	524		61	58	
Mean		3.53	3.21	749	119.2	76.4	608.0	591.6	149.9	338.9	253.0	104.6	32.2	65.1
± Sem		0.43	0.51	1	18	22.1	80.6	76.1	19.1	41.4	34.5	16.3	6.2	4.9
N		8	8	10	7	10	12	8	10	12	8	8	8	6

Table V. Prepubertal girls of 7–9 years: LH, FSH, Prl and steroid plasma levels.

Name	Chron. Age	LH mU/ml	FSH mU/ml	Prl ng/ml	Cortisol ng/ml	DHA-S ng/ml	DHA pg/ml	Δ_5-P pg/ml	P pg/ml	17-P pg/ml	A pg/ml	T pg/ml	DHT pg/ml	E_2 pg/ml
S.E.	7 yrs	3.9	3		160	108	1274	960	80	349	244	201	–	60
S.M.R.	7 yrs	3.3	4.5	5		115	647	540	92	579	241	64	25	47.5
R.P.	7 yrs	2.3	2	6.3	160	70	431	650	223		285	50	55	30
S.R.	7 yrs			5.5	80	75	508		150	719		89	43	52
D.M.E.	8 yrs	3.2	2	7.5			441	655	103	250	229		16	465
C.S.	8 yrs	3.85	3.7	10	130	460	1295	720	278	620	307	101	66	87
S.D.	9 yrs	5.9	3.9	8.5		180			210	758			62	
T.L.	9 yrs	3.8	3.7	8.9	100	130	785				153	64	36	45
M.S.	9 yrs	3.1	3.6		80	105	115	830	180	362			96	
Mean		3.66	3.30	7.38	118.5	155	812	725.8	164.5	519.6	243.2	94.8	49.9	52.6
± Sem		0.39	0.34	0.71	16.5	48	138.6	66.6	26.7	81.2	23.8	24.7	9 .6	7.2
N		8	8	7	6	8	8	6	8	7	6	6	8	7

other hand, FSH plasma levels (Fig.1) increased significantly ($P < 0.02$) from 1.79 mU/ml (Table III) in the first group, to 3.21 mU/ml in the second group (Table IV). No further increases were found in the third group (Table V).

No significant variations were found in plasma prolactin levels between 1 and 9 years of age (Fig.1); single values ranged from 2.3 to 13.8 ng/ml.

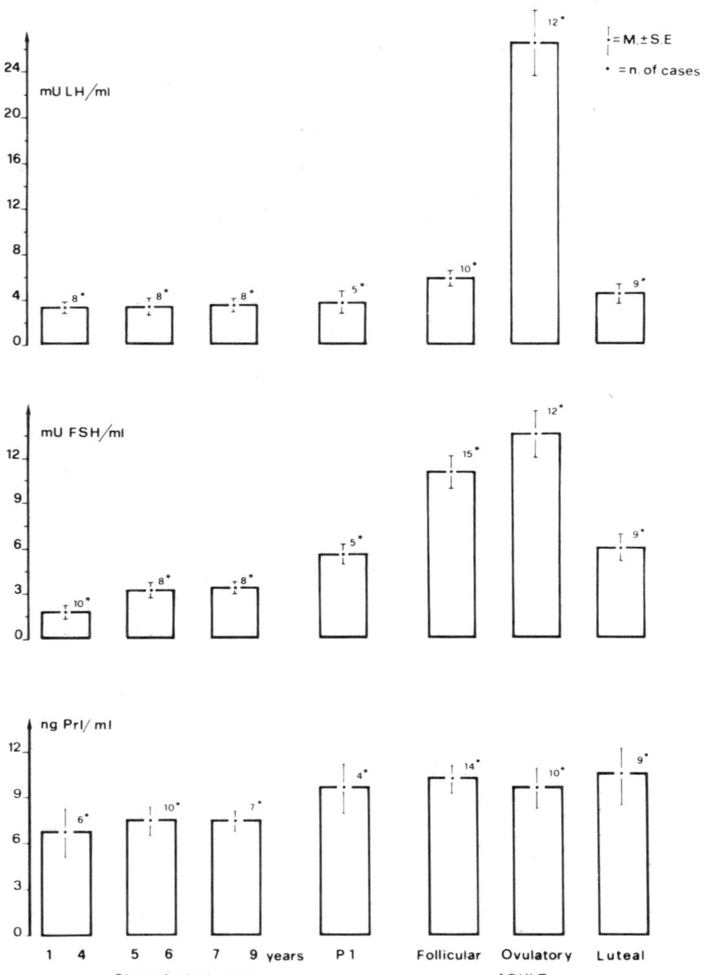

Fig.1 Plasma levels (Mean ± Sem) of LH, FSH and Prl in prepubertal girls subdivided in groups according to chronological age, in pubertal girls at Tanner's first stage and in adult women at the three phases of the menstrual cycle.

2. *Cortisol, dehydroepiandrosterone and dehydroepiandrosterone sulphate*

Cortisol plasma levels failed to show any significant variations in prepubertal girls (Fig.2). Single values ranged from 60 to 200 ng/ml (Tables III–V).

DHA plasma levels were 388.3 pg/ml (Table III) in the girls of the first group, and increased significantly ($P < 0.05$) in the third group (Table V), where a wide range (1295 – 431 pg/ml) was found.

DHA-S plasma levels showed similar behaviour, increasing from 25.2 ng/ml in the first group (Table III) to 76.4 ng/ml ($P < 0.05$) in the second (Table IV) and to 155.3 ($P < 0.001$) in the third group of 7-9 year olds (Table V). In view

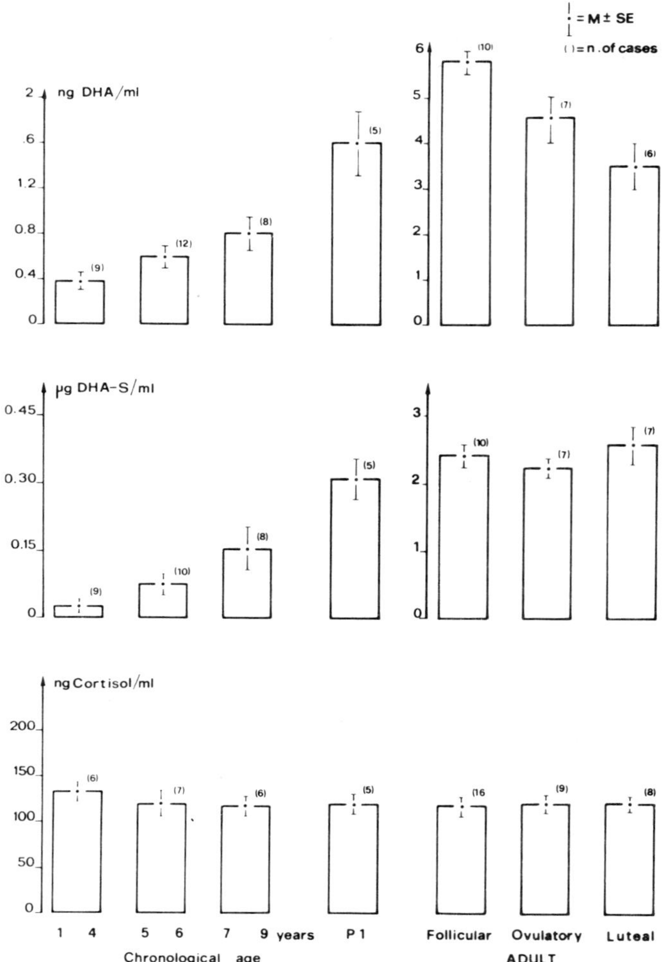

Fig. 2 Plasma levels (Mean ± Sem) of DHA, DHA-S and Cortisol in prepubertal girls subdivided in groups according to chronological age, in pubertal girls at Tanner's first stage and in adult women at the three phases of the menstrual cycle.

of the wide range of values found in these last two groups of cases (Tables IV–V) no significant difference was found (Fig.2).

3. *Pregnenolone, progesterone and 17-hydroxyprogesterone*

Δ_5-P varies in the first group from 131 to 326 pg/ml (Table III), with a mean value of 214.1 pg/ml; these values increase significantly ($P < 0.001$) in the second group to reach 591.6 pg/ml (Table IV, Fig.3). In the last group, a further increase to reach 725.8 pg/ml was found (Table V).

P plasma levels rose from 65.4 pg/ml in the first group (Table III) to 142.9 pg/ml in the second ($P < 0.005$) (Fig.3) and to 164.5 pg/ml in the third group. No significant difference was found by comparing the two latter groups (Fig.3).

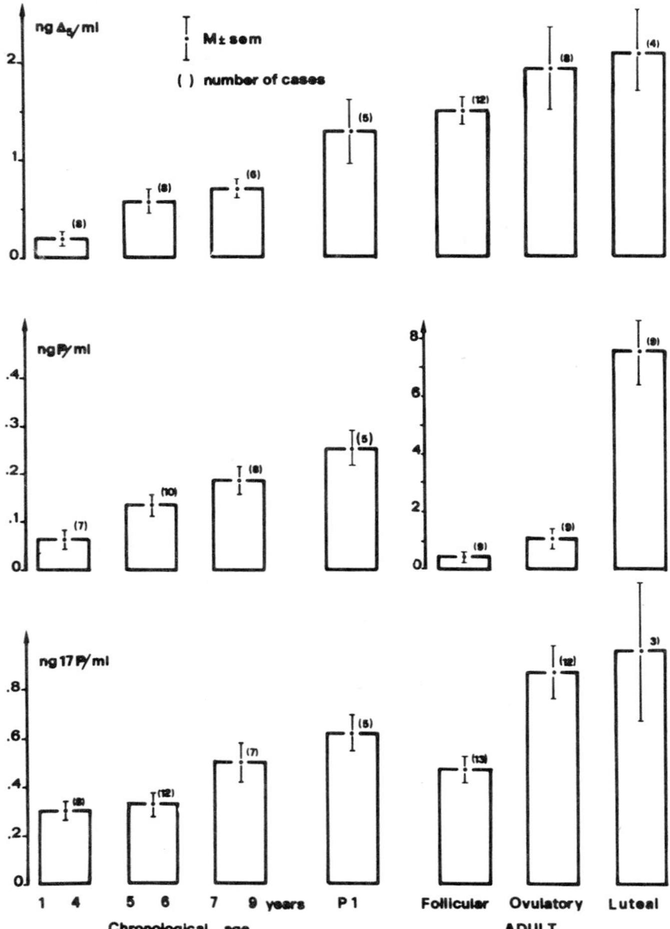

Fig.3 Plasma levels (Mean ± Sem) of Δ_5-P, P and 17-P in prepubertal girls subdivided in groups according to chronological age, in pubertal girls at Tanner's first stage and in adult women at the three phases of the menstrual cycle.

The 17-P plasma levels were 304.8 pg/ml in the first group (Table III) and remained unchanged in the second. A significant rise was found in the third group (519.6 pg/ml; Table V), both when compared to the first group ($P < 0.02$) and to the second ($P < 0.05$; Fig.3).

4. Androstenedione, testosterone, dihydrotestosterone and estradiol

No significant difference was found between any of the groups examined in the A plasma levels (Fig.4) (Tables III–V). Similarly, T plasma levels failed to show any significant difference between the three groups (Fig.5). However, DHT plasma values increased from 21.2 pg/ml (Table III) in the first group, to 32.2 (Table IV) in the second, and to 49.9 pg/ml ($P < 0.005$) in the last group (Table V, Fig.4). E_2 plasma levels passed from 33.4 pg/ml (Table III) in the 1-4 year old

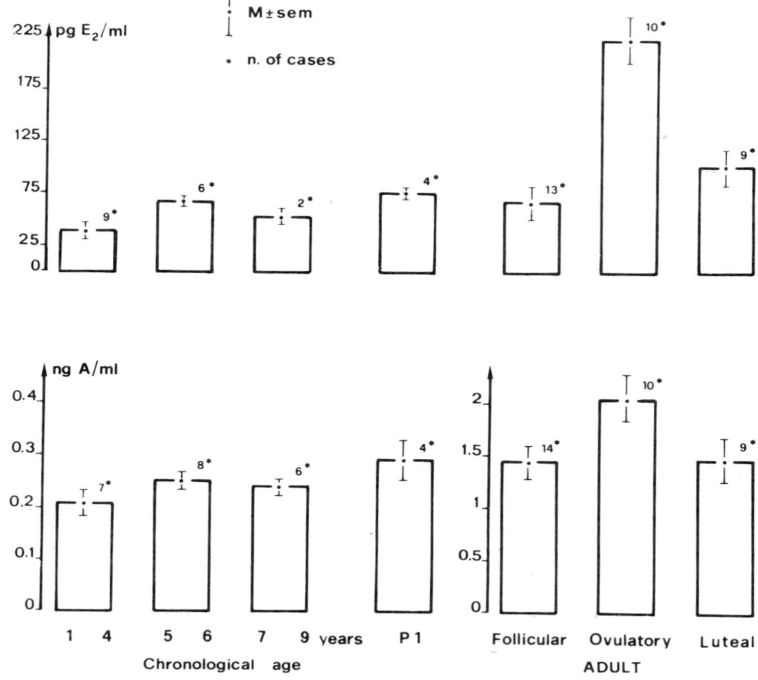

Fig.4 Plasma levels (Mean ± Sem) of E_2 and A in prepubertal girls subdivided in groups according to chronological age, in pubertal girls at Tanner's first stage and in adult women at the three phases of the menstrual cycle.

girls, to 65.1 pg/ml ($P < 0.005$) (Fig.IV) in the 5-6 year olds (Table III), thereafter remaining constant in the third group (52.6 pg/ml; Table V).

B. Pubertal Girls

1. Gonadotropins and prolactin

No variations were found in the LH plasma levels in P_1 girls (Table VI) when compared to those of prepubertal subjects (Fig.1). In the other cases of more advanced sexual maturation (Table VII) the LH values ranged from 2.15 to 4.6 mU/ml.

FSH plasma levels were found to be significantly increased ($P < 0.025$) in P_1 group (Table VI) when compared to the prepubertal girls (Fig.1). Slightly higher values were found in the cases at P_2—P_5 stages (Table VII).

In the P_1 group, prolactin plasma levels were slightly higher than in the prepubertal girls (Table III) but the difference was not significant at the statistical analysis (Fig.1). In the P_2-P_5 groups, the Prl values were in the same range as those of the P_1 group.

2. Cortisol, dehydroepiandrosterone and dehydroepiandrosterone sulphate

In both the P_1 and the P_2-P_5 groups of girls, the same plasma cortisol levels were found, ranging from 70 to 250 ng/ml (Fig.2).

DHA was characterized by a significant increase in P_1 (1657. 2pg/ml; Table

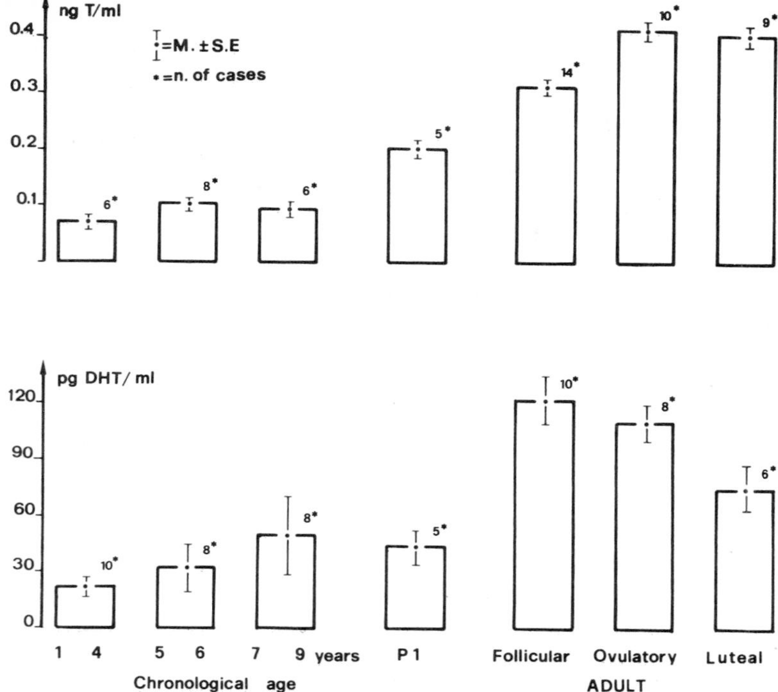

Fig.5 Plasma levels (Mean ± Sem) of T and DHT in prepubertal girls subdivided in groups according to chronological age, in pubertal girls at Tanner's first stage and in adult women at the three phases of the menstrual cycle.

VI) when compared to the DHA levels found in the last group of prepubertal girls ($P < 0.005$) (Fig.2). In the other cases of more advanced puberty (Table VII) the DHA values were also higher, and in some cases (S.R. and U.M.) within the normal limits for the follicular phase in young adult women (Fig.2). Similarly, DHA-S was significantly higher ($P < 0.05$) in P_1 (310.0 ng/ml)(Table VI) than in the older prepubertal girls (Fig.2). Further increases were found in the other stages of puberty, and the DHA-S ranged from 250 to 850 ng/ml (Table VII).

3. Pregnenolone, progesterone and 17-hydroxyprogesterone

Δ_5-P plasma levels in P_1 (1336.4 pg/ml; Table VI) were significantly higher than in the prepubertal girls ($P < 0.05$) (Fig.3); no marked further increases were observed in the P_2-P_5 cases (Table VII).

P also increased significantly in the P_1 group ($P < 0.02$) (Table VI) when compared to the 7-9 year old prepubertal girls (Fig.3). No further increases were observed in the other cases of more advanced puberty (Table VII). 17-P plasma levels ranged from 496 to 781 pg/ml in the P_1 girls (Table VI), the mean value not being significantly higher than in the third group of prepubertal girls, but it was significant when compared to the values found in the younger girls ($P < 0.001$) (Fig.3). No further increases were observed in the other cases of more advanced puberty (Table VII).

Table VI. Pubertal girls at Tanner's first stage: chronological age, LH, FSH, Prl and steroid plasma levels.

Name	Chron. Age	LH mU/ml	FSH mU/ml	Prl ng/ml	Cortisol ng/ml	DHA-S ng/ml	DHA pg/ml	Δ_5-P pg/ml	P pg/ml	17-P pg/ml	A pg/ml	T pg/ml	DHT pg/ml	E_2 pg/ml
S.R.	10	3.1	4.5	7.8	140	385	1317	1070	347	496	215	251	42	78.5
M.G.	10	2.9	7.4	4.1	175	430	2084	1760	325	502	152	282	33	72
M.C.	10	2.8	3.5		110	250	1071	620	217	642	461	163	47	
F.N.	12	3.2	4.5	16.2	80	205	1514	2280	202	781		235	49	85
M.L.	12	7.5	9	10	90	280	2300	952	170	770	345	176	53	71.5
Mean		**3.90**	**5.78**	**9.52**	**11.55**	**310**	**1657**	**1336.4**	**252.2**	**638.2**	**293.2**	**236**	**44.2**	**76.8**
± Sem		1.00	1.03	2.9	1.7	42	259.9	335.5	39.3	69.2	79.5	25.7	4.4	3.7
N		5	5	4	5	5	5	5	5	5	4	5	5	4

Table VII. Pubertal girls at Tanner's second–fifth stage and adult women in the three phases of the menstrual cycle: LH, FSH, Prl and steroid plasma levels.

Name	Chron. Age	Pub. Stage	LH mU/ml	FSH mU/ml	Prl ng/ml	Cortisol ng/ml	DHA-S ng/ml	DHA pg/ml	Δ_5-P pg/ml	P pg/ml	17-P pg/ml	A pg/ml	T pg/ml	DHT pg/ml	E_2 pg/ml
M.E.	11	2	3.2	2.8	13.5	250	250	2180	1100	217	480	461	163	47	64
S.A.	12	2	4.9	2.15	5.4	110	500	1514	1380	204	540	159	162	42	85
P.T.	13	3	6.3	2.15	7.8	70	650	2054	1420	168	636	496	258	63	96
S.R.	12	3	8.8	3.2	6.7	90	850	5074	1260	132	535	630	303	54	105
U.C.	12	3	8.5	4.4	7.2	120	760		1440	128	611	552	207		76
O.N.	11	4–5	10	4.6	6.5	105	600	4856	1580	212	683	506	177	39	58
Adults															
Follicular phase (from day −11 to day −6 according to E_2 mid-cycle peak)															
Mean			**5.91**	**11.36**	**10.08**	**117.0**	**2430**	**5800**	**1510**	**536.4**	**485.3**	**1410**	**312.9**	**123.80**	**68.6**
S.D.			1.14	2.26	3.89	27.7	1160	1390	560	233.4	171.3	320	61.3	37.1	45.9
N			10	15	14	12	10	10	12	14	13	14	14	10	13
Ovulatory Phase (from day −1 to day +1 according to mid-cycle peak)															
Mean			**26.85**	**13.61**	**11.28**	**132.5**	**2220**	**5050**	**2150**	**1093.2**	**878.6**	**2170**	**475.6**	**99.22**	**200.2**
S.D.			17.58	5.14	5.0	38.7	700	1570	940	700.1	413.2	750	147.1	44.31	81.9
N			12	12	12	12	9	8	10	12	12	12	12	9	11
Luteal phase (from day +5 to day +9 according to E_2 mid-cycle peak)															
Mean			**4.5**	**6.80**	**10.30**	**102**	**1867**	**3621**	**2058**	**7815**	**1724**	**1548**	**375.5**	**78.16**	**120.2**
S.D.			1.15	2.35	4.90	35	475	1257	604	3040	668	224	113.4	15	57.2
N			9	9	9	9	7	7	9	9	9	9	9	6	9

Table VIII. Delayed puberty: plasma steroid levels.

N	Name	Chron. Age	Cortisol ng/ml	DHA-S ng/ml	DHA pg/ml	P pg/ml	17-P pg/ml	A pg/ml	T pg/ml	DHT pg/ml	E_2 pg/ml
1	R.L.	17	110	1.4	2087	312	256	464	113		62
2	A.C.	18	70	0.8	1347	54	103	286	65		34
3	B.M.	20	150	1.4	1375	108	379	836	222	177	18
4	P.L.	21	110	0.9	412	23	270	127	62	100	30
5	S.A.	25	120	1.75	7650	90	933	635	136		7
6	D.F.M.	20	85	1.40		198	700	1088	319		40
	"	21	105	1.05		155		270			145
7.	N.O.	16	120	0.75	6680	27	478	1311	347	124	44
	"	17	135	0.62	7220	42	433	2123	454	136	17
	"	18	115	1.20	7050	78	371	1848	342	120	17
8	P.M.C.	18	90	0.98	6800	46	300	1971	488	221	48
	"	19	85	1.65	6400	209	289	2580	270		103
9	M.A.	17	80	1.42	3570	52	277	339	142	87	10
	"	18	110	1.65		31		410	121		10
	"	18½	95	0.72		45	191	345	130		19
10	F.G.	21	130	2.5	2889	173	543	944	253	173	23

4. *Androstenedione, testosterone, dihydrotestosterone and estradiol*

As absolute values, A plasma levels were higher in the P_1 group than in the third group of prepubertal girls, but this difference was not significant (Fig.4). Moreover, a futher increase was found in the other cases of puberty (Table VII).

On the other hand, T values were significantly higher in P_1 (Table III, $P < 0.005$) than in the older prepubertal group (Fig.5). In the other cases of puberty, the T levels were similar to those found in P_1 (Table VII). As far as DHT is concerned, no significant variations (Table VI) were found in P_1 when compared to the older prepubertal group (Fig.5), but the DHT levels were significantly higher ($P < 0.001$) when compared to the other prepubertal girls. A slight, further increase was found in the few cases in groups P_2–P_5 of more advanced puberty, where DHT ranged from 47 to 63 pg/ml (Table VII). E_2 levels were significantly higher ($P < 0.05$) (Fig.4) in P_1 (Table VI) than in the last prepubertal group. No further increases in E_2 were found in the other cases of more advanced puberty.

C. *Delayed Puberty*

1. *Gonadotropins and prolactin*

The results are reported in the section 'Materials and Methods' (Table I).

2. *Cortisol, dehydroepiandrosterone and dehydroepiandrosterone sulphate*

In all cases the cortisol plasma levels were within the normal range (Table I).

DHA plasma levels were found to be lower than in girls of 5-6 years, in case no.4; five cases (1, 2, 3, 9 and 10) showed DHA levels similar to those found in normal girls with corresponding pubertal maturation. Cases 5 , 7 and 8 showed values higher than those found in normal menstruating women (Table VIII). The latter two cases, followed up for more than a year, always showed DHA values higher than those of the controls. All cases had DHA-S plasma levels which were lower than those to be expected from the chronological age, except the case of F.G. (No.10), apparently at the P_4 stage, who had normal adult levels (2.5 μg/ml) (Table VIII).

3. *Progesterone and 17-hydroxyprogesterone*

Progesterone plasma levels ranged between 23 and 312 pg/ml (Table VIII) and were significantly lower ($P < 0.001$) than in the controls (Table VII). On the other hand, 17-P plasma concentrations varied from case to case: higher than normal values were found in cases 5 and 6, values within the normal range in cases 7 and 10, and more or less depressed values in the remaining subjects (Table VIII).

4. *Androstenedione, testosterone, dihydrotestosterone and estradiol*

A plasma levels (Table VIII) were similar to those measured in girls (Table VII) at the corresponding stage of puberty, in almost all cases. Patients No. 7 and 8 were, on the contrary, characterized by A plasma levels higher than those measured in normal adults (Table VII); moreover, these patients had T levels which were also higher than in control subjects (Table VIII), while the other cases of delayed puberty had T levels similar to those observed in girls with the same pubertal development (Table VII). DHT plasma levels did not show homogeneous results in the group of delayed puberty. The values ranged from normal (87 pg/ml) to such high values as 221 pg/ml in case 8 (Table VIII).

The E_2 plasma levels were normal in case 1, and also in cases 6 and 8 at the second analysis, while they were lower than normal, corresponding to the prepubertal range, in the other cases (Table VIII).

DISCUSSION

A cumulative analysis of the present results found in prepubertal and pubertal girls suggests some interesting observations, both on the particular behaviour pattern and on the relationship between the various hormones, in this period of life.

The FSH plasma levels increase significantly and progressively in prepuberty, while LH does not show a similar prepubertal pattern. At puberty, both FSH and LH rise progressively to reach adult values, in agreement with data reported by Sizonenko *et al.* (1970), Jenner *et al.* (1972), Angsusingha *et al.* (1974), Sizonenko and Paunier (1975). It is thus clear that different inhibitory and stimulatory mechanisms are involved in the control of gonadotropic plasma levels. Furthermore, the physiological significance of the progressive FSH prepubertal increase and its effects on the ovarian follicle and stroma should be further investigated.

Prolactin plasma levels also increase progressively, even though not significantly, from prepuberty, and this behaviour is in agreement with the data recently reported by Aubert *et al.* (1976). The small rise in prolactin seems due to the estradiol increase (Robyn *et al.*, 1976), as was also recently demonstrated, in man, by Wiedeman *et al.* (1976).

While in prepuberty the ovarian contribution to the different steroid plasma levels is of much less importance than in puberty or in adults, it is interesting to examine our results, subdividing the various hormones according to their most important source (Abraham, 1974; Genazzani *et al.*, 1976).

As regards the hormones of exclusively adrenal origin, cortisol levels do not vary throughout prepubertal life or during sexual maturation, according to the data of Ducharme *et al.* (1976). However, DHA-S plasma levels, also of totally adrenal origin, increase progressively and significantly from the first to the ninth year of age, undergoing a sharp rise during sexual maturation until full development is reached. The DHA-S data found in prepuberty differ from those reported by Hopper and Yen (1975), who found no differences in DHA-S plasma levels in girls from 8 to 12 years of age; our observations on behaviour of DHA-S levels during sexual maturation are, however, in agreement with these authors and with Lee and Migeon (1975). The results found in the case of DHA confirm the particular pattern found throughout puberty, as reported by Hopper and Yen (1975), Sizonenko and Paunier (1975), Ducharme *et al.* (1976) and Korth-Schutz *et al.* (1976), but our observations also show that the DHA increase begins during the first year of life and progresses until the start of pubertal maturation. At that stage, the DHA rise becomes more marked, reaching the plasma levels of the adult at stage P_4.

The particular behaviour pattern of plasma Δ_5-P, showing a progressive increase throughout prepubertal life, starting from the youngest age group studied, and a marked rise at the onset of sexual maturation, also confirms the major role of the adrenal steroids in determining the onset of puberty. Furthermore, P levels, as in the case of Δ_5-P, are also characterized by a progressive increase from the earliest period of life up to stage P_1 of maturation; on the contrary, 17-P plasma levels were constant in the first two groups of prepubertal girls, increasing significantly just prior to and at the onset of puberty, reaching levels even higher than those observed in adult controls (Genazzani *et al.*, 1976).

A difference in behaviour has been found between prepubertal and pubertal life, when measuring those androgens of ovarian origin: A and T. According to the data of Forest *et al.* (1974), Gupta *et al.* (1975), Sizonenko and Pauner (1975), Ducharme *et al.* (1976) and Korth-Schutz *et al.* (1976), the plasma levels of A and T do not vary in prepubertal life, but show strong increases throughout puberty. From our data, a sudden marked increase in plasma T is evident at P_1 stage. DHT levels increase gradually but progressively until the onset of sexual maturation, as has also been reported by Ducharme *et al.* (1976), and show a more pronounced rise throughout puberty until full maturation, as also reported by Gupta *et al.* (1975), Ducharme *et al.* (1976) and Korth-Schutz *et al.* (1976).

The behaviour of E_2 in prepuberty indicates a moderate but significant increase from 1 to 9 years followed, as reported by Jenner *et al.* (1972), Angsusingha *et al.* (1974), Gupta *et al.* (1975) and Ducharme *et al.* (1976) by a secondary progressive rise during sexual maturation.

In conclusion, it seems evident from our and others' data that in prepuberty and during sexual maturation, the various steroids of adrenal origin show different patterns of behaviour.

The stability of cortisol, the differences in behaviour of 17-P and P mentioned previously, the similar pattern of P, Δ_5-P, DHA and DHA-S which all increase progressively until the start of sexual maturation and present some differences only during puberty, all lead us to sustain that the adrenal cell population responsible for the production of androgens may multiply between one year of age and complete sexual maturity. Moreover, the androgens of chiefly ovarian origin (A and T) increase only after, and not prior to the onset of puberty. DHT, the steroid which is a peripheral androgen metabolite, increases from early to mid-prepuberty, but shows the most important modifications during sexual maturation, when A and T also show particular increases.

The effects of these modifications on the feedback levels of sexual steroids and gonadotropins remain to be elucidated, Until now, in fact, no data have become available to explain either the greater sensitivity to the negative feedback of estradiol in prepubertal female rats (Eldridge *et al.*, 1974), or the absence of positive feedback between estrogen and luteinizing hormone found in prepubertal girls by Reiter *et al.* (1974). Both these conditions might be modified by the chronic effects of ever-increasing amounts of androgens on hypothalamic receptors, as demonstrated throughout prepubertal life.

As far as delayed puberty is concerned, the data presented here do not indicate the existence of homogeneous results for all parameters, in all cases. In fact, while DHA-S plasma levels are always lower than expected from the chronological age, and within the limits expected for the pubertal development, the DHA plasma values permit division of the patients into two groups: the first (cases 1, 2, 3, 9 and 10) where the steroid concentration was adequate according to the stage of puberty, and the second (cases 5, 7 and 8) where DHA plasma levels were higher than in normal adult women. Other steroids were also found to be higher than normal in these last cases, i.e. A, T and DHT in cases 7 and 8, and 17-P in case 5. The first group of patients present plasma DHA as described in cases of delayed adrenarche by Sizonenko and Paunier (1975). Another interesting observation in our cases of delayed puberty is the finding of DHT plasma levels at upper limit of the normal range or higher. This fact appears to indicate the existence of an increase in 5-a reductase activity in this syndrome. The increased amounts of DHT, which were also found in case 4 where all the other androgens were strongly depressed, might be very important in maintaining the "gonadostat" (McCann and Ramriez, 1964) in this type of patient.

ACKNOWLEDGEMENT

The present research was partially supported by the CNR project "Biology of Reproduction".

REFERENCES

Abraham, G.E. (1973). *In* "Modern Methods of Steroid Analysis" (E. Heftman, ed) pp.451-470. Academic Press.

Abraham, G.E. (1974). *J. clin. Endocr. Metab.* **39**, 340-346.

Albright, F. (1947). *In* "Recent Progress in Hormone Research" **I**, pp.293-314. Academic Press.

Angsusingha, K., Kenny, F.M., Nankin, H.R. and Taylor, F.H. (1974). *J. clin. Endocr. Metab.* **39**, 63-68.

Aubert, M.L., Sizonenko, P.C., Kaplan, S.L. and Grumbach, M.M. (1976). *In* "Prolactin and Human Reproduction" (P.G. Crosignani and C. Robyn, eds) pp.9-20. Academic Press, London.

Boyar, R., Finkelstein, J.W., David, R., Roffwarf, H., Kapen, S., Weitzman, E.D. and Hellman, L. (1973). *New Engl. J. Med.* **9**, 282-286.

Boyar, R., Finkelstein, J.W., Roffwarg, H., Kapen, S., Weitzman, E. and Hellman, L. (1972). *New Engl. J. Med.* **21**, 582-586.

Cattaneo, S., Forti, G., Fiorelli, G., Barbieri, U. and Serio, M. (1975). *Clin. Endocrinol.* **4**, 505-512.

Del Pozo, E., Hiba, J., Lancranian, I. and Künzig, H.J. (1976). *In* "Prolactin and Human Reproduction" (P.G. Crosignani and C. Robyn, eds) pp.61-69. Academic Press, London.

Dohler, K.D. and Wuttke, W. (1974). *Endocrinology* **94**, 1003-1008.

Ducharme, J.R., Forest, M.G., Deperetti, E., Sempe, M., Collu, R. and Bertrand, J. (1976). *J. clin. Endocr. Metab.* **42**, 468-476.

Ehara, Y., Yen, S.S.C. and Siler, T.M. (1975). *Am. J. Obstet. Gynec.* **121**, 995-997.

Eldridge, J.C., McPherson, J.C. and Mahesh, V.B. (1974). *Endocrinology* **94**, 1536-1540.

Facchinetti, F., Romagnino, S., Cacchini, V. and Genazzani, A.R. (1976). *In preparation.*

Forest, M.G. and Cathiard, A.M. (1975). *J. Endocr. Metab.* **41**, 977-980.

Forest, M.G., Sizonenko, P.C., Cathiard, A.M. and Bertrand, J. (1974). *J. clin. Invest.* **53**, 819-828.

Genazzani, A.R. (1975). *Horm. Res.* **6**, 299-300.

Genazzani, A.R., Lemarchand-Beraud, Th., Aubert, M.L. and Felber, J.P. (1975). *J. clin. Endocr. Metab.* **41**, 431-437.

Genazzani, A.R., Magrini, G., Facchinetti, F., Romagnino, S., Pintor, C., Felber, J.P. and Fioretti, P. (1976). *In* "Androgens and Antiandrogens" (Neumann and Martin, eds) *(in press)*. Raven Press, N.Y.

Gupta, D. (1974). *Clin. Endocr. Metab.* **4**, 27-55.

Gupta, D., Attanasio, A. and Raff, S. (1975). *J. clin. Endocr. Metab.* **40**, 636-643.

Hopper, B.R. and Yen, S.S.C. (1975). *J. clin. Endocr. Metab.* **40**, 458-461.

Jenner, M.R., Kelch, R.P., Kaplan, S.L. and Grumbach, M.M. (1972). *J. clin. Endocr. Metab.* **34**, 521-530.

Kantero, R.L., Wide, L. and Widholm, O. (1975). *Acta endocr. (Copenh.)* **78**, 11-21.

Kapen, J., Boyar, R.M., Finkelstein, J.W., Hellman, L. and Wetzman, E.D. (1974). *J. clin. Endocr. Metab.* **39**, 293-299.

Korth-Schutz, S., Levine, L.S. and New, M.I. (1976). *J. clin. Endocr. Metab.* **42**, 117-124.

Lee, P.A. and Migeon, C.J. (1975). *J. clin. Endocr. Metab.* **41**, 556-562.

Magrini, G., Lemarchand-Beraud, Th., Reudi, B., Felber, J.P. and Vannotti, A. (1973). *Acta endocr. (Copenh.)* **Suppl.177**, 56.

McCann, S.M. and Ramirez, V.D. (1964). *In* "Recent Progress in Hormone Research" **XX**, pp. 131-181. Academic Press.

Melis, G.B., Facchinetti, F., Genazzani, A.R. and Fioretti, P. (1976). *J. Nucl. Biol. Med. (submitted).*

Parer, D.C., Judd, H.L., Rossman, L.G. and Yen, S.S.C. (1975). *J. clin. Endocr. Metab.* **40**, 1099-1109.

Reiter, E.O., Kulin, H.E. and Hamwood, S.M. (1974). *Pediat. Res.* **8**, 740-745.

Robyn, C., Delvoye, P., Van Exter, C., Vekemans, M., Caufriez, A., De Nayer, P., Delogne-Desnoeck, J. and L'Hermite, M. (1976). *In* "Prolactin and Human Reproduction" (P.G. Crosignani and C. Robyn, eds) pp.71-96. Academic Press, London.

Sizonenko, P.C. (1974). *Clin. Endocr. Metab.* **4**, 173-206.

Sizonenko, P.C., Burr, I.N., Kaplan, S.L. and Grumbach, M.M. (1970). *Pediat. Res.* **4**, 36-45.

Sizonenko, P.C. and Paunier, L. (1975). *J. clin. Endocr. Metab.* **41**, 894-904.

Tanner, J.M. (1962). "Growth and Adolescence". Blackwell Scientific Publications, Oxford.

Wiedeman, E., Schwartz, E. and Frantz, A.G. (1976). *J. clin. Endocr. Metab.* **42**, 942-952.

Winter, J.S.D., Hughes, I.A., Reyes, F.I. and Faiman, C. (1976). *J. clin. Endocr. Metab.* **42**, 679-686.

INHERITED TRUE SEXUAL PRECOCITY IN MALES: A CASE REPORT OF A FATHER AND HIS SON

M. Pierson, G. Fortier, L. Wuilbercq, J.R. Caudrelier and B. Cantus
Department of Pediatrics, University of Nancy I, France

In 1952, we had the opportunity of examining a two-year-old boy presenting a case of true sexual prococity and, twenty-two years later, this patient's son suffering from the same sexual disorder. A survey of the literature published so far on the subject shows that this hereditary form of precocious puberty is very rare and that the mode of transmission of the responsible gene is most uncommon.

CASE STUDY 1

Willy T... was born at full term, in good condition, and the first year of his life was uneventful. On and after the 15th month, however, an acceleration in his development, growth of pubic hair and an abnormal enlargement of his genitalia were to be noted.

When examined at the Children's Hospital at the age of two, he already had an impressive appearance, revealing unusual somatic and sexual development. He weighed 18 kg (+ 3 s.d.) and was 98 cm tall, with abnormally developed muscles, a low-pitched voice, an acneic complexion and genital organs corresponding to puberty stage II according to Tanner's scale. His penis was almost constantly erected and he was rather restless, boisterous, although not aggressive. His bone age, assessed according to Pyle's standards was about 5 years.

Laboratory tests gave the following results:
urinary 17 ketosteroids for 24 h : 8 mg
urinary gonadotrophin activity : 5 U.R.

A testicular biopsy showed that the development of the tubuli and of the leydig tissue corresponded to the adolescent stage. Neurological, ophthalmological and radiographical examinations led to the assumption that no pathological organic process was at the origin of the complaint.

The follow-up confirmed that the "idiopathic" type of pubertal precocity was the correct diagnosis, and the boy continued growing rapidly until he reached his adult stature, i.e. 143 cm, with all appearance of an adult at the age of 8.

He was seen for the last time at the age of 12, with psychological problems but in good somatic condition. Later on, he got married with an unrelated woman and they had two children. The first child, a girl now aged five, has had no problem; as for the second one, a boy, his case is related below.

CASE STUDY 2

Fabrice T ... was born at full term, weighing 3 200 g, measuring 51 cm, and the delivery was uneventful. His growth seemed to be quite normal till the end of his first year. His father, particularly careful, noticed the appearance of pubic hair and the abnormal growth of his genitalia at the age of 20 months. At the same time there was an obvious growth spurt.

When we first examined Fabrice, then aged 2, he was the very image of his father at the same age: marred male appearance, developed musculature acneic face, hard voice, rough behaviour and external genitalia corresponding to stage II or III in Tanner's scale.

Clinical, radiological and biological tests confirmed that we had to deal with a case of complete sexual development with no organic process either in the gonad or in the hypothalamo-hypophyso-gonadal axis.

The results of these tests were as follows:

urinary excretion of 17 ketosteroids	:	1.5 mg/d
urinary FSH and LH (bioassay)	:	1.5 μU/ml – 2 μU/ml
plasma testosterone (radioimmunoassay)	:	200 ng/100 ml
plasma FSH	:	1.5 mUI/ml
plasma LH	:	3.5 mIU/ml.

So the diagnosis was true sexual precocity of genetic origin, and the treatment performed was cyproterone acetate 100 mg weekly. It had a dramatic effect both on the penis erections, which completely stopped, and on the child's behaviour but unfortunately it did not affect his growth and in the following year the height gain was 21 centimetres.

In brief, the father and his son developed the same process of complete sexual maturation starting at the age of 15 months.

The father's follow-up shows that the mechanism has been quite innocuous and has enabled him to lead a normal life in spite of a rather short stature and some behavioural difficulties in childhood,

DISCUSSION

Very few such records have been published since 1852: only 16 families have been studied with genealogic trees available (the collection of cases can be seen in Table I), and reservations must be made regarding Jolly's and Ferrier's reports, for in both cases the first symptoms appeared in the father only at the age of 9, i.e. the borderline of pubertal onset.

So it is quite obvious that this is a very rare complaint: the 16 families concerned amount to 103 patients and no new case has been reported at least in

Table I.

Stone	1852	Father and his son
Reuben and Manning	1922	Father and his son
Orel	1928	Two brothers
Rush	1937	Father and 2 sons (pedigree restudied by Jacobsen)
Sigrist	1940	Two brothers
Engström and Munson	1951	Father and 2 sons
Walker	1952	Father, 2 sons and 5 other boys in 5 generations
Jacobsen	1952	Twenty-seven males affected in 7 generations
Talbot	1954	Seven males (not published)
Mortimer	1954	Eight males in 3 generations
Jungck	1956	Three different trees: 1–5 males in 3 generations 2–7 males in 3 generations 3–19 males in 4 generations
Keizer	1956	Four males in 3 generations
Beas	1962	Eight males in 3 generations
Pierson	1952–1976	Father and his son

major medical reviews since 1962, although, given the singularity of the clinical picture and the fact that this complaint affects the whole family, no case could have been passed over.

Particular emphasis must be laid on the *genetic aspect* and on the mode of transmission of the complaint. The most expressive pedigrees are presented in Figs 1 to 6.

Each of them could be analyzed in turn, but it is more economical to summarize the findings taking Jacobsen's family as a model since it constitutes the most important tree. Besides, the other trees have been studied in the same manner and the conclusions that are listed below apply perfectly to each of them:

1. The most original finding is that *only males* are affected, with no exception recorded to this day.

2. In every family with three or more generations, the mode of transmission is *vertical* and this *dominant*, as one more patient is affected in each generation.

3. No consanguinous marriages are reported in any of the 16 families, which excludes the possibility of a recessive gene.

4. The fact that this complaint is restricted to males could suggest the possibility of a gene located on the sex chromosomes. It is true that three pedigrees are consistent with X linked transmission (Jungck's family 1 and family 2: Walker's family), but this mode is not the only one possible. Besides, the other pedigrees are by no means compatible with X linked modality since some fathers affected by the disease have off-print the gene directly to one or more of their females as well as males.

Now, if the gene was located on the Y chromosome, every male ought to be affected and more of them could be normal if we exclude the possibility of a very

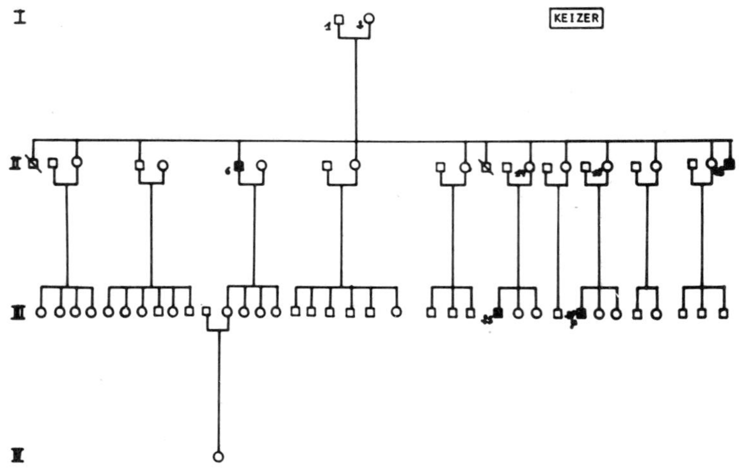

Fig. 1

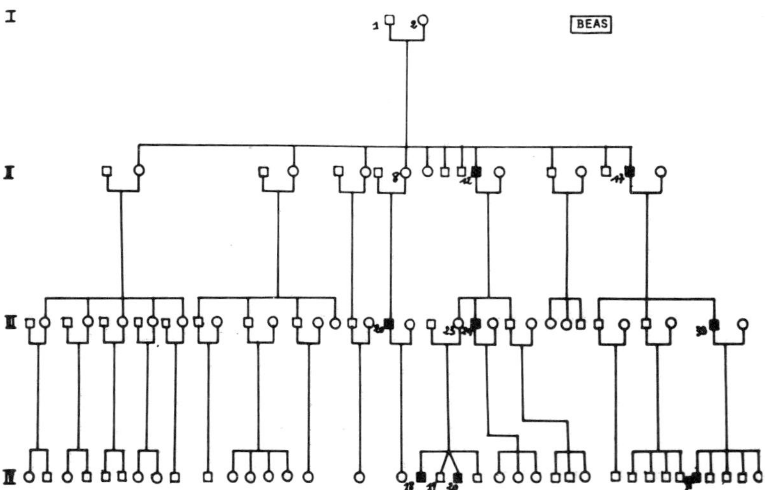

Fig. 2

low penetrance of the gene.

So, to sum up, the responsible gene is not located on a gonosome but on an autosome. It is dominant and not recessive, and it does not manifest itself in females. This peculiarity cannot be accounted for by some lethal property of the gene, since no deviation of the sex ratio has been noted in Jacobsen's family and we have arrived at the same result in studying the other families from that standpoint (Walker's, Mortimer's, Jungck's, Keizer's and Beas's).

The mode of inheritance is mendelian autosomal dominant: the responsible gene is sex limited or sex influenced. These two terms might in fact refer to the same phenomenon.

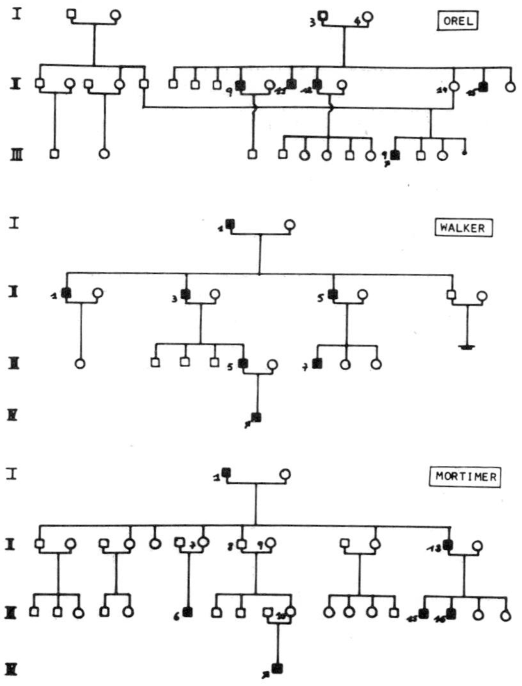

Fig. 3

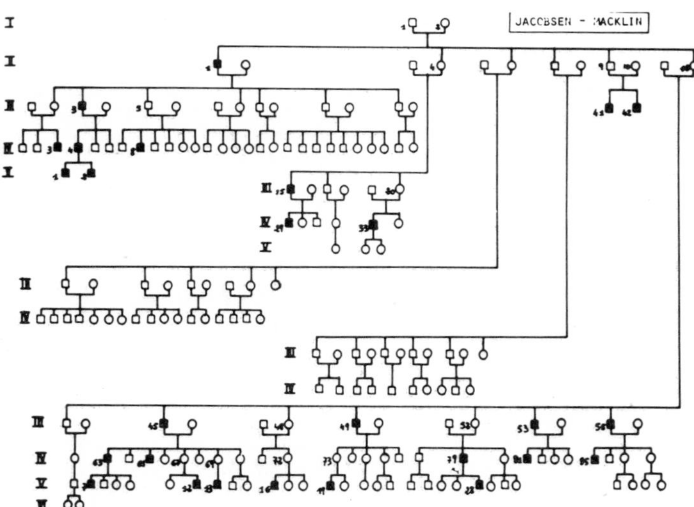

Fig. 4

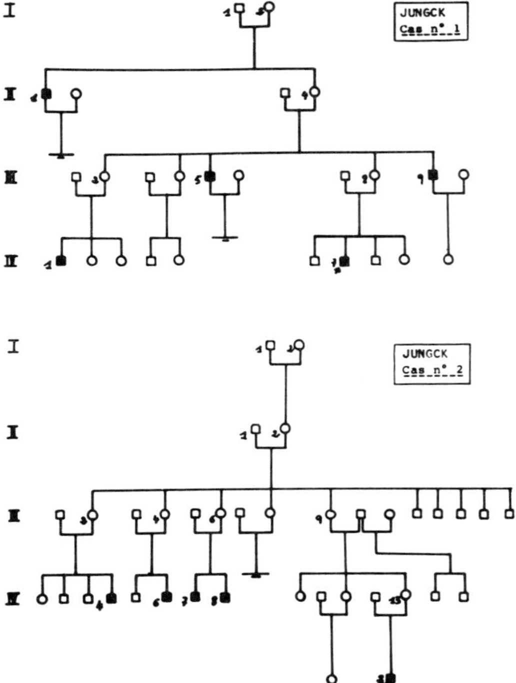

Fig. 5

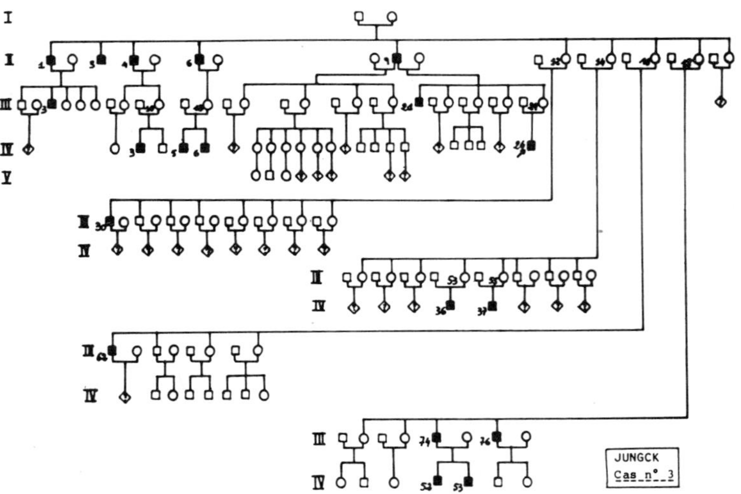

Fig. 6

MODE OF ACTION OF THE GENE AT THE CELLULAR AND MOLECULAR LEVELS

a) Although the gene may be present in either males and females, it cannot express itself, but only be transmitted by, the latter sex.

One explanation of this phenomenon is that the gene is inhibited by a repressor effect at the chromosomal level (ADN), or at the cytoplasmic level (ARN), which would put an end to its information. This inhibitory effect could be related to some specific antihormone or some estrogen.

Another exploration, more in agreement with recent findings about the control of the hypophyso-gonadal axis, assumes that previous imprinting of the hypothalamus by male hormones is necessary for the gene to have any action, which is precisely what is to be found in the case of male fetuses and neonates, but not in that of females.

b) How does this gene function in males?

By analogy with the concept of the organic etiology of sexual precocity in females, one could hypothesize that male patients develop microscopic harmatomae in the hypothalamus. Such a possibility, however, has never been corroborated by any of the case reports published so far and it seems very unlikely that a dysplasic process should be confirmed to the sexual control nuclei. A biochemical mechanism – to be more precise, a neurohormonal mechanism – might provide a more satisfactory explanation.

From recent studies on the regulation of the gonadal axis and on pubertal development (Grumbach and Kaplan, Sizonenko, Job, Bertrand), we know that the mechanism of sexual development implies several concomitant regulations.

1. The progressive maturation of cellular structures and neuro-amine secretions.

2. In the case of males, a fairly high production of testosterone, which is responsible for the specific imprinting of hypothalamus nuclei in the perinatal period.

3. During infancy and childhood, the maintenance of a certain quantity of sexual hormone secretion in order to continue allowing the sexual tract to mature without disturbing the equilibrium of the hypothalamo-hypophyso-cortico-gonadal axis.

4. Finally, the progressive increase in sensitivity of the hypothalamic receptors to the feedback mechanism as an initiator of pubertal development.

The gene determining hereditary precocious puberty can intervene at different times and at different levels. It is likely that the gene acts as an initiator of pubertal changes very early in life, perhaps in the fetal period, and by keeping the sensitivity threshold of the gonadostat to circulating testosterone at a very high level.

This phenomenon can take place in male fetuses only because there is no previous imprinting by testosterone in females.

Other hypotheses on the direct mechanism of genetic action cannot be excluded: i.e. enzymatic anomaly of peripheral testosterone metabolism, changes in the sensitivity of the hypothalamus to neuro-amino-factors, changes in the production of releasing factors, etc..

But, up to now, no specific case of this genetic endocrine disease has been reported in sufficient detail and with sufficient patterns to help throw light on this problem.

REFERENCES

Beas, F., Zurbrugg, R.P., Leibow, S.G., Patton, R.G. and Gardner, L.J. (1962). *J. clin. Endocr. Metab.* **22**, 1095-1102.
Bertrand, J. (1973). *Prob. actuels Endocrinol. Nutrit. Fr.* **16**, 73-100.
Burr, J.M., Sizonenko, P.C., Kaplan, S.L. and Grumbach, M.M. (1970). *Pediatr. Res.* **4**, 25.
Engström, W.W. and Munston, P.L. (1951) *Am. J. Dis. Child.* **81**, 179-192.
Ferrier, P., Shepard, T.H. and Smith, E.K. (1961). *Pediatrics* **28**, 258-275.
Jacobsen, A.W. and Macklin, M.T. (1952). *Pediatrics* **9**, 682-695.
Job, J.C. (1967). *Méd. Infant.* **74**, 699-706.
Jolly, H. (1955). "Sexual Precocity", p.276. Thomas, Springfield.
Jungck, F.C., Brown, N.H. and Carmona, H. (1956). *Am. J. Dis. Child.* **91**, 138-143.
Keizer, D.P.R. (1956). *Arch. Fr. Pédiat.* **13**, 986-992.
Lowrey, G.H. and Brown, T.G. (1951). *J. Pediat.* **38**, 325-340.
Mortimer, E.A. (1954). *Pediatrics* **13**, 174.
Orel, J. (1928). *Z. Konstitutional.* **14**, 244-252.
Pierson, M. (1953). Thèse Méd. Nancy, No.73.
Reuben, M.S. and Manning, G.R. (1922). *Arch. Pediatr.* **39**, 769-785.
Royer, P. (1967). *Rev. Franç. Endocrin. Clin.* **8**, 217-230.
Schachter, M. (1949). *Ann. Paediat. Basel* **6**, 173-183.
Sigrist, V.E. (1940). *Ann. Paediat.* **155**, 84-106.
Sizonenko, J.B., Burr, I.M., Kaplan, S.L. and Grumbach, M.M. (1969). *Ann. Endocrinol.* **30**, 702-703.
Sizonenko, P.C., Lewin, M. and Burr, I.M. (1972). *Arch. Fr. Pédiat.* **29**, 185-201.
Sizonenko, P.C. and Burr, I.M. (1972). *Arch. Fr. Pédiat.* **29**, 203-230.
Stone, R.K. (1852). *Am. J. med. Sci.* **24**, 561.
Tanner, J.M. (1969). "Growth and Endocrinology in the Adolescent ". *In* "Endocrine and Genetic Disease of Childhood". Saunders, Philadelphia.
Walker, J.H. (1952). *J. Pediat.* **41**, 251-257.
Wilkins, L. (1950). "The Diagnosis and Treatment of Endocrine Disorders in Childhood and Adolescence", pp.152-160, 280-290. Thomas Springfield.

COMPENSATORY TESTICULAR HYPERTROPHY IN PREPUBERTAL BOYS

L. Tatò, A. Corgnati, A. Boner, L. Pinelli and D. Gaburro
Department of Pediatrics, Clinical Chemistry, University of Verona, Italy

The phenomenon of compensatory testicular hypertrophy (CTH) in unilateral cryptorchidism in children and in adolescents was described by Laron and Zilka (1969). Oversecretion of follicle-stimulating hormone (FSH) either on basal level or after stimulation with LRH , and to a greater extent of luteinizing hormone (LH) only after stimulation, was reported on these subjects at pubertal age. A tentative explanation of the phenomenon was given by Laron *et al.* (1975) on this basis.

We have revaluated the hypothesis in the CTH prepubertal boys with orchidometry, LRH test and human chorionic gonadotropin (HCG) test.

SUBJECTS AND METHODS

Two groups of patients were studied. The first group consisted of five prepubertal (8—11 years old) boys with unilateral undescended testis who showed compensatory testicular hypertrophy (CTH). All these patients were examined for two years, before and after operation; all the biological tests were performed only before orchidopexy. The second group consisted of nine prepubertal (8—11 years old) boys with normal testicular development. All boys underwent a complete physical examination which included rating of sexual development, measurement of testicular volume by orchidometer (Prader, 1966) and measurement of penis length and width. The bone age was assessed according to the atlas of Greulich and Pyle (1959); the testicular volume was estimated with an orchidometer by comparative palpation.

The LH-RH test was performed after an overnight fast. A 21-Butterfly needle was inserted into a cubital vein and the lumen was kept open by attaching a syringe with a 5% sodium citrate solution.

After one hour of rest, blood was withdrawn for determination of the basal plasma level of LH, FSH and Testosterone (time 0) and LH-RH (Serono) 100 μg/

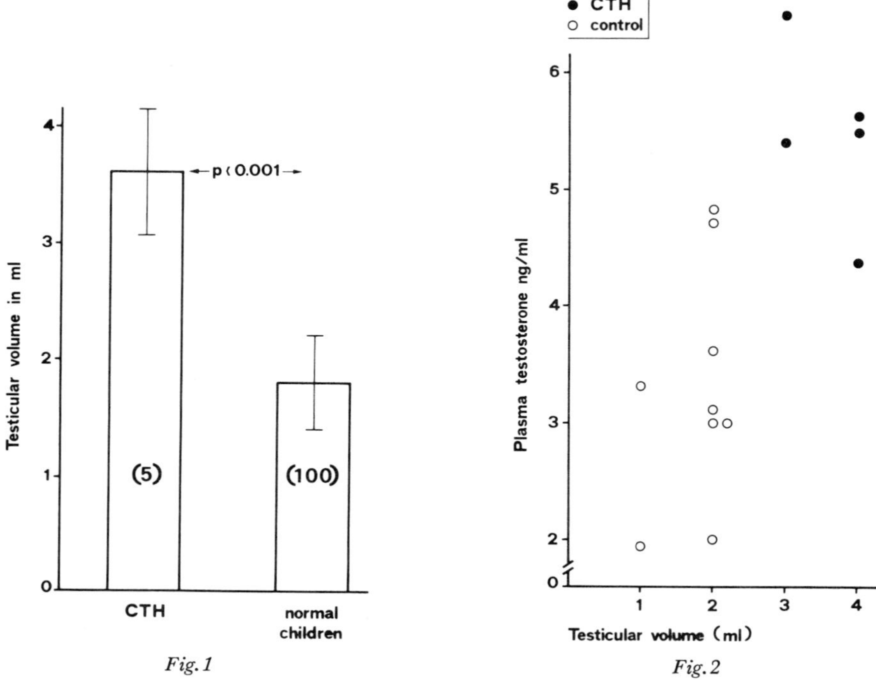

Fig. 1 Testicular volume in CTH and normal boys. Volume in normal boys is the mean of the two testicles.

Fig. 2 The peak plasma testosterone concentration after HCG plotted against testicular volume (in normal boys the volume is the mean of the two testicles).

m^2 was injected intravenously in one bolus. At time 15, 30, 40, 60, 90 and 180 min after LH-RH injection the additional blood samples were withdrawn. The plasma was separated immediately and kept frozen at $-20°C$ until assayed.

Two days after the LH-RH test to all subjects was administered e.m. 1500 UI/m^2 of HCG (Serono); the same injection was made at days 3 and 5 and at days 2, 4 and 6 venous blood samples were collected for testosterone and plasma kept frozen at $-20°C$ until assayed.

The plasma FSH and LH were measured with double antibody radioimmunoassay according to Franchimont (1969). LH and FSH results are expressed as ng/ml based on the LER 907 reference preparation. Testosterone in plasma was measured by radioimmunoassay according to Furuyama (1970).

Statistical evaluations were made using the Student's *t* test.

RESULTS

When the size of the enlarged testicles was compared to that found in 100 boys of the same age and of the same country (Fig. 1), the difference in volume was statistically significant ($p < 0.001$).

The basal and peak levels of plasma LH and FSH during the LH-RH test are given in Table I. The basal levels of testosterone are given in Table II; no significant

Table I. Plasma LH, FSH concentration during the LH-RH test (100 μg/m² e.v.) in boys with CTH and boys with normal testicular development.

Patients		Chronol. age	Bone age	Testic. volume (ml)		Plasma LH (ng/ml)		Plasma FSH (ng/ml)	
No.	Name	yr.	yr.	Rt.	Lt.	Basal	Peak	Basal	Peak
Compensatory testicular hypertrophy									
1	Z.G.	10	10 4	—		0.2	1.0	1.0	2.8
2.	R.B.	11	11 -	4		0.9	4.0	0.3	1.6
3	C.A.	9	9 3	—		1.6	3.5	1.4	2.8
4	G.M.	12	12 4	—		0.6	5.0	1.3	2.6
5	S.P.	8	8 -	3		0.8	3.2	1.0	4.2
Mean						**0.82±0.26**	**3.3±2.18**	**1.0±0.18**	**2.8±0.86**
Normal boys									
Mean		**(8–11)**		**1.66**	**1.77**	**0.54±0.09**	**1.57±1.09**	**0.67±0.01**	**1.99±0.98**

Table II. Plasma testosterone concentration after HCG stimulation in the CTH boys and boys with normal testicular development.

Patients		Chronological	Plasma testosterone ng/ml	
No.	Name	Age	Basal	Peak
Compensatory testicular hypertrophy				
1	Z.G.	10	0.24	5.6
2	R.B.	11	0.14	5.47
3	C.A.	9	0.37	6.52
4	G.M.	12	0.13	4.35
5	S.P.	8	0.08	5.40
Mean			**0.19±0.05**	**5.46±0.59**
				↑
Normal boys				$p < 0.01$
				↓
Mean		**(8 – 11)**	**0.17±0.01**	**3.27±0.91**

change in testosterone concentration was observed during the test.

Table I reveals that in four of the five boys with CTH the plasma peak levels of LH were higher than in their control of the same age; nevertheless, the mean difference of the two groups was not significant. The peak values of FSH of the CTH boys were, on the contrary, only in the highest range of the control group.

In the CTH boys, there was a greater increase of plasma testosterone after HCG stimulation than in normal control (Table II and Fig.2) and the peak mean difference of the two groups was significant ($p < 0.01$).

DISCUSSION

In all CTH patients examined the undescended testis was found smaller than the descended and the follow-up after operation of the testicular growth showed that these testicles continued to develop in larger dimensions than the testicles in normal children too.

Four of the five CTH subjects showed a greater LH response than the boys with normally-developed testicles. The FSH response to LH-RH was only in the higher range of the normality for the age. These findings may be interpreted as an inconstant hyperfunction of the pituitary gonadotropin-secreting cells. Gonadotropin oversecretion has been demonstrated in the CTH pubertal boys and, moreover, all the testis of our CTH patients appeared hyperstimulated, not only clinically for the larger volume but also for the oversecretion of testosterone after injection of HCG.

These findings in CTH boys point to the still controversial problem of the gonadotropin feedback in the male and the role that the testosterone is supposed to play in it (Sherins and Loriaux, 1973). In these last years, it has been described that the FSH secretion in the male may also be influenced by a substance "inhibin", which supposedly originates in the Sertoli cells of the testis (Johnsen, 1970) and which is insufficiently produced if one testis is maldeveloped.

In conclusion, our data support the hypothesis that the hypertrophied testis of the CTH boys is also overstimulated in prepubertal age may be by a discontinuous oversecretion of gonadotropins.

REFERENCES

Franchimont, P. (1969). *Ann. Endocrin.* **29**, 403.
Furuyama, S. (1970). *Steroids* **16**, 415.
Greulich, W.W. and Pyle, S.L. (1959). "Radiographic Atlas of Skeletal Development of the Hand and Wrist", 2nd Ed. Stanford University Press, Stanford, California.
Johnsen, S.G. (1970). *In* "The Human Testis" (E. Rosenberg and C.A. Paulsen, eds), p.231. Plenum Press, New York – London.
Laron, Z. and Zilka, E. (1969). *J. clin. Endocr. Metab.* **29**, 1409.
Laron, Z., Dickerman, Z., Prager-Lewin, R., Keret, R. and Halabe, E. (1975). *J. clin. Endocr. Metab.* **40**, 977.
Prader, A. (1966). *Triangle* **7**, 240.
Sherins, R.J. and Loriaux, D.D. (1973). *J. clin. Endocr. Metab.* **36**, 886.

HYPOTHYROIDISM AND DEFICIENCIES OF SPECIFIC IMMUNITY

F. Severi

Department of Pediatrics, University of Pavia, Italy

For a time long investigators have focused attention on the relationship between hormones and specific immunity. As early as 1952, Dougherty reviewed the effects of hormones on lymphatic tissue. In 1970 a Symposium of the Ciba Foundation Study Group was dedicated to this topic and, very recently, in July, 1976, one of the Symposia of the V International Congress of Endocrinology.

While the rapid evolution of knowledge in both endocrinology and immunology paradoxically makes the problem more and more complicated, it also provides new highlights for further investigation; it is sufficient to recall the recent advances regarding production by the thymus of one or more hormones (Astaldi, 1976; Goldstein, 1976) which currently led us to consider the thymus an endocrine gland, or to recall observations, still of uncertain biological significance, like that of the affinity of the Fc immunoglobulin fragment for a constituent present both on the membrane and in the cytoplasm of ACTH cells in human anterior pituitary (Pouplard *et al.*, 1976).

Aside from the effects of adrenal-pituitary-axis hormones on specific immunity, about which the most information is available, experimental evidence also indicates the existence of relationships between thymus and gonads (Nishizuka and Sakakura, 1969, 1971a&b; Sakakura and Nishizuka, 1972; Besedowski and Sorkin, 1974), between insulin and cell-mediated immunity (Mahmoud *et al.*, 1975, 1976; MacCuish *et al.*, 1974) and, above all, between GH and specific immunity. According to Bentley *et al.* (1974), GH probably interferes with specific immunity by stimulating the synthesis of somatomedin, perhaps even a somatomedin specific for the thymus. The most extensive studies on growth hormone are those, by now classical, carried out using a particularly suitable animal model , Snell-Bagg (see Pierpaoli *et al.*, 1970) and Ames (see Duquesnoy, 1975) strains of autosomal recessive pituitary dwarf mice, which have been shown to develop severe immunodeficiency primarily affecting the thymus-dependent immune system; in addition, decreased thymic hormone activity has been demonstrated in the serum of such mice (Pelletier *et al.*, 1976). The same experimental model has allowed furthering knowledge of the relationship between thyroid and specific immunity, of particular interest here. To evaluate the findings regarding such relationships is not yet possible; so far experimental studies are too few and the results sometimes contradictory; however, some of major interest will be cited briefly. Treatment of Snell-Bagg dwarf mice with thyroxin and GH is followed by normalization of thymic structure as well as of peripheral lymphoid tissue histology; immune responses also revert to normal. Administration of anti-thyrotropic hormone sera to normal mice has been shown to suppress antibody formation (Pierpaoli *et al.*, 1969; Baroni *et al.*, 1969). A remarkable reduction in serum thyroxin levels has been demonstrated both in nude mice and in mice thymectomized at birth (Pierpaoli and Besedowsky, 1975). The latter results apparently contrast with Gyllensten's (1953) previous findings of increased mean thyroid weight and mean acinar cell height as well as of increased functional activity and response of the gland to thyrotropic hormone in guinea pigs subtotally thymectomized at birth.

Human studies, carried out for the most part in hyperthyroidism (Brody and Greenberg, 1972; Aoki *et al.*, 1973; Farid *et al.*, 1973; Wara *et al.*, 1973; Urbaniak *et al.*, 1974; Maciel *et al.*, 1976) do not aid in clarifying the problem since there is no agreement in the literature. Hypothyroidism has been reported in a patient with thymic hypoplasia and immune deficiency primarily affecting cell-mediated immunity (Hong *et al.*, 1970); anti-thyroglobulin antibodies were present in serum. To explain the association of defective cellular immunity and hypothyroidism the authors discuss the possibilities of an embryologic defect involving the derivatives of the second and third pharyngeal pouches, a GvH reaction, and an autoimmune thyroid disease related to a developmental abnormality of the thymus. With regard to the latter hypothesis, it is useful to underline the importance of the thymus in controlling autoantibody formation (Waldmann *et al.*, 1974; Allison, 1974); it has been suggested that the appearance of autoantibodies may be secondary to lack of a thymus-derived lymphocyte subpopulation (suppressor T lymphocytes) which has been shown to control the antibody response to several antigens (Gershwin and Steinberg, 1973; Irvine, 1976). These considerations may also apply to those endocrine disorders, including hypothyroidisms, associated with serum autoantibodies and mucocutaneous candidiasis, which is often also associated with defective cellular immune function. In fact in one case of chronic mucocutaneous candidiasis with impaired cell-mediated immunity and hypothyroidism a dramatic improvement of the infection, previously resistant to prolonged anticandidal treatment, was observed by Montes *et al.* (1972) only after initiating hormone-replacement therapy; the hypothesis of the latter authors that normal thyroid function is essential for the integrity of the thymus-dependent immune system, probably for the production of lymphokines, seems justified; in fact, defective production of MIF can be associated with chronic mucocutaneous candidiasis (Chilgren *et al.*, 1969; Valdimarsson *et al.*, 1970; Kirkpatrik *et al.*, 1971).

Such a brief outline obviously does not allow any definite statement on the relationships between hypothyrodisim and deficiency of specific immunity; however, it probably confirms their existence which also emerges from our in-

Table I. Results relative to the thymus-dependent system in the hypothyroid patients.

Name	Age	T* %	PHA** %	ConA** %	PHA/ ConA***
M.E.	4 m.	37 – 43.5	199 – 65	226 – 47	1.5 – 5.1
D.M.	7 m.	41.5 – 44	155 – 68	197 – 66	1.3 – 3.9
F.D.****	1 y. 3/12	58	42	33	3
A.T.	1 y. 4/12	57 – 55.6	25 – 118	5 – 67	8.6 – 6.6
S.B.	1 y. 11/12	59.5 – 47	79 – 82	160 – 79	0.8 – 3.9
F.F.	2 y. 1/12	62.6 – 53.6	122 – 85	90 – 41	2.3 – 7.7
S.A.****	2 y. 10/12	67.5	78	126	2.2
M.B.	4 y.	58 – 67	7 – 104	47 – 82	0.25 – 4.8
R.S.	4 y. 4/12	60.6	83	85	3.6
R.B.C.	4 y. 9/12	57.5 – 52.5	14 – 100	142 – 69	0.2 – 5.5
G.E.	5 y. 4/12	55.5	92	57	6.1
A.P.	5 y. 6/12	62.5 – 53.5	7 – 81	64 – 88	0.18 – 3.5
A.S.	7 y.	57 – 32	15 – 53	126 – 93	0.20 – 2.1
G.O.	9 y. 6/12	60.5 – 62.5	56 – 91	116 – 53	0.8 – 6.5
C.C.	9 y. 7/12	72 – 68	9 – 77	21 – 56	0.75 – 5.1
P.F.	10 y. 3/12	66.6 – 47.5	24 – 67	35 – 60	1.1 – 4.2
S.R.	10 y. 4/12	57.5 – 41.5	91 – 62	77 – 31	2 – 7.6
R.M.	14 y. 7/12	74 – 68.5	161 – 82	168 – 74	1.6 – 4.2
D.C.	14 y. 10/12	62 – 58	25 – 73	102 – 98	0.4 – 2.8

* Normal values for our laboratory: 50–75%. Normal controls tested simultaneously gave results within these limits. ** Percentage with respect to the simultaneously tested controls (normal values: ⩾ 40%). *** Normal values for our laboratory: 4.7 ± 1.4 (S.D.). Normal controls tested simultaneously gave results within these limits. **** Not yet treated.

vestigation presently in course, the preliminary results of which are reported below.

Specific immunity was tested in 19 children, 4 males and 15 females, from 4 months to 14 and 10/12 years old with primary hypothyroidism. Seventeen patients were in treatment with dessicated thyroid, while two had not yet begun treatment.

The following studies were done in all patients: serum IgG, IgA and IgM (simple radial immunodiffusion according to Mancini *et al.*, 1965), isohemagglutinin levels, blood lymphocyte counts, percentages of B lymphocytes (immunofluorescent technique according to Pernis *et al.* (1970), as modified by Ugazio *et al.* (1974)) and of T lymphocytes (spontaneous rosette formation with sheep erythrocytes according to a previously reported method: Nespoli *et al.* (1975)), response of lymphocytes to phytohemagglutinin (PHA) and Concanavalin A (ConA) (microtechnique according to Burgio *et al.* (1975)). For every group of 3-4 hypothyroid patients at least 2 healthy control subjects matched for age and sex were also tested.

In 11 patients, all in treatment, skin tests were also carried out: tuberculin (1:1000)*, candidin (Dermatophytin 0.1:100)**, streptokinase-streptodornase (SK-SD) (Varidase, 40 U SK and 10 U SD/ml)***.

* Behringwerke. ** Hollister-Stier. *** Lederle.

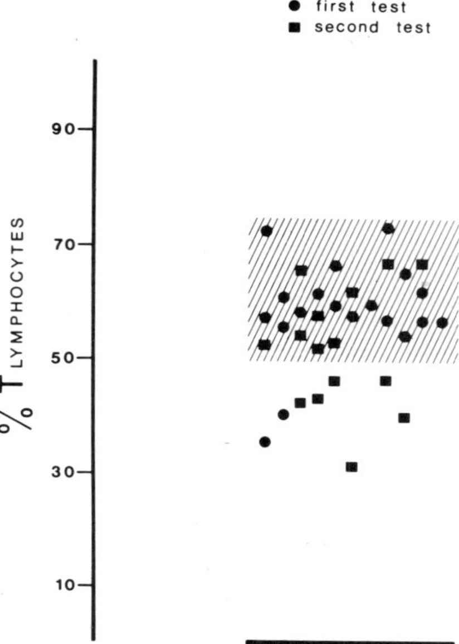

Fig. 1 Percent of peripheral blood lymphocytes forming spontaneous rosettes with sheep erythrocytes (T lymphocytes) in the hypothyroid patients. 50% is the lower limit of the normal range (shaded area) for our laboratory. The first and second tests were carried out at different times.

In 15 cases, all in treatment, complete immunologic work-up, except skin tests, was repeated at an interval of a few months.

Results are reported considering the two determinations carried out at different times. The serum immunoglobulin levels, isohemagglutinin titers and percentages of circulating B lymphocytes obtained in both the hypothyroid and control groups fell within the range of normal age-matched values for our laboratory.

Blood lymphocyte counts were always in the normal range for age. The percentage of circulating T lymphocytes, the response to mitogen stimulation (Table I) and the results of the skin tests, can be summarized as follows:

1. Low percentage of T lymphocytes (less than 50%, the lower limit of normal in our laboratory) in 6/19 (31.5%) patients, all in treatment; a low percentage was observed both times in 2 patients (Fig.1).

2. Dimished response of the lymphocytes to PHA stimulation *in vitro* (less than 40% of the mean of the simultaneously tested controls) in 8/19 (42.1%) patients; in 1 of the 2 untreated subjects the result was at the lower limit (42%) of the control values; no diminished responses were recorded when the same patients were tested again (Fig.2).

3. Diminished response of the lymphocytes to ConA stimulation (less than 40% of the mean of the simultaneously tested controls) in 5/19 (26.3%) patients; of the 5 diminished responses 4 were recorded only at the first testing, including 1 of the 2 untreated cases, and 1 only at the second testing (Fig.2).

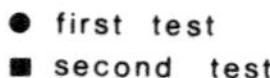

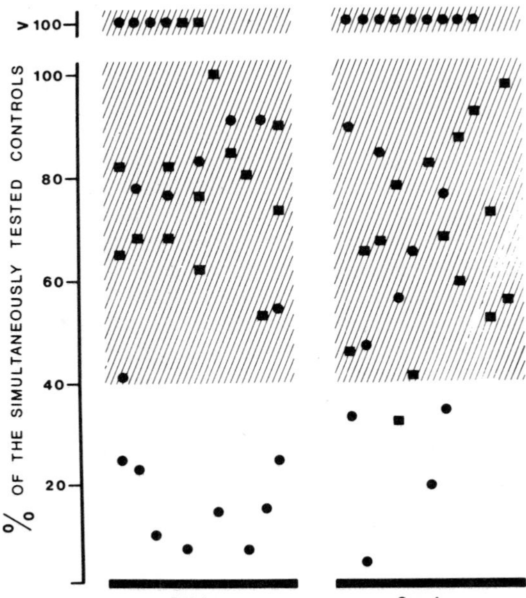

Fig. 2 PHA and ConA responsiveness of the peripheral blood lymphocytes of the hypothyroid patients. Results are expressed as percent of the simultaneously tested controls. Shaded area represents the normal range. The first and second tests were carried out at different times.

4. Decreased PHA/ConA ratio in 16/9 (84.2%) patients including the 2 untreated cases, as compared to the normal values for our laboratory (4.7 ± 1.4 S.D.) and to controls simultaneously tested. A decreased PHA/ConA ratio was observed both times in 2 patients (Fig.3).

These results were not constant; the only alterations observed both times were a low percent of T lymphocytes in 2 cases and a decrease in the PHA/ConA ratio in 2 others.

5. Skin tests with tuberculin were all negative but this was considered of little significance; skin tests with candidin were positive in 1/11 (9.1%) patients, whereas the percentage of positive responses is about 90% in normal children of comparable age and sex; similarly, only 3/11 (27%) patients were positive to skin testing with SK-SD as compared to an expected percentage of about 60% (Burgio *et al.*, 1970) (Fig.4).

Given the normality of serum immunoglobulins, isohemagglutinins and percent of circulating B lymphocytes it appears that the Bursa-equivalent system was not affected in our patients; however, a reduced response to antigenic stimuli cannot be excluded; in fact, we plan to explore the antibody response to vaccination in these patients.

As regards the thymus-dependent system, in more than 80% of our patients some deviation from normal was observed in at least one of the parameters

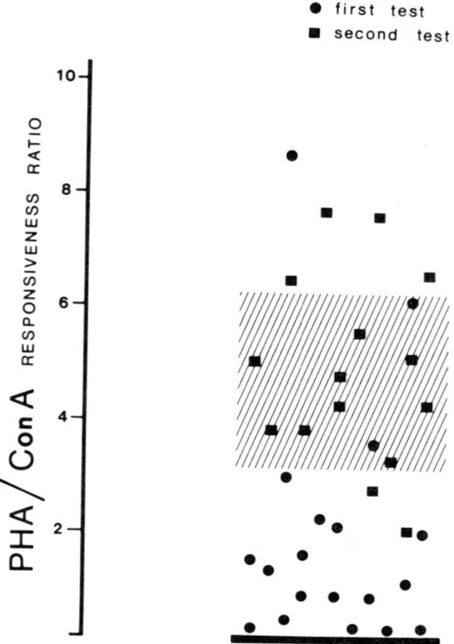

Fig.3 Ratio of PHA- to ConA-responsiveness of the lymphocytes of the hypothyroid patients. The shaded area represents 2SD of the mean value of the ratio for normal lymphocytes in our laboratory. The first and second tests were carried out at different times.

studied, although almost always inconstant. Technical errors could be reasonably excluded, given also the normal results of the simultaneously tested controls; furthermore all patients were free of clinically evident infections that might have interfered with the results of the tests. The possibility of changes in time of the thyroid status of the patients, perhaps related to dosage variations in the replacement therapy were considered, but only in a few patients they explained the differences observed. Furthermore, no differences were observed between treated and untreated patients. GH was not measured but, on the basis of our experience with some pituitary dwarfs, we do not think that the variations observed can be due to modifications in growth hormone secretion.

Discussion of the individual results would probably prove of little help in interpreting our findings. Alterations of the same type, although more marked and less variable, are found in primary deficiencies of the thymus-dependent immune system (DiGeorge and Nezelof syndromes, etc.) and may be interpreted as disturbances in T lymphocyte differentiation: the details of this maturation process are still far from being completely known. On the basis of clinical and experimental evidence it is thought that some of the hemopoietic stem cells differentiate into lymphoid precursors of T lymphocytes (Pre-T); these cells migrate to the thymus where, under the influence of the "microenvironment" and of thymic hormonal activity, differentiate into T1 cells (reversible differentiation if thymic hormone is withdrawn), which leave the thymus to reach peripheral lymphoid organs, in particular the

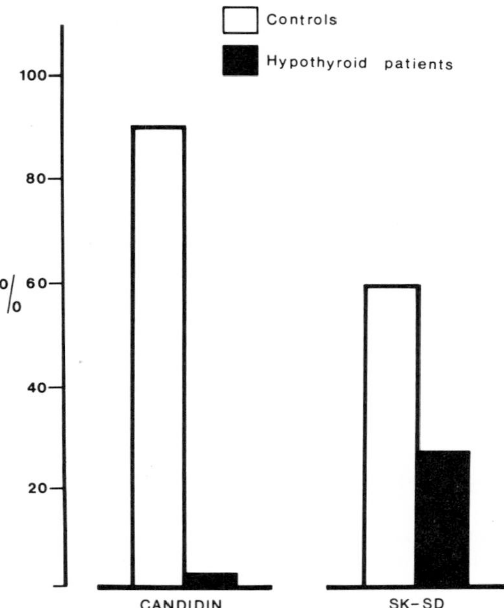

Fig.4 Percent of hypothyroid patients with positive skin tests to candidin and SK-SD, as compared to that of age- and sex-matched controls.

spleen. By interaction with antigen and in the presence of circulating thymic hormonal factors, T1 lymphocytes differentiate in part to effector cells (transplant rejection, destruction of cells infected with viruses or intracellular bacteria, etc.) and in part to memory cells of cell-mediated immunity (T2 lymphocytes) (irreversible differentiation) (Fig.5). Some properties of Pre-T, T1 and T2 lymphocytes, demonstrated mostly in the mouse, but in part also in man, are indicated in Table II.

To what extent is this information useful, at least for a preliminary interpretation of the data obtained in primary hypothyroidism?

It is interesting to recall that of 13 cases with a diminished response to at least one of the two mitogens used (PHA, ConA) in only 5 was it to ConA alone; in 1 of these the response to PHA was at the lower limits of normal (42%). Comparing these data with the information summarized in Table II, it seems reasonable to hypothesize that the circulating lymphocytes of these patients were in some way "immature" (failure of transition from T1 to T2?). If we refer to an accepted animal model (Stobo, 1972; Shortman *et al.*, 1975; Droege and Zucker, 1975) the hypothesis of a maturation defect is further reinforced by the frequent, although not constant, reduction up to the inversion of the normal ratio between the proliferative response to PHA and ConA, even in some patients whose responses to the two mitogens were within normal limits. The finding of low percentages of circulating T lymphocytes in some cases can be interpreted in a similar fashion.

The question can be raised as to whether the defect is at the T1 lymphocyte

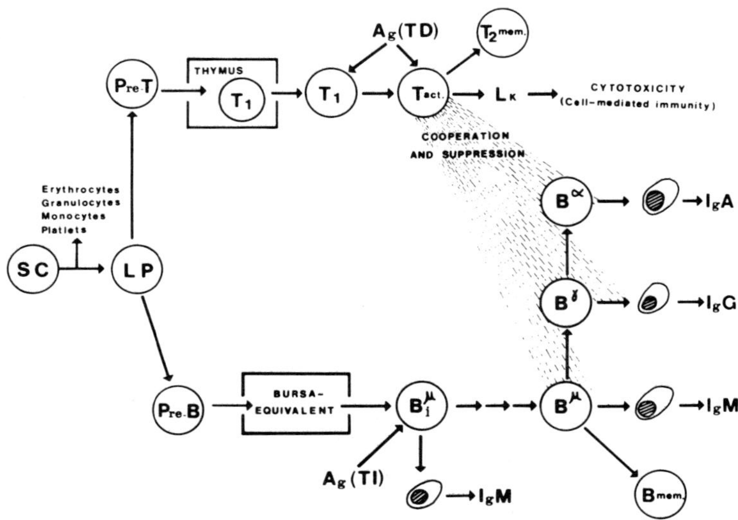

Fig.5 Differentiation pathways of the T and B cell lines from the hematopoietic stem cell. Ag (TD): thymus-dependent antigen; Ag (TI): thymus-independent antigen; B^{μ}, B^{γ}, B^{d}: precursors of the IgM, IgG and IgA secreting plasma cells; B_i: immature B lymphocyte which can only differentiate to IgM-secreting plasma cells when triggered by an Ag (TI); $B_{mem.}$: memory B lymphocyte; LK: lymphokines; LP: lymphoid precursor; Pre-B and Pre-T: precursors of the immunocompetent B and T lymphocytes; SC: stem cell; $T_{act.}$: activated T lymphocyte; T_2 mem.: memory T lymphocytes.

Table II. Some biological properties of T lymphocytes.

	Pre-T	T_1	T_2
Recirculation	±	±	+++
Predominant T cells in:	Bone marrow Spleen	Thymus Spleen	Lymph node Peripheral blood
Life span	Short	Short	Long
Rosette-forming capacity with sheep erythrocytes	—	+	+
PHA-responsiveness	—	+	+++
ConA-responsiveness	—	+++	+++

level (insensitivity to the stimulus) or in the afferent phase, that is, antigen stimulation.

If a maturation defect of thymus-dependent lymphocytes is confirmed in primary hypothyroidism, at least 2 pathogenetic hypotheses could be suggested: an embryologic defect or an endocrine-functional defect.

In fact, since the sites of embryologic origin of thymus and thyroid are quite close, the "noxa" responsible for thyroid hypoplasias may also produce failure of thymus development in some cases. It is worth mentioning in this context that the most typical of the hypoplasic thymus syndromes, the DiGeorge syndrome or the 3rd and 4th pharyngeal pouch syndrome may be associated with hypothyroidism (see Hitzig (1973)).

The hypothesis of an endocrine-functional defect mostly relies on experimental findings which, although contradictory and fragmentary, seem to indicate that thyroid function is in some way necessary for the normal maturation of immunocompetent lymphocytes. It has also been shown that lymphocytes possess receptors with a high affinity for thyroid hormones, particularly T3 (Holm *et al.*, 1975).

Since thyroid hormone activity on target cells is known to be mediated by an increase in the intracellular synthesis of cAMP, it is probably worth mentioning that various substances capable of increasing intracellular synthesis of cAMP, like prolactin, glucagon and prostaglandin E1, have been shown to induce maturation of mouse thymocytes *in vitro* (Sing and Owen, 1976); furthermore, it has been demonstrated that the differentiation processes induced by thymic hormone are accompanied by an increased intracellular level of cAMP.

For the moment these observations are not more than suggestive; however, to hypothesize that the thyroid has some influence on lymphocyte differentiation appears useful especially since such a hypothesis can be verified experimentally.

ACKNOWLEDGEMENTS

I am indebted to Dr. Alberto G. Ugazio whose cooperation made this study possible and to Dr. Virginia Monafo for assistance with the manuscript.

REFERENCES

Allison, A.C. (1974). *In: Proceedings of the Immunological Conference Pavia*, Villa D'Este, May 27-29 (G.R. Burgio, G. Astaldi and A. De Barbieri, eds) pp.123-130.

Aoki, N., Wakisaka, G. and Nagata, I. (1973). *Lancet* 2, 49-50.

Astaldi, A. (1976). *Pathologica* **68**, 1-8.

Baroni, C.D., Fabris, N. and Bertoli, G. (1969). *Immunology* **17**, 303-314.

Bentley, H.P., Hughes, E.R. and Peterson, R.D.A. (1974). *Nature* **252**, 747-748.

Besedowsky, H.O. and Sorkin, E. (1974). *Nature* **249**, 356-358.

Brody, J.I. and Greenberg, S. (1972). *J. clin. Endocr. Metab.* **35**, 574-579.

Burgio, G.R., Biscatti, G., Rizzoni, G., Genova, R. and Severi, F. (1970). *Mschr. Kinderheilk.* **118**, 267-271.

Burgio, G.R., Ugazio, A.G., Nespoli, L., Marcioni, A.F., Bottelli, A.M. and Pasquali, F. (1975). *Eur. J. Immunol.* **5**, 600-603.

Chilgren, R.A., Menwissen, H.J., Quie, P.G., Good, R.A. and Hong, R. (1969). *Lancet* 1, 1286-1288.

Dougherty, T.F. (1952). *Physiol. Rev.* **32**, 379-401.

Droege, W. and Zucker, R. (1975). *Transplant. Rev.* **25**, 3-25.

Duquesnoy, R.J. (1975). *In* "Immunodeficiency in Man and Animals" (D. Bergsma, ed) **Vol. XI**, pp.536-543. The National Foundation – March of Dimes. Sinauer Associates, Inc., Publishers, Sunderland, Mass.

Farid, N.R., Munro, R.E., Row, V.V. and Volpé, R. (1973). *New Engl. J. Med.* **289**, 1145.

Gershwin, M.E. and Steinberg, A.D. (1973). *Lancet* 2, 1174-1176.

Goldstein, G. (1976). *V International Congress of Endocrinology*, Hamburg, July 18-24, **(Abstract).**

Gyllensten, L. (1953). *Acta Anat.* **Suppl.18 = 1 ad.vol. XVII**, 1-163.
Hitzig, W.H. (1973). *In* "Immunologic Disorders in Infants and Children" (E.R. Stiehm and V.A. Fulginiti, eds) pp.215-235. W.B. Saunders Company, Philadelphia, London, Toronto.
Holm, A.C., Lemarchand-Béraud, T., Scazziga, B.R., Cuttelod, S. (1975). *Acta endocr. (Copenh.)* **80**, 642-656.
Hong, R., Gatti, R., Rathbun, J.C. and Good, R.A. (1970). *New Engl. J. Med.* **282**, 470-474.
Kirkpatrick, C.H., Rich, R.R. and Bennett, J.E. (1971). *Ann. Intern. Med.* **74**, 955-978.
Irvine, W.J. (1976). *V International Congress of Endocrinology*, Hamburg, July 18-24. **(Abstr.)**.
MacCuish, A.C., Urbaniak, S.J., Campbell, C.J., Duncan, L.J.P. and Irvine, W.J. (1974). *Diabetes* **23**, 708-712.
Maciel, R.M.B., Miki, S.S., Nicolau, W. and Mendes, N.F. (1976). *J. clin. Endocr. Metab.* **42**, 583-587.
Mahmoud, A.A.F., Cheever, A.W. and Warren, K.S. (1975). *J. infect. Dis.* **131**, 634-642.
Mahmoud, A.A.F., Rodman, H.M., Mandel, M.A. and Warren, K.S. (1976). *J. clin. Invest.* **57**, 362-367.
Mancini, G., Carbonara, A.O. and Heremans, J.F. (1965). *Immunochemistry* **2**, 235-254.
Montes, L.F., Pittman, C.S., Moore, W.J., Taylor, C.D. and Cooper, M.D. (1972). *J.A.M.A.* **221**, 156-159.
Nespoli, L., Ugazio, A.G. and Altamura, D. (1975). *Riv. Ital. Pediat.* **1**, 17-29.
Nishizuka, Y. and Sakakura, T. (1969). *Science* **166**, 753-755.
Nishizuka, Y. and Sakakura, T. (1971a). *Endocrinology* **89**, 886-893.
Nishizuka, Y. and Sakakura, T. (1971b). *Endocrinology* **89**, 902-909.
Pelletier, M., Montplaisir, S., Dardenne, M. and Bach, J.F. (1976). *Immunology* **30**, 783-788.
Pernis, B., Forni, L. and Amante, L. (1970). *J. exp. Med.* **132**, 1001-1018.
Pierpaoli, W., Baroni, C., Fabris, N. and Sorkin, E. (1969). *Immunology* **16**, 217-230.
Pierpaoli, W., Fabris, N. and Sorkin, E. (1970). *In* "Hormones and the Immune Response" (G.E.W. Wolstenholme and J. Knight, eds) pp.126-153. Ciba Foundation Study Group No. 36. Churchill, London.
Pierpaoli, W. and Besedowski, H.O. (1975). *Clin. exp. Immunol.* **20**, 323-338.
Pouplard, A., Bottazzo, G.F., Doniach, D. and Roitt, I.M. (1976). *Nature* **261**, 142-144.
Sakakura, T. and Nishizuka, Y. (1972). *Endocrinology* **90**, 431-437.
Shortman, K., Boehmer von, H., Lipp, J. and Hopper, K. (1975). *Transplant. Rev.* **25**, 163-210.
Sing, U. and Owen, J.J.T. (1976). *Eur. J. Immunol.* **6**, 59-62.
Stobo, J.D. (1972). *Transplant. Rev.* **11**, 60-86.
Ugazio, A.G., Marcioni, A.F., Astaldi, A. and Burgio, G.R. (1974). *Acta Paediatr. Scand.* **63**, 205-208.
Urbaniak, S.J., Penhale, W.J. and Irvine, W.J. (1974). *Clin. exp. Immunol.* **18**, 449-459.
Valdimarsson, H., Holt, L., Riches, H.R.C. and Hobbs, J.R. (1970). *Lancet* **1**, 1259-1261.
Waldmann, T.A., Durm, M., Broder, S., Blackman, M., Blaese, R.M. and Strober, W. (1974). *Lancet* **2**, 609-613.
Wara, D.W., Reiter, E.D., Ammans, J.A. and Kaplan, S.L. (1973). *New Engl. J. Med.* **289**, 1145.

EXPERIENCE WITH THYROTROPIN RELEASING HORMONE (TRH): TEST IN SUSPECTED THYROID DISORDERS IN CHILDHOOD

J. Girard, J.J. Staub*, P.W. Nars, U. Bühler, P. Studer and J.B. Baumann

Endocrine Department, University Children's Hospital

and

**Medizinische Universitäts-Poliklinik Basel, Switzerland*

ABSTRACT

Hypothalamo-pituitary-thyroid function can be assessed with great sensitivity by measuring the plasma TSH, Tri-iodothyronine and Thyroxin, response to the intravenous or oral administration of the synthetic tripeptide thyrotropin-releasing hormone (TRH). For the intravenous test 200 μg of TRH (infants below 6 months of age 100 μg) were injected and the plasma TSH was measured before injection and 30 (and ev. 60) minutes later. The maximum TSH response occurs at 20--30 minutes. TSH rises under normal conditions from a basal value of 3 μU/ml (1.5–4.9 μU/ml, 10th–90th percentile) to a mean maximum of 11.3 μU/ml (6.1–22.3 μU/ml, 10th–90th percentile) in children and to a mean maximum of 16.7 ± 7.4 μU/ml in infants. Tri-iodothryronine increases from a mean value of 1.17 ng/ml after 120 minutes to a mean maximum of 1.62 ng/ml. The increase in Tri-iodithyronine is statistically significant, but not reliable for a definitive interpretation of an individual test. Thyroxin increases only slightly.

Oral stimulation with TRH (20 mg/m^2 body surface) has a depot effect and leads to a prolonged and extended rise of plasma TSH to a mean maximum of 14.4 (95% conf. lim. = ±2 SD_{log} 5.5–37.7) μU/ml, after three hours. T_3 increases to a mean maximum of 2.19 (± 0.62) ng/ml. TRH tests have been performed with 130 newborns, infants and children, from 2 days to 18 years of age. In suspected hypothalamo-pituitary disorders TRH stimulation has been used in combination with LH-RH and insulin-induced hypoglycemia or arginine infusion. Hyperthyroidism can be excluded by a significant TSH response to TRH. A low or absent response to i.v. stimulation was however observed in obesity, anorexia nervosa, and rarely in euthyroid young adults.

Obvious hypothyrodism can usually be diagnosed on clinical grounds. Grossly elevated non-stimulated plasma TSH levels confirm the diagnosis. In case of subclinical primary thyroid dysfunction a TSH stimulation above 2 SD of the normal response, is however, a sensitive indicator of a developing hypothyroid state. Furthermore, the test has been used for control of substitution therapy in hypothyroidism and of adequate suppression in Graves' disease. In the follow-up of hyperthyroidism a relapse is detectable before the clinical expressions of the symptoms. In secondary and tertiary (hypothalamic) hypothyroidism, TSH response to TRH can be misleading. Apparently normal TSH responses to TRH have been observed in clearly clinically hypothyroid subjects. The oral or intravenous TRH test has proved to be the most sensitive parameter of thyroid function. The test is harmless and easy to perform on the out-patients and can detect preclinical hyper- and hypothyroidism.

INTRODUCTION

Synthetic thyrotropin releasing hormone (TRH) has been widely used for assessing the TSH reserve of the thyrotrophs of the anterior pituitary. In a euthyroid state, plasma TSH increases in response to TRH within 20 to 30 minutes of a mean maximum of about 10 micro-units/ml. Reports on TSH response in physiological and pathological states are numerous for adults (Sawin and Hershamn, 1976; Hall *et al.*, 1972; Hershman, 1974; Faglia *et al.*, 1972; Shenkman *et al.*, 1973; Vagenakis *et al.*, 1974; Azizi *et al.*, 1975; Besser and Mortimer, 1974; Beckers *et al.*, 1972; Fleischner *et al.*, 1972) but few for children (Girard *et al.*, 1973; Brock Jacobsen *et al.*, 1976; Job *et al.*, 1971; Folley *et al.*, 1972). In contrast to adult endocrinology, hyperthyroidism is not the predominant problem in pediatric endocrinology. In disturbance of growth and development an impaired thyroid function must be excluded. Furthermore, the thyroid state in patients with goiters has to be defined and finally any suspicion of hypothyroidism in the newborn period is of outstanding individual and social economic importance. A suspicion of hypothyroidism in infancy should therefore be excluded or confirmed with certainty in the shortest possible time. In the following our experience with the highly sensitive TRH test of pituitary thyroid function in children is reported.

PATIENTS, MATERIALS AND METHODS

TSH was assayed with a double antibody radioimmunoassay using human TSH (Kabi) for labeling, MCR 68/38 as a reference preparation and a rabbit antiserum raised against human TSH. For T_3 and T_4 a radioimmunoassay using I^{125} labeled T_4 and T_3 respectively (Hoechst) and a charcoal separation was used. Antisera to T_3 and T_4 were raised in rabbits.

For the intravenous test TRH (Hoffman-La-Roche) was injected in a single dose of 200 μg. Children below one year of age received 100 μg TRH. Blood samples were drawn before injection, (20) – 30 – 60 – (90) and 120 minutes after administration of TRH. Stimulation with oral TRH: ingestion of 20 mg/m^2 body surface TRH after fasting for at least 2 hours. Blood samples were taken before ingestion and three hours later (Girard *et al.*, 1973; Staub and Girard, 1975).

The patients investigated and the age distribution are given in Table I. In patients with suspected hypothalamo-pituitary insufficiency, i.e. in most patients

Table I. TRH – Tests.

Patients	No.	Age
Stunted growth	65	(2 9/12 – 17)
Anorexia nervosa	7	(12 – 18)
Obesity	16	(3 9/12 – 16)
Goiter	9	(6 – 15 10/12)
Hyperthyroidism	21	(10 9/12 – 16)
Hypothyroidism	30	(– 17)
Hypothalamo-pit.	18	(6/12 – 20)

with stunted growth, TRH has been combined with insulin-induced hypoglycemia and LH-RH tests (Girard *et al.*, 1974). Children with goiters and clinical signs of thyroid dysfunction are divided into hyper- and hypothyroidism respectively. Two of the patients with hyperthyroidism had repeated TRH tests during treatment. The youngest mean age is found within the group of suspected hypothyroidism. A noticeable side effect has never been observed in any of the tests performed.

RESULTS IN EUTHYROID STATES IN INFANTS AND CHILDREN

In children of preschool and school age the TSH response to intravenous injection of 200 μg of TRH does not differ from that observed in adults. TSH usually increases from undetectable basal levels to a median maximum level of 11.0 μU/ml within 30 minutes. Over a period of two hours the level falls again to the basal value. The basal median value is 3.0 μU/ml (10th percentile to 90th percentile = 1.5 – 4.9 μU/ml). The maximum value at 30 min lies within 6.1 μU/ml (10th percentile) and 22.3 μU/ml (90th percentile). This normal response was calculated from 65 clinically euthyroid children with a mean age of 10.8 years (Fig.1). A significant difference in the values between the 40 boys and the 25 girls was not observed. For the diagnosis of hypothyroid states – the major problem in pediatrics – it is the upper limit of TSH response to TRH which is relevant. It must be noted, therefore, that in infancy a more pronounced effect is seen than in children (Fig.2).

Within the group of 15 infants with a mean age of 15.7 months TSH increased within 30 min from an undetectable value to a mean maximum of 16.7 ± 7.4 microunits/ml. Two hours after injection of 100 μg of TRH the mean TSH concentration (7 ± 1.8 μU/ml) had not returned to basal levels.(Because the number of infants investigated was rather small, mean and standard deviation is used instead of percentiles in spite of the non-normal distribution.) The values of Figs 1 and 2 correspond well with those reported previously in infancy and childhood (Girard *et al.*, 1973; Job *et al.*, 1971; Chaussain and Job, 1972). The TSH stimulation is somewhat higher than in adult patients investigated in this same laboratory.

Over 2 hours T_3 increased in euthyroid children from a mean value of 1.17 ± 0.25 to a mean of 1.6 ± 0.36 ng/ml. The mean maximum increase is thus 0.4 ± 0.51 ng T_3/ml (Fig.3). This increase is statistically significant, but the wide variation does not allow an interpretation in individual cases.

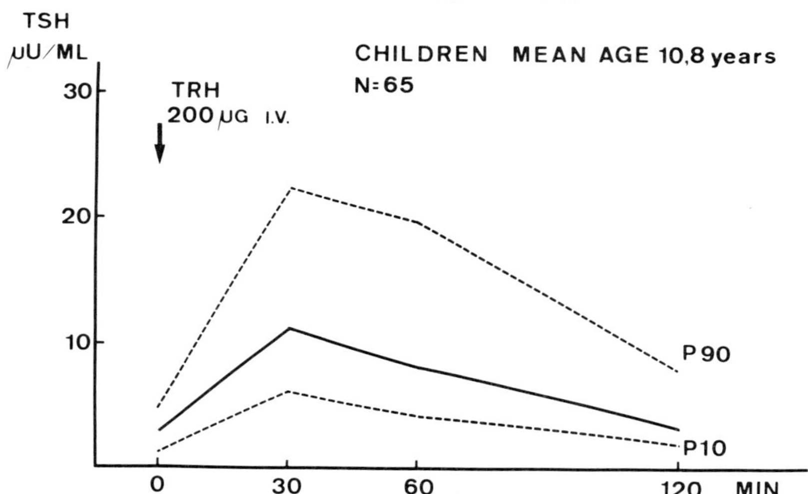

Fig. 1 TSH response to TRH in children.

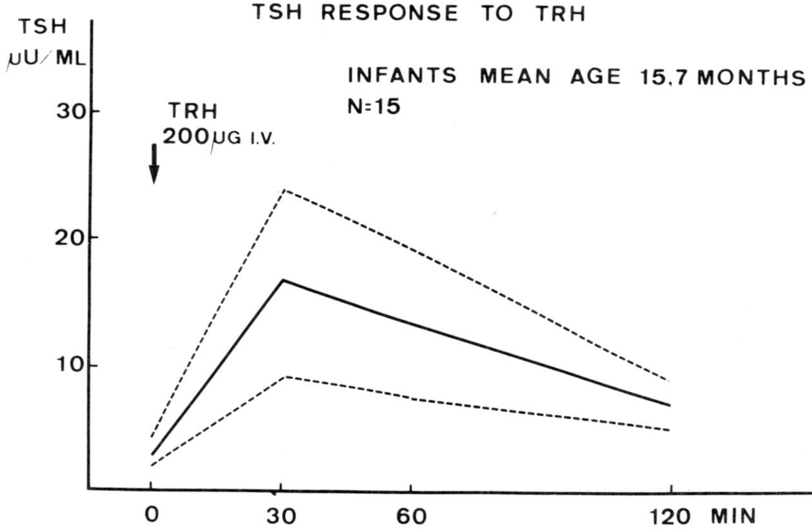

Fig. 2 TSH response to TRH in infants.

After oral stimulation with 20 mg/m^2 body surface of TRH, the mean TSH maximum reached is somewhat higher than after 0.2 mg of intravenous stimulation and reached 14.4 μU/ml.

The most striking difference between oral and intravenous stimulation is however the pattern of TSH response. After oral stimulation the maximum TSH level is observed 3 h after ingestion and after 8 h the mean level is still somewhat above the basal concentration. This depot effect of oral stimulation is reflected in

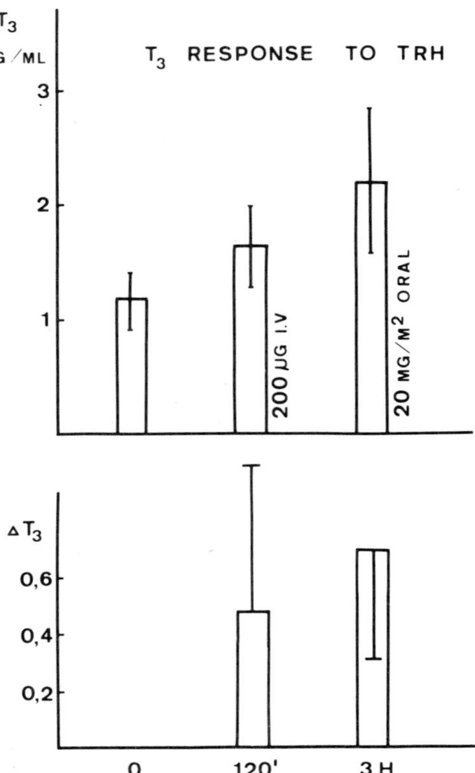

Fig.3 T_3 response to i.v. TRH (120 min) and oral TRH (3 h).

a more pronounced increase in T_3. The maximum level of 2.1 ± 0.62 ng/ml was observed after 3 hours. This corresponded to an increase of 0.69 ± 0.39 ng/ml (Fig.3).

The oral test offers thus the main advantage of assessing the pituitary and thyroid "reserve". It is a more potent stimulus and might be helpful in distinguishing a suspected TSH suppression, which is an important differential diagnosis in the elderly where the TSH response to TRH is normally low (Snyder and Utiger, 1972; Wenzel *et al.*, 1972).

Obesity and Anorexia Nervosa

Obesity. In 16 obese children (definition: body weight at least 20% above weight for height percentile) the pattern of TSH response to TRH did not differ from normals, but the mean maximum was somewhat lower (Fig.4). The lower mean response in obese children is due to the 2 out of 16 patients with a very low, just detectable increase in TSH and to the 1 out of 16 patients with no measurable TSH response whatsoever.

All obese patients were clinically euthyroid with normal T_3 and T_4 levels. In obese patients a reduction in the growth hormone response to various stimuli and an impaired cortisol response to insulin-induced hypoglycemia has been observed (Girard *et al.*, 1972). The absent or low TSH response can not be explained

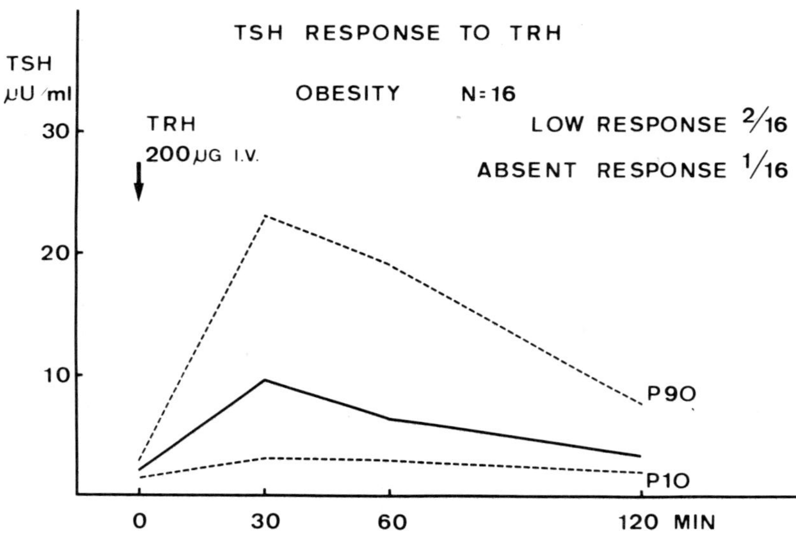

Fig. 4 TSH response to TRH in obese children.

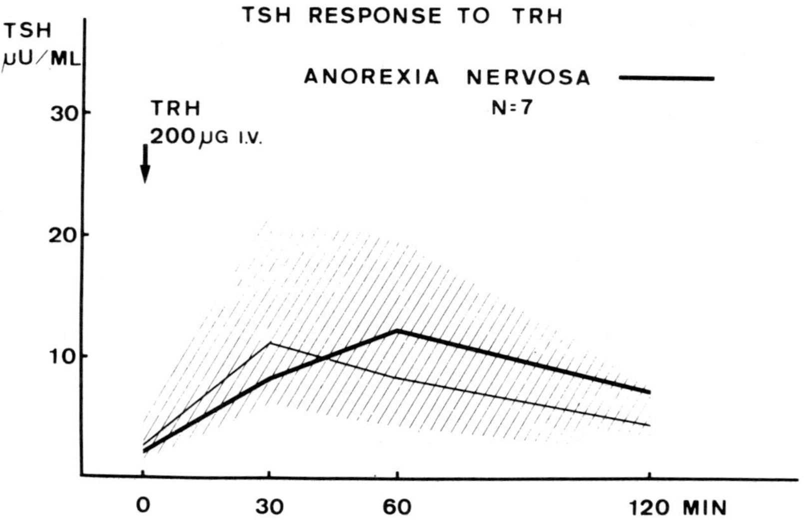

Fig. 5 TSH response to TRH in children with anorexia nervosa.

by the relatively lower dose (related to body weight), but must be taken as indication of an abnormality of hypothalamic function, which can be demonstrated in some of the obese patients. An increased cortisol production rate could explain the impaired TSH response (Poloa *et al.*, 1972; Otsuki *et al.*, 1973).

Anorexia nervosa. In anorexia nervosa the best known hypothalamo-pituitary dysfunction is a diminished LH and FSH secretion leading to secondary

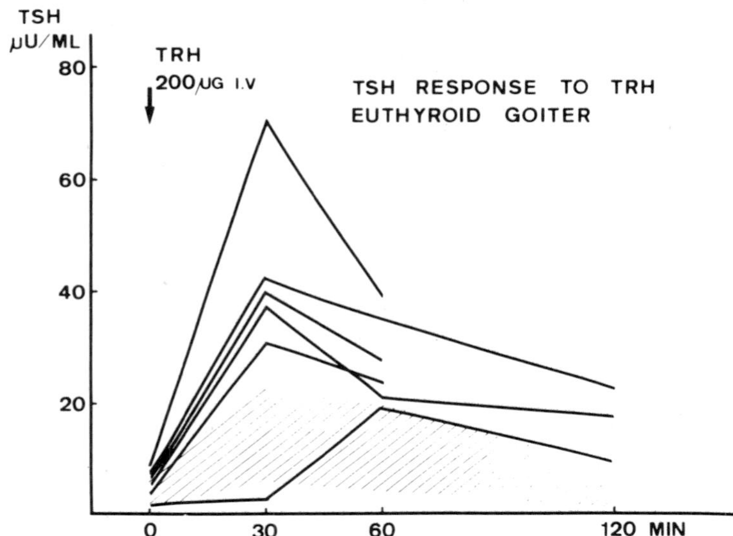

Fig. 6 TSH response to TRH in 6 children with euthyroid goiters. Shadowed area 10th to 90th percentile of normal response.

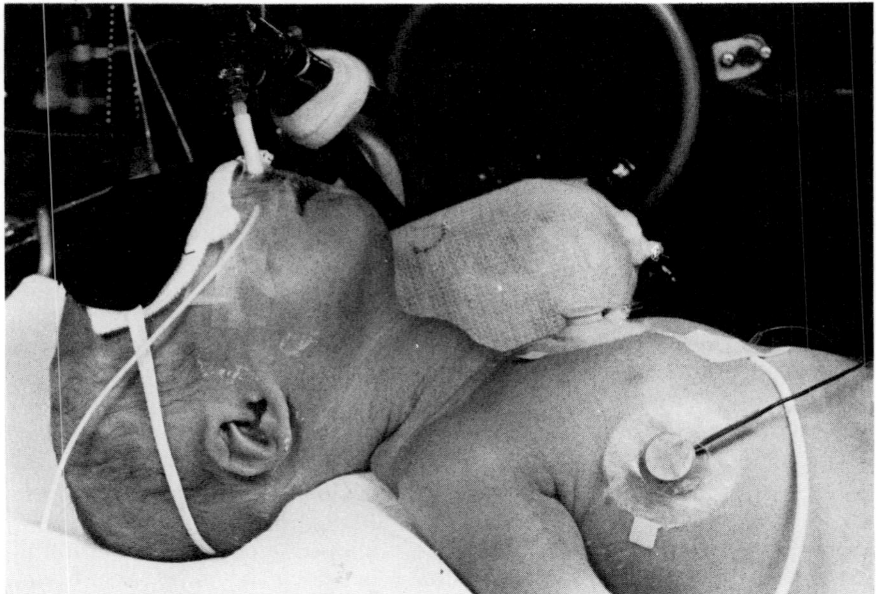

Fig. 7 Lithium-induced goiter in a premature.

amenorrhea (Frankel and Jenkins, 1975). Under-nutrition can lead to a fall in total T_4 and T_3 and to an increase in reversed T_3. TSH response to TRH in these cases is normal and indicates a euthyroid state during a phase of overall low "metabolism". In our 7 patients the mean TSH rises to a normal maximum level

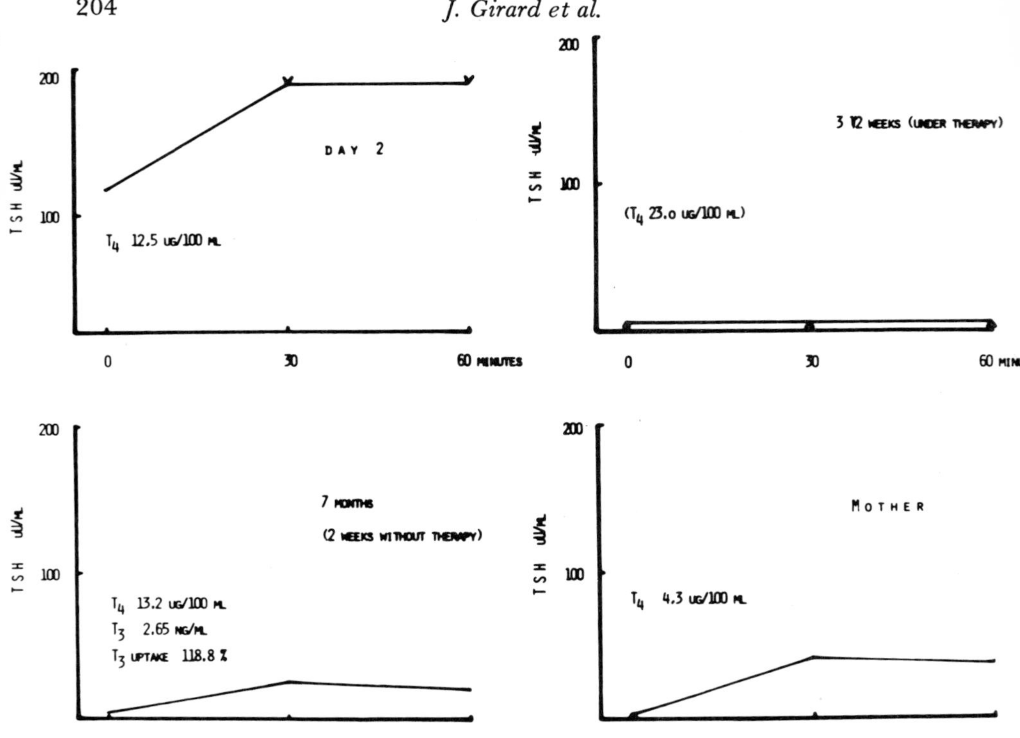

Fig.8 TSH response to TRH in newborn with lithium-induced goiter. At 2 days, during therapy, after withdrawal of therapy and in the mother.

of 12.2 μU/ml. The maximum is, however, observed at 60 min only. This delayed response is reflected in a still elevated level of 7.4 μU/ml after 2 h (Fig.5). This pattern of pituitary hormone response to hypothalamic releasing hormones has been interpreted as characteristic for a hypothalamic lesion.

SUSPECTED THYROID DISORDERS

Euthyroid Diffuse Goiter

In order to decide on a therapy the "activity" of the hypothalamo-pituitary thyroid axis should be documented in patients with diffuse enlargement of the thyroid gland. Figure 6 shows the individual TSH values in 6 patients with euthyroid goiter and normal basal TSH concentrations. All children were clinically euthyroid. The maximum response to TRH is increased above the upper normal limit in 5 of the 6 patients.

This observation underlines the sensitivity of the test, which is superior to a single basal TSH. It furthermore points to an increased pituitary TSH reserve in this condition and thus supports the necessity for a replacement therapy in spite of normal T_4 and T_3 levels. The following unusual case history of a lithium-induced goiter illustrates the possible importance of TRH tests.

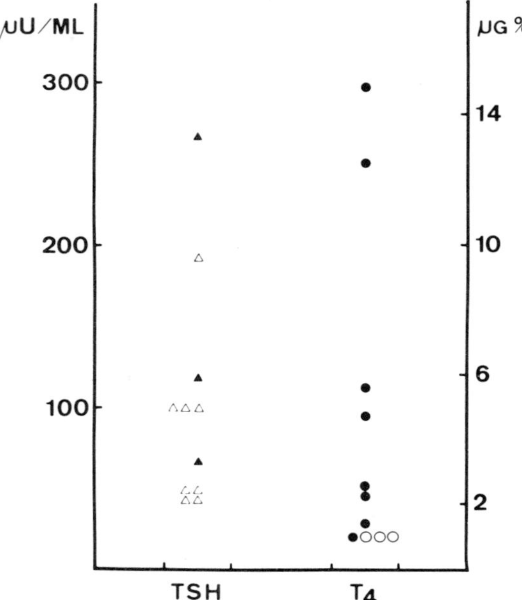

Fig.9 T_4 and TSH values without stimulation in primary hypothyroidism.

Case History

Throughout pregnancy a mother was under therapy with lithium (750 mg/d). A prematurely (35th week of gestation) born girl presented with a large goiter (Fig.7). Bone age was not retarded and overt clinical signs of hypothyroidism were not observed. T_4 was 12.5 µg% but TSH elevated to 118 µU/ml at the second day of life. TSH increase in response to 100 µg TRH to levels above 300 µU/ml (Fig.8). Replacement therapy was started with Eltroxin. At the second TRH test after 3½ weeks of therapy, TSH was undetectable throughout the test. At 7 months of age therapy was withdrawn for 2 weeks and a TRH test performed. Basal TSH was undetectable and the pattern of response well within normal limits. A euthyroid state was thus documented and replacement therapy could definitively be withdrawn.

PRIMARY HYPOTHYROIDISM

TSH secretion rises rapidly in response to a lowered T_4. T_4 values below the lower limit of normal and grossly elevated basal TSH values are usually sufficient for the diagnosis of primary hypothyroidism. It is of great importance to note, however, that normal or even elevated T_3 concentration can be observed in primary hypothyroidism with elevated basal TSH concentrations.

Figure 9 shows TSH and T_4 values in children with primary thyroid insufficiency. TSH concentrations are in all instances above 40 µU/ml. In 7 patients T_4 levels are clearly hypothyroid. Two patients have T_4 values which are at the lower limit of normal. In 1 patient, a newborn with lithium-induced goiter (see above),

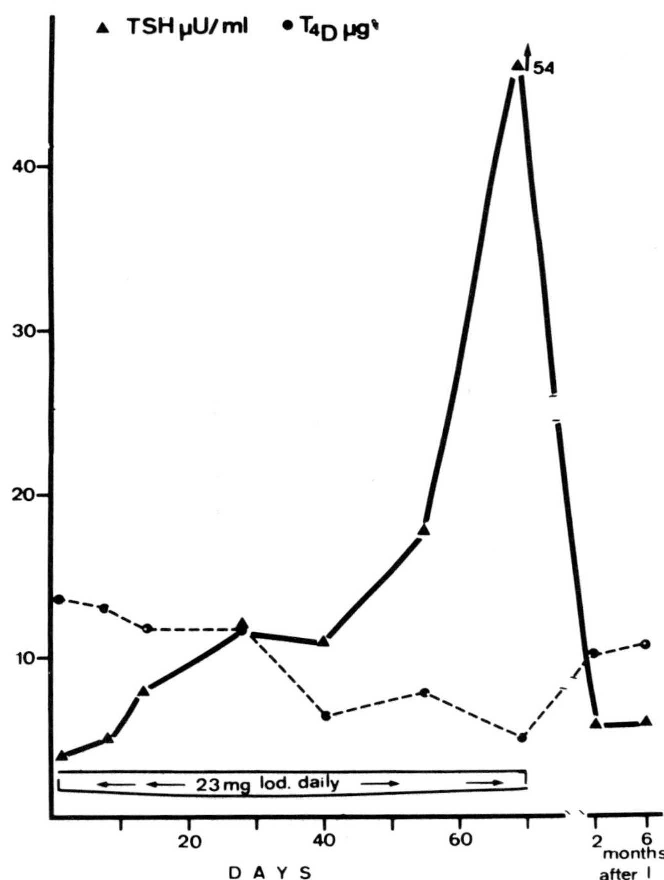

Fig. 10 TSH and T_4 during iodine load in iodide-induced goiter.

normal thyroxin could be measured and in 1 patient thyroxin is elevated due to substitution therapy.

The sensitivity of the feedback system is well documented by a patient with an iodide-induced goiter. During intrauterine life this child received two intra-uterine transfusions (29th week and 32nd week 10 ml Lipiodol into the amniotic sac and Endographine intraperitoneally) and was thus exposed to a total iodine dose of 12 g. Three weeks after delivery hypothyroidism was diagnosed and replacement therapy started. In order to confirm the diagnosis the child was challenged at 1 year of age with an iodine load. Figure 10 shows that TSH clearly rises above the upper normal limit into an abnormal range well before thyroxin concentration falls below the lower limit of normal.

It is obvious, therefore, that TSH rises very rapidly during a developing hypothyroidism and is a sensitive indicator of impaired thyroid function. In some cases a TRH test can be necesssary to confirm a suspected impaired thyroid function. This is illustrated by a girl 7 6/12 years of age, who had been investigated

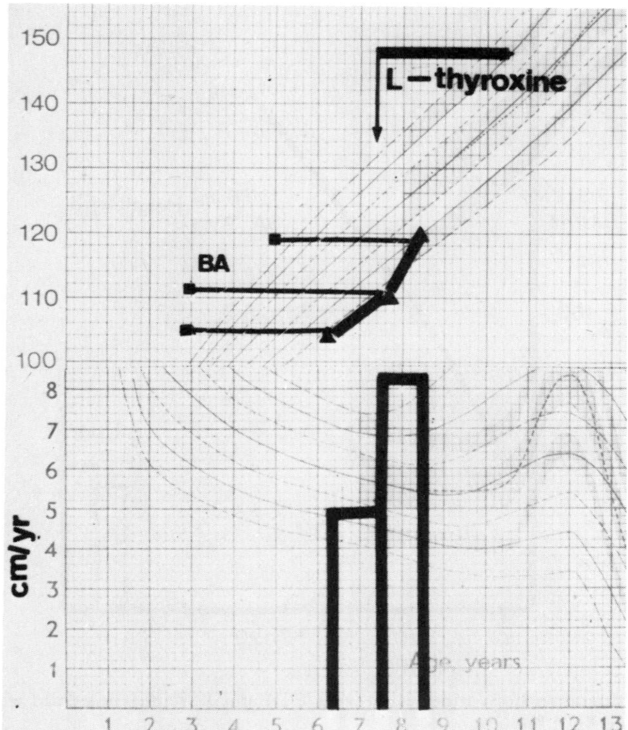

Fig.11 Ectopic thyroid gland: height, bone age and height velocity before and during therapy.

for stunted growth. Clinical signs of hypothyroidism could not be found. The height was just below the 3rd percentile and bone age severely retarded (Fig.11). Thyroxin was in the normal range and basal TSH elevated. Subsequently, a TRH test was performed, which again showed an increased basal TSH and an exaggerated response to TRH. Thyroxin was at the lower limit of normal (Fig.12). Scintigram and iodine uptake revealed an ectopic thyroid gland with a diminished uptake. Substitution therapy was started and the catch-up growth and development of bone age is shown in Fig.11.

In hypothyroid states the increased TSH reserve is present for several days and weeks after adequate thyroxin therapy. In Fig.13 TSH and T_4 values in a case of primary hypothyroidism are shown during therapy. TSH induced an exaggerated TSH response 16 days after commencement of substitution therapy. At that time thyroxin levels in plasma were above upper normal limits.

HYPOTHALAMO-PITUITARY DISORDERS

It was hoped that, with the introduction of synthetic hypothalamic releasing hormones, a distinction between hypothalamic and pituitary disorders would be possible. Accumulating experience shows, however, that secondary or tertiary

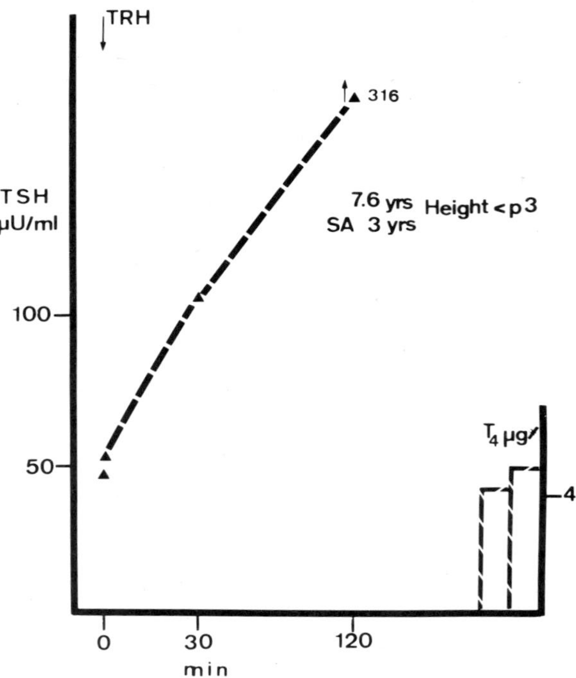

Fig.12 TSH with and without stimulation with TRH and T_4 values in a child with ectopic thyroid gland (see Fig.11).

lesions are not reflected by a well-defined pattern of hormone response (Staub and Girard, 1975; Faglia *et al.*, 1973; Patel and Burger, 1973). Figure 14 shows the TSH response to 200 µg TRH in 7 children with hypothalamo-pituitary disorders. The TSH response was absent in 2 of the 3 clinically euthyroid patients with normal T_4 and T_3 concentration: a boy with an adrenal insufficiency due to a hypothalamic failure, a boy (twin premature) with cerebral palsy and minimal brain damage and a boy with a familial hypothalamic lesion and an isolated growth hormone deficiency.

Two children with a craniopharyngioma, 1 girl with a large pinealoma and 1 boy with a septico-ocular syndrome (Brook *et al.*, 1972) were clearly clinically hypothyroid, with low T_4 values. The hypothyroid state could hardly be diagnosed from the TSH response. In 1 patient an absent response confirmed an area of complete destruction in the pituitary. In 3 patients, however, a definitive increase of TSH from 0 min to 30 min could be observed. In 2 of these patients a delayed maximum response to the high peak level was seen.

HYPERTHYROIDISM

In hyperthyroid states the TSH response to TRH is most useful in the differential diagnosis as well as for follow-up during therapy. Figure 15 shows T_3, T_4 and TSH values in a case of hyperthyroidism in a girl 15 years of age. At

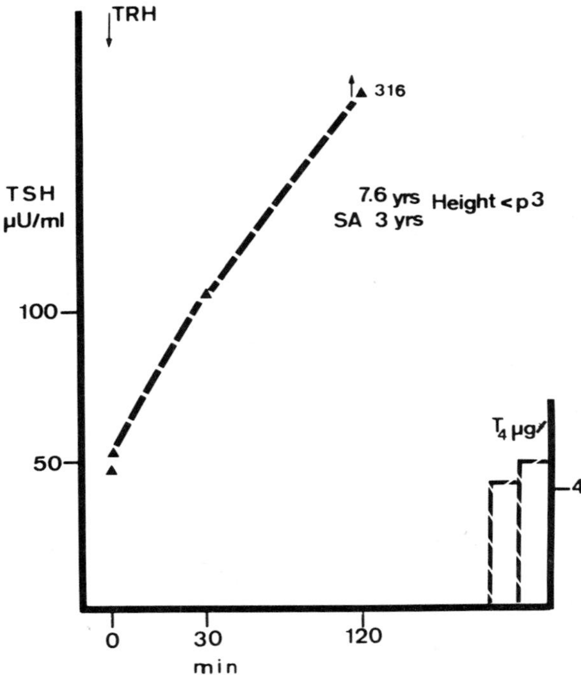

Fig.13 **TSH and T_4 with and without stimulation with TRH during therapy in primary hypothyroidism.**

diagnosis thyroxin was above 16 μg% and TSH did not respond to TRH. During therapy with PTU, thyroxin fell rapidly to the normal range. During slight increase in T_4 within the first 7 months of treatment TSH responded well to the TRH stimulation. At 14 months the therapy was reduced, T_4 and T_3 were in the normal range, TSH still responded well to TRH. Therapy was further reduced during the following period, but T_4 gradually increased. Twenty-eight months after initiating therapy, T_4 and T_3 were above the upper normal limit. TSH was unmeasurable and did not respond anymore to the stimulation of TRH. At that time a relapse could only be suspected from various slight clinical symptoms, but clearly diagnosed from the TRH test. During the next period basal TSH increased and an exaggerated response to TRH indicated a hypothyroid state. PTU was then reduced and plasma T_4, T_3, basal TSH and response to TRH recorded for control of therapy.

In conclusion, TRH test has proved to be helpful in diagnosis of "compensated" hypothyroidism. It is a most sensitive test for assessing the thyroid state in goiter patients (Gemsenjäger *et al.*, 1975a&b). In the newborn period it might be necessary to start a preventive therapy, when hypothyroidism could not be excluded with certainty. A normal TSH response to TRH after a therapy-free period of at least 2 weeks allows a clear decision on withdrawal of such a preventive therapy. The test has a definitive place in the differential diagnosis and follow-up of hyperthyroidism (Staub *et al.*, 1975). In secondary or tertiary hypothyroidism the TSH response to TRH is of limited value.

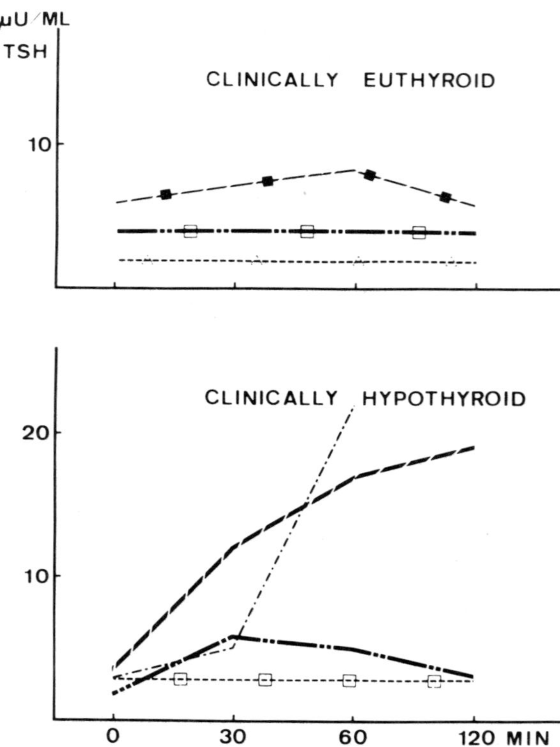

Fig. 14 TSH response in hypothalamo-pituitary disorders.

ACKNOWLEDGEMENT

This work was supported by Schweizerischer Nationalfonds 3.0690.73.

REFERENCES

Azizi, F., Vagenakis, A.G., Portnay, G.I., Rapoport, B., Ingbar, S.H. and Braverman, L.E. (1975). *New Engl. J. Med.* **292**, 273.

Beckers, C., Maskens, A. and Cornette, C. (1972). *Eur. J. clin. Invest.* **2**, 220.

Besser, G.M. and Mortimer, C.H. (1974). *J. clin. Path.* **27**, 173.

Brock Jacobsen, B., Andersen, H., Dige-Petersen, H. and Hummer, L. (1976). *Paediatr. Scand.* **65**, 433.

Brook, C.G.D., Sanders, M.D. and Hoare, R.D. (1972). *Br. med. J.* **3**, 811.

Chaussain, J.L. and Job, J.C. (1972). *Ann. Endocr.* **33**, 6, 557.

Faglia, G., Beck-Peccoz, P., Ambrosi, B., Ferrai, C. and Travaglini, P. (1972). *Acta endocr. (Copenh.)* **71**, 209.

Faglia, G., Beck-Peccoz, P., Ferrari, C., Ambrosi, B., Spada, A., Travaglini, P. and Paracchi, S. (1973). *J. clin. Endocr. Metab.* **37**, 595.

Fleischner, N., Lorente, M., Kirkland, J., Kirkland, R., Clayton, G. and Calderon, M. (1972). *J. clin. Endocr. Metab.* **34**, 4, 617.

Folley, T.P., Jr., Owings, J., Hayford, J.T. and Blizzard, R.M. (1972). *J. clin. Invest.* **51**, 431.

Frankel, R.J. and Jenkins, J.S. (1975). *Acta endocr. (Copenh.)* **78**, 209.

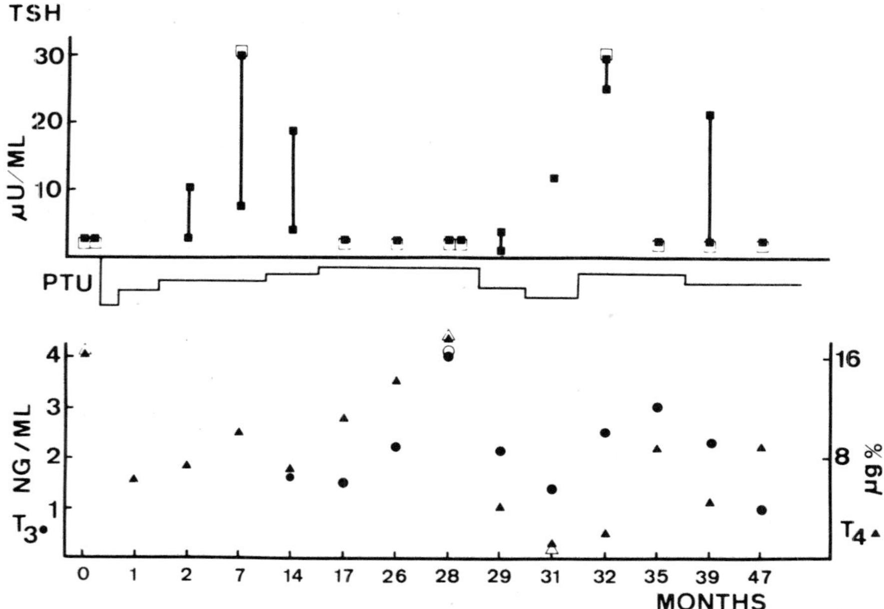

Fig.15 T_3, T_4 and TSH with and without stimulation with TRH during treatment of hyperthyroidism.

Gemsenjäger, E., Staub, J.J. and Girard, J. (1975a). *Helv. chir. Acta* **42**, 81.

Gemsenjäger, E., Staub, J.J. and Girard, J. (1975b). *Lancet* **II**, 371.

Girard, J., Stahl, M., Nars, P.W. and Baumann, J.B. (1972). *Klin. Wschr.* **50**, 706.

Girard, J., Staub, J.J., Buhler, U., Nars, P.W., Stahl, M. and Baumann, J.B. (1975). *Acta endocr. (Copenh.)* **Suppl. 177**, 301.

Girard, J., Staub, J.J., Baumann, J.B., Stahl, M. and Nars, P.W. (1974). *Acta endocr. (Copenh.)* **Suppl. 184**, 22.

Hall, R., Werner, I. and Holgate, H. (eds) (1972). "Thyrotropin-releasing Hormone", Front. Hormone Res., Karger, Basel.

Hershman, J.M. (1974). *New Engl. J. Med.* **290**, 886.

Job, J.C., Milhaud, G., Binet, E., Rivaille, P. and Moukhtar, M.S. (1971). *Rev. Europ. études clin. et biol.* **XVI**, 537.

Otsuki, M., Dakoda, M. and Baba, S. (1973). *J. clin. Endocr.* **36**, 95.

Patel, Y.C. and Burger, H.G. (1973). *J. clin. Endocr. Metab.* **37**, 2, 190.

Polossa, P., Vigneri, R., Papalia, D., Squatrito, S. and Motta, L. (1972). *Ann. Endocr.* **33**, 6, 593.

Sawin, C.T. and Hershman, J.M. (1976). *J. clin. Endocr. Metab.* **42**, 5, 809.

Shenkman, L., Mitsuma, T. and Hollander, C.S. (1973). *J. clin. Endocr. Metab.* **36**, 1074.

Snyder, P.J. and Utiger, R.D. (1972). *J. clin. Endocr.* **34**, 1096.

Staub, J.J. and Girard, J. (1975). *In: International Symposium on Growth Hormone and Related Peptides*, University of Milan, p.94.

Staub, J.J., Barthe, P.L., Werner, I. and Girard, J. (1975). *Lancet* **II**, 661.

Vagenakis, A.G., Rapoport, B., Azizi, F., Portnay, G.I., Braverman, L.E. and Ingbar, S.H. (1974). *J. clin. Invest.* **54**, 913.

Wenzel, K.W., Meinhold, H., Herpich, M., Adlkofer, F. and Schleusener, H. (1972). *Klin. Wschr.* **52**, 722.

RELATIONSHIP OF BREAST FEEDING TO CONGENITAL HYPOTHYROIDISM

A. Tenore, J.S. Parks and A.M. Bongiovanni

Department of Pediatrics, University of Pennsylvania, School of Medicine Philadelphia

Children's Hospital of Philadelphia, USA

Hypothyroidism is among the most common endocrine diseases of children and mental retardation has long been recognized as one of its more important consequences. However, there appears to be general agreement that early diagnosis and treatment confers a more favorable prognosis. Collip *et al.* (1965), Raiti *et al.* (1971) and Klein *et al.* (1972) have separately provided evidence for improved prognosis in congenital hypothyroidism treated before 3 months of age. Unfortunately, early detection is difficult and only 39 (26%) of the 158 patients in this series were diagnosed before 3 months of age. Futhermore, even among those diagnosed before 3 months, there are still approximatley 20% who do not attain normal mental development. At present, there are no published accounts of the results obtained when replacement medication was begun within the first week of life; therefore, it has not been possible to determine that complete salvage would occur if the athyreotic patient could be treated sufficiently early in post-natal life.

Recent observations in our clinic have suggested that human breast milk may provide sufficient thyroid hormone to ameliorate congenital hypothyroidism. If breast milk is a source of thyroid hormone, then breast-fed hypothyroid infants could be considered as a model for initiation of therapy within the first week of life. We have therefore undertaken this study to assess whether breast feeding the athyreotic newborn confers protection against the early and late manifestations of hypothyroidism and, if so, to what degree.

For this purpose, we have retrospectively reviewed over 100 cases of congenital hypothyroidism with the aim of evaluating various parameters known to be influenced by lack of thyroid hormone. These paramters included: (1) linear growth, (2) degree of skeletal maturation, (3) developmental milestones and (4) present intellectual functions.

Initially the study group consisted of 109 cases diagnosed in the 25 year span between 1950 and 1975. However, since the information recorded in the charts or long-term follow-up was insufficient for this study, questionnaires were sent to each family requesting the needed information. This included: (1) type and duration of nourishment in the first months of life, (2) time of additional food supplementation, (3) attainment of developmental milestones with regard to language, social, gross and fine motor functions, and (4) present mental status as assessed by recent IQ tests, type and schools attended, school performance and extent of education. Of the 109 cases originally reviewed, 51 questionnaires were returned containing sufficient information to be used in the study.

Table I. Characteristics of the study group.

	Breast Fed	Formula Fed
n	16	35
Females	12	26
Males	4	9
Age at Diagnosis		
mean	9 months	10 months
(range)	(0.25 months – 52 months)	(1.5 months – 65 months)
Duration of Breast Feeding:		
mean	5.7 months	–
(range)	(1 month – 9 months)	–
Present Age:		
mean	8.8 yrs	14.5 yrs
(range)	(9 months – 22 yrs)	(2 yrs – 25 yrs)

Table I characterizes the study group. Sixteen, or approximately 1/3 of the 51 subjects were breast fed. The female to male ratio in both the breast fed infants (BFI) and formula fed infants (FFI) was 3:1. The age at the time of diagnosis in the BFI was 9 months as compared with 10 months in the FFI. This difference was not significant. The mean length of breast feeding was 5.7 months with a range of 1 to 9 months. The present ages of the BFI ranged from 9 months to 22 years with a mean of 8.8 years, while those of the FFI ranged from 2 years to 25 years with a mean of 14.5 years.

The first parameter to be investigated was the effect of breast feeding on linear growth. There were 12 individuals who were breast fed. Of these, there were 5 who were off breast milk at the time of diagnosis. Linear growth in all subjects was expressed as a percentage of the growth increment attained by a normal child growing along the 50th percentile on the Boston-Anthropometric Chart for the particular span of time being compared. As can be seen in Table II, the 12 subjects while being breast fed had a mean growth increment equivalent to 91% of normal and the 5 patients who had been weaned before diagnosis had a mean growth increment equivalent to 50% of normal following the cessation of breast feeding. This difference was found to be statistically significant at a P value of less than 0.0005. The same level of significance was obtained in comparing the 30 infants who were formula fed and growing at a mean increment of 44% of normal with the 91% of the BFI on breast milk. However, no difference was found between the 44% of normal growth increment of the FFI and the 50% of the BFI who had stopped breast feeding.

In the first few months of life, it is difficult to ascertain monthly bone age differences. However, the 6 breast-fed patients who were diagnosed after they were weaned had a mean age at diagnosis of 19.8 months, a mean age of weaning of 5.5 months and a mean skeletal age of 5 months. In these individuals, the skeletal age at the time of diagnosis coincided with the age at which breast feeding was discontinued.

Table II. Comparison of growth between breast fed infants (BFI) and formula fed infants (FFI).

		n	Mean % of Normal for Age ± SEM	P
1)	Growth of BFI on Breast Milk	12	91 ± 3	
	v.			< 0.0005
	Growth of BFI off Breast Milk	5	50 ± 9	
2)	Growth of FFI	30	44 ± 4	
	v.			< 0.005
	Growth of BFI on Breast Milk	12	91 ± 3	
3)	Growth of FFI	30	44 ± 4	
	v.			NS
	Growth of BFI off Breast Milk	5	50 ± 9	

Table III. Comparison of the degree of skeletal maturation in breast fed infants (BFI) and formula fed infants (FFI) diagnosed before 7 months of age to that of a normal newborn infant.

	n	Age (months) at diagnosis (Mean ± SEM)	No. of subjects with all 5 newborn centres	No. of subjects with no newborn centres	No. of ossification centres at time of Dx (Mean ± SEM)
FFI	15	3.1 ± 0.4	0	8	1.0 ± 0.3
BFI	11	3.6 ± 0.6	5	1	3.7 ± 0.5
"P"	—	NS	—	—	< 0.0005

Approximately 90% of all newborns have 5 ossification centers distributed between the knee and foot. In order to determine whether skeletal maturation was affected by breast feeding, all patients diagnosed before 7 months of age were selected and the degree of skeletal maturation at the time of diagnosis was compared to that of a normal newborn (Table III). Fifteen FFI were diagnosed before 7 months of age compared to 11 of the BFI. The mean age of diagnosis of 3.1 months in the FFI and 3.6 months in the BFI did not differ significantly. There was not a single FFI who had all 5 newborn centers present at the time of diagnosis, whereas 5 of 11 BFI had all 5 centers present. Eight of the FFI were missing all 5 centers as opposed to 1 of the BFI at the time of diagnosis. Collectively, the FFI averaged 1 ossification center at the time of diagnosis as opposed to 3.7 centers for the BFI. This difference was significant at a P value of less than 0.0005.

In an attempt to determine whether there was a difference between FFI and BFI in early development, each patient was scored a value of "1" for delay in each of the categories of infant development so that a child with a score of "4" had

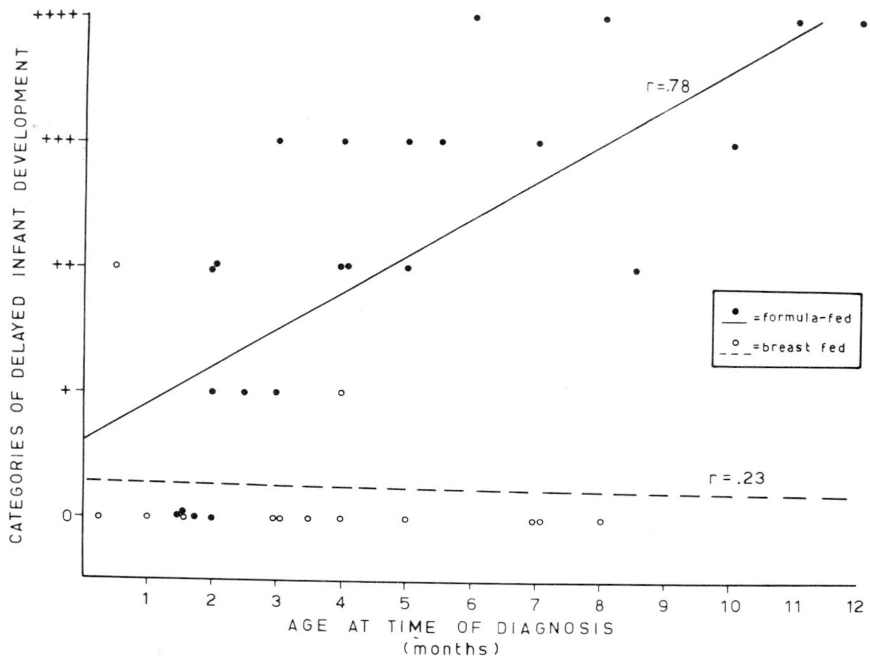

Fig. 1 **Correlation between delayed infant development and age at time of diagnosis of breast-fed and formula-fed infants.**

delay in language, social, gross and fine motor functions.

A positive correlation was obtained in the 30 FFI between categories of delayed infant development and age of diagnosis. Delay in infant development was greater in those individuals who were diagnosed the latest. On the contrary, no such correlation was found in the 16 BFI, even though there were 11 infants diagnosed after 3 months of age (Fig. 1).

We then examined these relationships in later life. Subjects were categorized according to IQ testing and past and present school performance into: (1) Above Average (IQ > 105), (2) Average (IQ 95–105), and (3) Below Average (IQ < 95). Three of the BFI were "Above Average", 12 were "Average" and none "Below Average", whereas in the formula-fed group only 1 was "Above Average' 11 were "Average" and 20 "Below Average" (Table IVA). Fifteen of the 20 subjects graded "Below Average" had formal IQ testing with a mean IQ of 67 ± 4.7. A break-down of the 20 as a function of the time of diagnosis (Table IVB) shows that 37.5% of all FFI diagnosed before 3 months who fell in this group had a mean IQ of 80. Sixty-seven percent of those diagnosed between 3 and 6 months of age had a mean IQ of 76 and 73.4% of subjects diagnosed after 6 months had a mean IQ of 60.

The evidence thus far presented supports the contention that breast-fed athyreotic infants do significantly better than FFI with regard to the discussed parameters which are known to be influenced by lack of thyroid hormone.

The full blown picture of severe neonatal hypothyroidism unfolds gradually within the first few critical months of life and the speed and severity with which

Table IV. *A.* Comparison of intellectual function between breast fed infants (BFI) and formula fed infants (FFI).

		BFI	FFI
Above Average	(n)	3	1
Average	(n)	12	11
Below Average	(n)	0	20*

**B.* Mean IQ in subjects graded "Below Average" as a function of the time of diagnosis.

Age at Diagnosis	Total Number Dx.	No. of Subjects "Below Average"	% of Total	No. Tested	Mean IQ ± SEM
3 months	8	3	37.5	3	80 ± 11
3–6 months	9	6	66.6	3	76 ± 13
6 months	15	11	73.4	9	60 ± 5

Table V. Comparison of PBI values between breast fed infants (BFI) and formula fed infants (FFI).

		n	μg/dl Mean ± SEM	P
1)	PBI of BFI on Breast Milk	7	2.4 ± 0.2	
	v.			< 0.01
	PBI of FFI	21	1.7 ± 0.1	
2)	PBI of BFI off Breast Milk	4	1.4 ± 0.1	
	v.			< 0.0025
	PBI of BFI on Breast Milk	7	2.4 ± 0.2	
3)	PBI of BFI off Breast Milk	4	1.4 ± 0.1	
	v.			NS
	PBI of FFI	21	1.7 ± 0.1	

it progresses has been said to be inversely related to the amount of thyroid activity present. We therefore looked to see if there were any differences between the PBI values of the FFI and those of the BFI both *on* or *off* breast milk. Twenty-one FFI had PBI's done (Table V). The mean value of this group was 1.7 μg/dl. Seven of the BFI who were still on breast milk at the time PBI's were done had a mean value of 2.4 μg/dl, whereas the 4 BFI who were off breast milk had a mean PBI value of 1.4 μg/dl. The mean PBI value of the BFI receiving breast milk was significantly greater than the mean value of either the FFI ($P < 0.01$) or the BFI who were not on breast milk ($P < 0.0025$).

It may therefore be logical to surmise that BFI do better than FFI because the former have higher circulating levels of iodide which may be hormonal iodide.

We shall now present preliminary, limited data to ascertain whether breast milk was the contributing source of the iodide. Human breast milk from healthy, euthyroid mothers was obtained from one week to 6 months post-partum and compared to standard commercial infant formulas and whole milk for thyroid hormone content. Thyroid hormones were extracted with ethanol and assayed

Table VI. Thyroxine levels in breast milk.

Months Post-Partum	n	T_4 (μg/dl ± SEM)
< 1	4	5.4 ± 0.8
1 – 2	6	4.0 ± 1.8
2 – 4	4	1.6 ± 0.6
4 – 6	4	1.3 ± 0.3

by radioimmunoassay. Neither the commercial infant formulas nor the whole milk had detectable hormone levels. On the contrary, breast milk contained variable amounts of hormones. Unfortunately, the limited number of human breast milk samples assayed, which were scattered over a 6 month span, were not of sufficient number to draw a precise conclusion correlating T_4 content with time post-partum. Table VI reports the thyroxine levels found in breast milk. Except for a mean level of 8 μg/dl at the end of the first week in two samples, the mean T_4 value by the end of the first month was 5.4 μg/dl. The T_4 level continued to decrease, reaching a mean of approximately 4.0 μg/dl by 2 months, 1.6 by 4 months and 1.3 μg/dl by 6 months.

Additional milk samples are presently being processed and data compiled for both thyroxine and triiodothyronine levels.

In conclusion, we have shown that BFI with congenital hypothyroidism grow better, show a more mature skeletal maturation, have better infant development and have a better intellectual prognosis than FFI. The finding of thyroid hormone in breast milk leads us to postulate that BFI do better because in essence they are "being treated" within the first week of life and for the greater part are being protected during the first few critical months of life in terms of both neurologic and mental development.

REFERENCES

Collip, P.J., Kaplan, S.A., Kogut, M.D. *et al.* (1965). *Am. J. Ment. Defic.* **70**, 432.
Raiti, S. and Newns, G.H. (1971). *Arch. Dis. Child.* **46**, 692.
Klein, A.H., Meltzer, S. and Kenny, F.M. (1972). *J. Pediatr.* **81**, 912.

A RADIOIMMUNOASSAY FOR REVERSE TRIIODOTHYRONINE IN THE TERM FETUS, IN THE NEWBORN AND IN VARIOUS THYROID DISEASES

C. Carella, G. Pisano, V. Tripodi*, V. Olivieri**, P. Carayon*** and M. Faggiano

Institutes of Endocrinology and of Obstetrics, I Faculty of Medicine University of Naples, Italy*
*Biodata Laboratories**, Rome, Italy*
*Institute of Biochemistry***, University of Marseille, France*

SUMMARY

In this chapter we report plasma rT_3 values in cord blood and maternal blood measured with a radioimmunoassay of high specificity and sensitivity recently developed in our laboratory. The aim of our study is to define better the role of rT_3 and therefore we report the plasma values in the term fetus, in the newborn and in various thyroid diseases compared with those of plasma T_3, T_4 and TSH. Plasma rT_3 values offer another approach to a precocious diagnosis of neonatal hypothryoidism and therefore it is desirable to obtain maternal and umbilical cord blood at the delivery.

It is known that reverse triiodothyronine is found in rat's blood (Roche *et al.*, 1956). Injecting radioactive thyroxine in the rat, T_4 monodeiodination may occur either on the phenolic ring, with the consequent formation of 3,5,3'-triiodothyronine (T_3), or on the tyrosil ring, with the formation of reverse triiodothyronine (Surks and Oppenheimer, 1971). To date, the scarce information on plasma rT_3 is the result of different methods either from extracted (Chopra, 1974; Meinhold *et al.*, 1975a,b) or unextracted plasma (Kodding *et al.*, 1976).

The aim of this chapter was to evaluate rT_3 levels in some physiological and pathological thyroid conditions. For this purpose, a radioimmunoassay for

rT_3 of high specificity and sensitivity was developed on unextracted plasma.

MATERIALS AND METHODS

The radioimmunoassay for reverse T_3 was as follows:

Reagents

L-3,3′-diodothyronine (reverse-T_2, rT_2) and D,L-3,3′,5-triiodothyronine were provided by Dr. H.J. Cahnmann of NIH, Bethesda, Maryland, and by Warner-Lambert Research Institute, Morris Plaines, New Jersey.

Antiserum against L-rT_3 was performed by Biodata Laboratories, Rome.

Iodination

Radioactive rT_3 was prepared in our laboratories by iodination of 5nM of rT_2 with 1 mCi of NaI^{125}. 2.85 μg of chloramine T was employed. The reaction was stopped with excess sodium metabisulphite.

Chromatography

Purification of the labeled rT_3 was performed on Sephadex G-25 fine (column size: 200 × 19 mm) with NaOH 0.02 N as eluant; 3 peaks were obtained: I^{125}, I^{125}-rT_2 and I^{125}-rT_3. Specific radioactivity was 450 μCi/μg (Fig.1).

Radioimmunoassay

Each sample was determined in triplicate. 0.08 M barbital buffer pH 8.4 with 0.25% BSA was used, as well as 500 μg/tube of ANS as TBP inhibitor.

The assay was performed on 100 μl of serum; 100 μl of plasma-free was added in the standard curve. Incubation volume was 500 μl and final dilution of the antibody was 1:8,000. Cross reaction of the antibody used was 0.08% with L-T_4 and 0.0024% with L-T_3. The tubes were incubated at 4°C for 48 h; separation was made with 20% PEG. The intraassay variation coefficient was 8.4%. Minimum sensitivity of this assay was 2 pg/ml with a correlation recovery assay of 0.997 (Fig.2).

Plasma T_3 and TSH were measured by a radioimmunoassay procedure with both a Richter Kit set and a Biodata Laboratories Kit set; plasma T_4 was measured by a competitive binding procedure with an Ames Kit set. Normal values (mean ± 2 SD) for plasma T_3, T_4 and TSH were 0.7–1.8 ng/ml, 3.8–12.2 μg/100 ml and 0.6–5 μU/ml, respectively.

Statistical analysis of the data was performed by the Student's *t* test.

CLINICAL STUDY

Plasma reverse T_3 level was measured in the blood plasma of 7 mothers and in the cord blood plasma of their respective term fetuses at the time of delivery.

In 3 out of 7 newborn, plasma rT_3 was evaluated also 24 and 72 h after birth. Reverse T_3 level was measured in 18 normal subjects, in 10 hyperthyroid and 6 hypothyroid patients. The diagnosis of hyper- and hypothyroidism was documented by clinical indices together with laboratory data (T_3, T_4 and TSH assays).

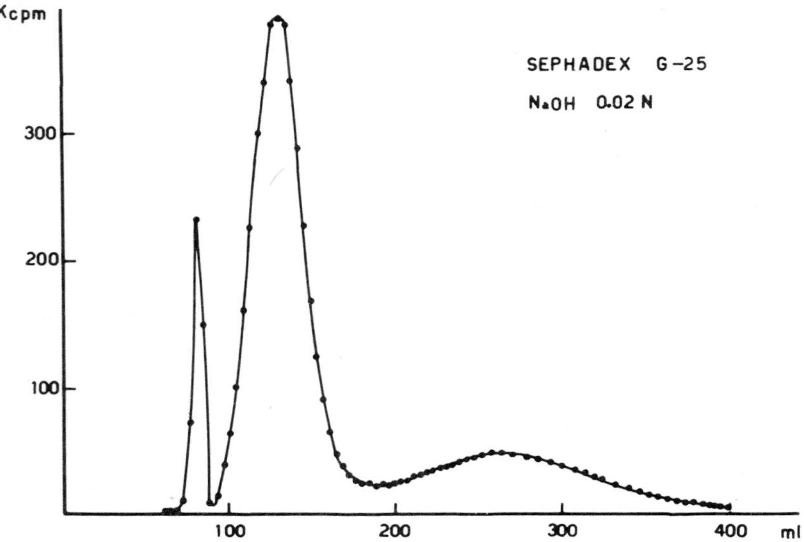

Fig. 1 Purification of L-3,3',5-triiodothyronine (reverse T_3, rT_3) by column chromatography on Sephadex G-25 fine (column size: 200 × 19 mm), with NaOH 0.02 N as eluant.

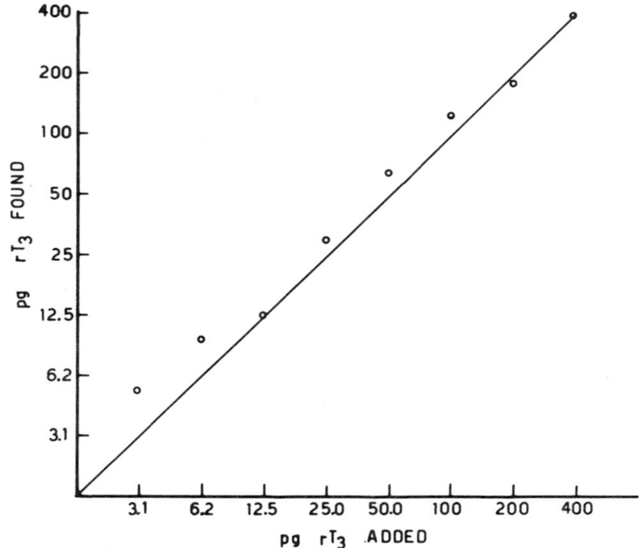

Fig. 2 Correlation coefficient (r = 0.997) found in a recovery assay.

Table I. Plasma reverse triiodothyronine (rT_3), triodothyronine (T_3), thyroxine (T_4), TSH in some physiological and pathological thyroid states.

Group		n	Mean	SD	Range
Normal Subjects	rT_3 ng/ml	18	0.29	0.07	0.16 – 0.44
	T_3 n/ml	18	1.17	0.23	0.75 – 1.55
	T_4 μg/100 ml	18	5.92	1.07	4.8 – 9.2
	TSH μU/ml	18	1.65	0.94	0.6 – 4.3
Hyperthyroidism	rT_3 ng/ml	10	1.01	0.50	0.56 – 2.16
	T_3 ng/ml	10	2.95	0.78	1.90 – 4.70
	T_4 μg/100 ml	9	14.49	1.87	11.6 – 18.0
	TSH μU/ml	10	0.70	0.22	0.6 – 1.2
Hypothyroidism	rT_3 ng/ml	6	0.11	0.02	0.03 – 0.18
	T_3 ng/ml	6	0.33	0.08	0.20 – 0.40
	T_4 μg/100 ml	6	2.15	0.87	1.0 – 3.3
	TSH μU/ml	6	123.0	73.5	12.0 – 220.0
Newborn	rT_3 ng/ml	7	3.50	1.07	1.70 – 4.00
	T_3 ng/ml	7	0.59	0.42	0.30 – 1.50
	T_4 μg/100 ml	7	9.00	3.50	4.4 – 13.8
	TSH μU/ml	7	6.00	3.80	2.5 – 12.5
Maternal Blood	rT_3 ng/ml	7	0.41	0.10	0.25 – 0.59
	T_3 ng/ml	7	2.48	1.10	0.80 – 4.50
	T_4 μg/100 ml	7	11.90	2.50	7.20 – 15.0
	TSH μU/ml	7	1.70	0.90	0.60 – 2.70

RESULTS

Table I summarizes rT_3, T_3, T_4 and TSH concentration data found in normal euthyroid subjects, in hyper- and hypothyroid patients, in the blood plasma of the 7 mothers and the cord blood plasma of their respective fetuses at the time of delivery.

Plasma rT_3 (mean ± SEM values 0.41 ± 0.04 and 3.50 ± 0.41 ng/ml in maternal and cord blood respectively, $p < 0.001$) and TSH concentration (mean ± 1.77 ± 0.36 and 6.09 ± 1.45 μU/ml in maternal and cord blood, respectively, $p < 0.001$) were higher in cord than in maternal blood. In contrast with this last data, plasma T_3 concentration was higher in maternal than in cord blood (mean ± SEM 2.58 ± 0.45 and 0.59 ± 0.16 ng/ml, respectively, $p < 0.001$). Plasma T_4 concentration was similar in cord and in maternal blood (mean ± SEM 9.07 ± 1.35 and 11.9 ± 0.98 μg/100 ml, respectively).

Plasma rT_3, T_3, T_4 and TSH values are reported in Table II.

The same parameters were evaluated in 3 out of the 7 newborn, also 24 and 72 h after birth (Fig.3). Reverse T_3 concentrations appeared progressively decreased in contrast with the increased values of plasma TSH, T_3 and T_4.

DISCUSSION

In the present study, plasma rT_3 values were in agreement with those of T_4 and T_3 in patients with hyper- or hypothyroidism, even if more in accordance with those of plasma T_4.

Table II. Plasma reverse triiodothyronine (rT_3), triiodothyronine (T_4), thyroxine (T_4) and thyrotropin (TSH) in 7 paired maternal and cord blood.

Pairs	Maternal				Cord Blood			
	rT_3 (ng/ml)	T_3 (ng/ml)	T_4 (μg/100 ml)	TSH (μU/ml)	rT_3 (ng/ml)	T_3 (ng/ml)	T_4 (μg/100 ml)	TSH (μU/ml)
I	0.40	2.00	13.3	2.0	3.80	0.50	9.3	8.3
II	0.59	4.50	15.0	2.7	3.00	0.50	6.8	8.9
III	0.49	0.80	7.2	0.2	3.05	0.25	6.4	2.8
IV	0.25	3.50	11.4	2.6	5.22	0.45	13.6	2.5
V	0.42	2.05	13.0	0.9	4.00	0.30	4.4	4.0
VI	0.38	2.40	10.4	1.5	3.70	1.50	13.8	12.5
VII	0.42	2.80	13.6	2.5	1.70	0.60	9.2	3.6
Mean	**0.41**	**2.58**	**11.9**	**1.7**	**3.50**	**0.59**	**9.0**	**6.0**
SEM	0.04	0.45	0.98	0.36	0.41	0.16	1.35	1.45
SD	0.10	1.10	2.50	0.9	1.07	0.42	3.50	3.8

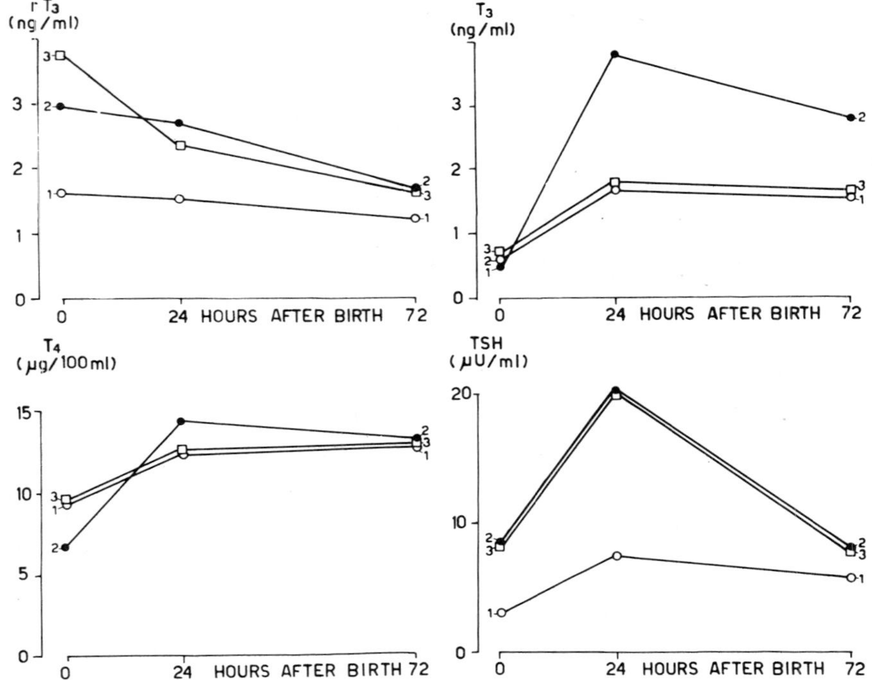

Fig.3 Plasma rT_3, T_3, T_4 and TSH values in newborn at birth and 24 and 27 h later.

Moreover, rT_3 concentrations found in our laboratory in normal controls and in opposite states of thyroid function (Table I) are in agreement with those of Meinhold *et al.* (1975a&b) but in disagreement with others (Chopra, 1974; Nicod *et al.*, 1976). The explanation for these discrepancies is probably attributable to technical differences between the used methods. In fact, some authors use extracted plasma (Chopra, 1974; Meinhold *et al.*, 1975a&b; Ködding *et al.*, 1976) while others use unextracted plasma (Nicod *et al.*, 1976); moreover, certain authors utilize D,L-rT_3 (Chopra, 1974), and others L-rT_3 (Meinhold *et al.*, 1975a&b) as standard or for immunization.

Plasma TSH values were significantly higher in cord blood than in maternal blood whereas plasma T_4 levels were similar (Table II). This observation is in agreement with that of other authors (Utiger, 1968; Fisher and Odell, 1969; Fisher, 1975a) and may be considered as an expression of the fact that the fetal hypothalamic-pituitary-thyroid axis is independent of and more active than that of the mother.

In contrast, rT_3 values were found markedly higher in cord blood than in 3 maternal blood. Considering that rT_3 is a product of T_4 conversion, this occurrence may be due to fetal differences of particular enzymatic activity (Chopra, 1974; Chopra *et al.*, 1975).

The parameters of thyroid function were also studied in 3 cases during the first 72 h of birth (Fig.3). A TSH increase was observed here similar to that found by Fisher and Odell (1969), probably due to the TRH increase resulting from cooling at birth, and a consequent increase of plasma T_3 and T_4 values in contrast to an opposite pattern shown by rT_3 values.

These findings are probably due to the setting up in adult subjects of metabolic routes of T_4 conversion to T_3 (Chopra *et al.*, 1975a&b; Erenberg *et al.*, 1974). Furthermore, rT_3 evaluation in the amniotic fluid, as recently reported by Chopra and Crandall (1975), offers another approach to a precocious diagnosis of neonatal hypothyroidism whose frequency is of 1:7,000 births (Fisher, 1975b) before the age of 3 months, thus preventing the neurologic and mental deficiencies due to thyroid hormone deprivation.

Finally, it is desirable to obtain maternal and umbilical cord blood at delivery in order to confirm the euthyroid status of the mother and infant, considering that for an appropriate interpretation, thyroid function indices in the newborn vary significantly with respect to the passage of time after birth.

ACKNOWLEDGEMENTS

The authors are grateful to Mr. T. Pepe for his invaluable technical collaboration and Miss G. Vigoriti for her impeccable secretarial assistance.

REFERENCES

Chopra, I.J. (1974). *J. clin. Invest.* **54**, 583-592.

Chopra, I.J. and Crandall, B.F. (1975). *New Engl. J. Med.* **293**, 740-743.

Chopra, I.J., Sack, J. and Fisher, D.A. (1975a). *In* "Perinatal Thyroid Physiology and Disease" (D.A. Fisher and G.N. Burrow, eds) pp.33-48. Raven Press, Pub., New York.

Chopra, I.J., Sack, J. and Fisher, D.A. (1975b). *J. clin. Invest.* **55**, 1137-1141.

Erenberg, A., Phelps, D.L., Lam, R. and Fisher, D.A. (1974). *Pediatrics* **53**, 211-216.

Fisher, D.A. and Odell, W.D. (1969). *J. clin. Invest.* **48**, 1670–1676.

Fisher, D.A. (1975a). *In* "Perintal Thyroid Physiology and Disease" (D.A. Fisher and G.N. Burrow, ed) pp.21-32. Raven Press, Publ., New York.

Fisher, D.A. (1975b). *New Engl. J. Med.* **293**, 770-771.

Ködding, R., Hesch, R.D. and von zur Mühlen, A. (1976). *Acta endocr. (Copenh.)* **Supp.202**, 47-49.

Meinhold, H., Wenzel, K.W. and Schürnbrand, P. (1975a). *Z. Klin. Chem. Klin. Biochem.* **12**, 571-574.

Meinhold, H., Schurnbrand, P. and Wenzel, K.W. (1975b). *Acta endocr. (Copenh.)* **199**, 343 **(Abst.)**.

Nicod, P., Burger, A., Staeheli, V. and Vallotton, M.B. (1970). *J. clin. Endocr. Metab.* **42**, 823-828.

Roche, J., Michel, R. and Nunez, J. (1956). *C.R. Séances Soc. Biol. Fil.* **150**, 20-24.

Surks, M.I. and Oppenheimer, J.H. (1971). *J. clin. Endocr. Metab.* **33**, 612-618.

Utiger, R.D., Wilber, J.F., Cornblath, M., Harm, J.T. and Mack, R.E. (1968). *J. clin. Invest.* **47**, 97 **(Abst.)**.

EFFECT OF OBESITY ON THE HYPOTHALAMO-HYPOPHYSO-GONADAL FUNCTION IN CHILDHOOD

E. Cacciari, A. Cicognani, P. Pirazzoli, F. Zappulla, P. Tassoni, F. Bernardi, S. Salardi and L. Mazzanti

Department of Pediatrics, University of Bologna, Italy

SUMMARY

In 22 normal and 21 obese boys a gonadal functioning test (2,000 IU of HCG i.m. a day for three days and assays of plasma testosterone and plasma 17β-oestradiol before and after the HCG administration) and an LH-RH test (50 μg i.v.) were carried out.

In 60% of the cases, both normal and obese boys, plasma 17β-oestradiol (both in basal conditions and after stimulus) turned out to be less than the method sensitivity (5 pg/ml). While basal testosterone was similar in the two groups of children, after HCG testosterone was significantly ($p < 0.01$) lower in the obese boys. In the normal children a significant positive correlation between bone age and basal and after HCG testosterone was demonstrated; this correlation was not found in the obese boys. The pituitary reserve of gonadotrophins did not show significant differences between the two groups of children. Finally, a significant positive correlation ($p < 0.01$) between the LH curve area during the LH-RH test and bone age was found only in the normal boys.

Gabrilove *et al.* (1974) found that Cushing's syndrome in the male is often associated with a decreased endocrine testicular efficiency, which then becomes normal after the treatment of the disease. Hajjar *et al.* (1975) showed that an ACTH excess, through the adrenal mediation, minimizes in the male the testosterone release of the gonads. Since it is known that the function of the hypophyso-adrenal axis is increased in obesity (Migeon *et al.*, 1963; Dunkelman *et al.*, 1964; Garces *et al.*, 1968), we have studied the endocrine function of the gonads and the pituitary reserve of gonadotrophins in the prepubertal obese child.

SUBJECTS AND METHODS

Twenty-two normal boys (chronological age ranged from 5 to 11 7/12 years, mean 8 7/12; bone age ranged from 4 8/12 to 11 7/12 years, mean 8 6/12) and 21 obese boys (chronological age ranged from 6 to 12 3/12 years, mean 10 1/12; bone age ranged from 6 to 12 years, mean 10 2/12) were studied. In all the children examined the difference between the chronological and the bone age was never greater than six months. In the second group obesity had existed for at least three years, and the mean weight was 58% over the ideal weight (from 41% to 98%) according to the Tonelli and Marinelli Tables (1960). No child had lost any weight in the year preceding this study. All the examined children were in the prepubertal stage of sexual development, i.e. the first stage according to Tanner (1962). The external genitalia aspect of the obese children did not induce suspicion of the existence of hypogonadism. The x-rays of the sella turcica of the same children were normal.

All of the children, following permission from the parents, underwent both a gonadal function and a LH-RH test. The gonadal function test was carried out in the following manner: HCG was administered at a dosage of 2,000 IU i.m. every day for three days. The dose was administered at 9 a.m. on the first two days, and at 6 a.m. on the third day. Immediately before the beginning, and at the end of the test, a blood sample was collected to assay plasma testosterone and plasma 17β-oestradiol. The LH-RH test was performed at 9 a.m. after an overnight fast, using venous injection of 50 μg of synthetic LH-RH (Farbwerke Hoechst AG). Venous blood for the evaluation of LH and FSH was collected at times 0, 15, 30, 60 and 90 minutes. Bone age was determined according to the Greulich and Pyle Tables (1959).

Plasma testosterone was determined according to the radioimmunoassay method of Collins *et al.* (1972). The antiserum we used was obtained from rabbits pretreated with an antitubercular vaccine as we have previously reported (Cacciari *et al.*, 1974). The antiserum was used at a dilution of 1:30,000. The method sensitivity was 0.5 ng% ml. The variation coefficient of duplicate samples was ± 4.2%. Plasma 17β-oestradiol was assayed according to the radioimmunoassay method of Emment *et al.* (1972) using an antiserum at a dilution of 1:30,000 as previously reported (Cacciari *et al.*, 1974). The sensitivity of the method was 5 pg/ml. The variation coefficient of duplicate samples was ± 10%. Serum LH and FSH were evaluated according to the double antibody radioimmunoassay method of Reuter *et al.* (1973) using human pituitary LH and FSH (the radioimmunological equivalent of LH is 2150 IU as compared to the 68/40 reference preparation of the National Institute for Medical Research (MRC), Mill Hill, London. For FSH it is 2800 IU compared to the 68/39 reference preparations of MRC. The results are expressed as mIU/ml MRC reference preparation. The method sensitivity was 0.5 mIU/ml, both for LH and FSH. The variation coefficient of duplicate samples was ±7.4% and ± 8.5% for LH and FSH respectively.

For the statistical analysis of the results, the Student's t test was used and the correlation coefficient r was calculated.

RESULTS

More than 60% of the cases, both among the normal children and the obese, showed plasma 17β-oestradiol values lower than 5 pg/ml, both in basal conditions and after stimulus.

Table I. **Plasma testosterone behaviour in basal conditions and after HCG in 22 normal and 21 obese children.**

	Basal Testosterone (ng/100 ml)		After HCG Testosterone (ng/100 ml)	
	Mean	SEM	Mean	SEM
Normal children	15.40	1.49	114.21**	9.91
Obese children	19.13	1.95	64.99**	6.98

** P < 0.01.

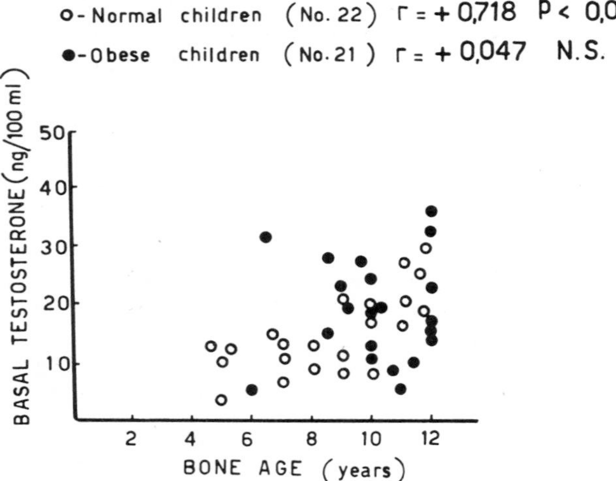

Fig. 1 **Correlation between basal testosterone values and bone age.**

The mean basal plasma testosterone value (Table I) did not present any significant differences between the two groups of examined children. After the HCG stimulus the plasma testosterone level in the obese children was significantly lower ($p < 0.01$) than that of the normal children (Table I). In the normal children there is a significant positive correlation between bone age and basal ($r = +0.718$; $p < 0.01$; Fig.1) and after HCG testosterone ($r = +0.472$; $p < 0.05$; Fig.2). This correlation is not found in the obese children.

The mean LH and FSH curve during the LH-RH test does not show any significant differences between the two groups (Table II; Fig.3). Moreover, the mean LH curve is constantly lower in the obese children, even if the difference is not significant (Fig.3). The pituitary reserve of gonadotrophins was also studied by

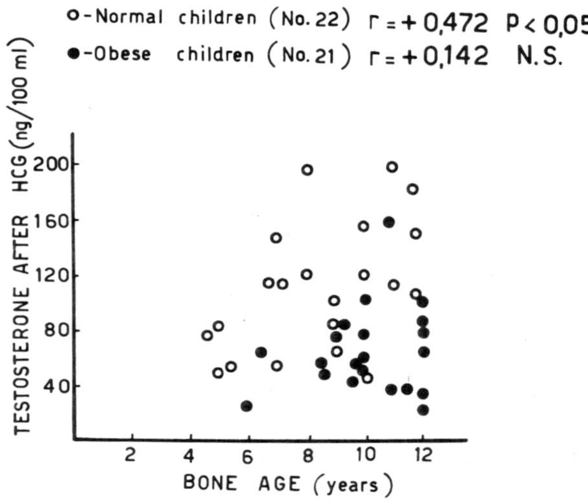

Fig. 2 Correlation between values after HCG testosterone and bone age.

Table II. Mean values ± SEM of serum LH and FSH (mIU/ml) in 22 normal and 21 obese boys who underwent the LH-RH test (50 μg i.v.).

	Time (min)	0	15	30	60	90	Peak	Maximum increase	Area of the curve
Normal children	LH	1.96 ±0.17	3.92 ±0.64	4.13 ±0.65	3.67 ±0.55	3.15 ±0.40	4.52 ±0.66	2.56 ±0.65	19.50 ± 1.97
	FSH	2.14 ±0.22	3.65 ±0.34	4.95 ±0.52	5.36 ±0.51	5.46 ±0.73	6.27 ±0.74	4.13 ±0.63	28.51 ± 2.87
Obese children	LH	1.83 ±0.25	3.51 ±0.70	3.68 ±0.67	3.17 ±0.69	2.82 ±0.45	4.19 ± 0.76	2.33 ±0.65	19.00 ± 3.45
	FSH	2.37 ±0.30	3.90 ±0.37	4.40 ±0.40	5.10 ±0.47	5.10 ±0.45	5.70 ±0.46	3.33 ±0.32	27.10 ± 2.37

evaluating the peak, the maximum increase and the area of the curve (Cacciari *et al.*, 1975)(Table II), and it did not show any significant differences between the two groups of children.

In both the normal children and the obese there is no correlation between bone age and the basal values or the FSH pituitary reserve. As far as the LH is concerned, we found a highly significant positive correlation ($r = +0.610$; $p < 0.01$; Fig.4) between the area of the curve and bone age only in the normal children. No correlation was found between LH and testosterone, both in basal conditions and after stimulus.

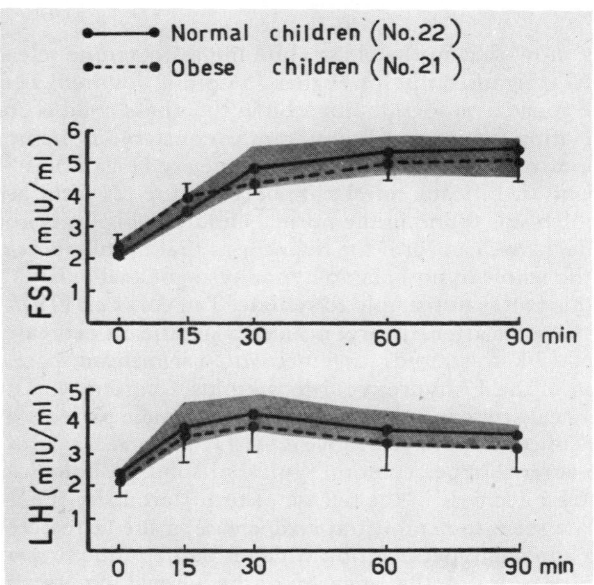

Fig.3 FSH and LH behaviour (mean ± SEM) in normal and obese boys submitted to the LH-RH test (50 μg i.v.).

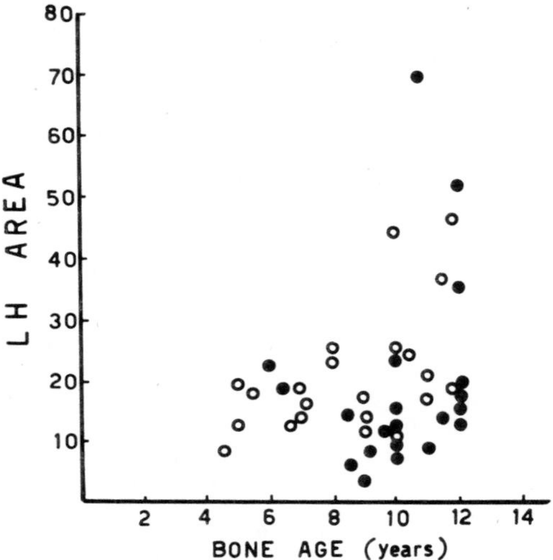

Fig.4 Correlation between the LH curve area and bone age in normal and obese boys submitted to the LH-RH test.

DISCUSSION

Our results show that in the obese child the testosterone release by the gonads after HCG is significantly lower than in normal children. The different behaviour of the gonadal endocrine function in the obese child is confirmed by the lack of correlation (which was found, on the contrary, in the normal child) between basal or after HCG testosterone and bone age (Figs 1 and 2). If we consider that the highly significant correlation between the LH pituitary reserve and bone age, which was found in the normal children (Fig.4), is not to be found in the obese subjects, we can form the hypothesis that in the obese child there is a disorder of the whole hypothalamo-hypophyso-gonadal axis.

However, this fact is not simple to valuate. Tanaka *et al.* (1970), when examining male patients after surgery, noticed a significant decrease in the urinary excretion of 17-keto-steroids, together with a significant increase in the urinary excretion of the 17-hydroxycorticosteroids. Charters *et al.* (1969) noticed after surgical stress in a group of male and female patients a lowered gonadotrophins concentration. Gabrilove *et al.* (1974) and Hajjar *et al.* (1975) showed that the adrenal hypersecretion typical of some pathological situations is accompanied by a decrease in the release of testosterone by the male gonads.

All these data seem to demonstrate a decrease in the testosterone release when there is an adrenal hypersecretion which is perhaps due to a suppression of the gonadotrophins secretion. Being aware of the adrenal hypersecretion in obesity (Migeon *et al.*, 1963; Dunkelman *et al.*, 1964; Garces *et al.*, 1968), our data seem to confirm the existence of a relationship between the adrenal function and the activity of the hypothalamo-hypophyso-gonadal axis.

The insignificant data we obtained on the release of estrogens do not add anything to the hypothesis made by Hajjar *et al.* (1975) who consider these hormones hypersecreted by the hyperfunctioning adrenal as being responsible for the gonadotrophin suppression and, consequently, for the lower endocrine efficiency of the male gonad.

ACKNOWLEDGEMENTS

We thank in particular Dr. F. Enzmann and Dr. M. Sesso (Farbwerke Hoechst AG) for the generous supply of synthetic LH-RH. The skilful technical assistance of Mr. L. Zannarini is gratefully acknowledged.

REFERENCES

Cacciari, E., Cicognani, A., Tassoni, P., Flamigni, P., Bolelli, F., Pirazzoli, P. and Salardi, S. (1974). *Helv. Paediat. Acta* **29**, 27.

Cacciari, E., Cicognani, A., Pirazzoli, P., Tassoni, P., Zappulla, F., Salardi, S. and Bernardi, F. (1975). *J. clin. Endocr. Metab.* **40**, 802.

Charters, A.C., Odell, W.D. and Thompson, J.C. (1969). *J. clin. Endocr. Metab.* **29**, 63.

Collins, W.P., Mansfield, M.D., Alladina, N.S. and Sommerville, I.F. (1972). *J. Ster. Biochem.* **3**, 333.

Dunkelman, S.S., Fairhurst, B., Plager, J. and Waterhouse, C. (1964). *J. clin. Endocr.* **24**, 832.

Emment, Y., Collins, W.P. and Sommerville, I.F. (1972). *Acta endocr. (Copenh.)* **69**, 567.

Gabrilove, J.L., Nicolis, G.L. and Sohval, A.R. (1974). *J. Urology, Baltimore* **112**, 95.

Garces, L.Y., Kenny, F., Drash, A. and Taylor, F. (1968). *J. clin. Endocr.* **28**, 1843.

Greulich, W.W. and Pyle, S.I. (1959). "Radiographic Atlas of Skeletal Development of the Hand and Wrist", 2nd Ed. Stanford University Press, Stanford.

Hajjar, R.A., Stratton Hill, C. and Samaan, N.A. (1975). *Acta endocr. (Copenh.)* **80**, 339.
Migeon, C.J., Green, O.P. and Eckert, J.P. (1963). *Metabolism* **12**, 718.
Reuter, A.M., Hendrick, J.C. and Franchimont, P. (1973). *Ann. Biol. Clin.* **31**, 479.
Tanaka, H., Manabe, H., Koshiyama, K., Hamanaka, Y., Matsumoto, K. and Uozumi, T. (1970). *Acta endocr. (Copenh.)* **65**, 1.
Tanner, J.M. (1962). "Growth at Adolescence", 2nd E., p.32. Blackwell Scientific Publications, Oxford.
Tonelli, E. and Marinelli, M. (1960). *Igiene e Sanità Pubblica* **16**, 736.

A HYPOTHALAMIC ISLET-STIMULATING FACTOR AND CHILDHOOD OBESITY

P. Lautala, H.K. Åkerblom, K. Kouvalainen and J.M. Martin

Department of Pediatrics, University of Oulu, Oulu, Finland
Research Institute, The Hospital for Sick Children, Toronto, Canada

Obesity is the most common nutritional disorder in developed countries, with a prevalence of approximately 10% according to various studies. This condition often starts already in childhood and usually continues into adulthood. Obesity in the latter period, in turn, increases the risk for cardiovascular diseases, diabetes mellitus, and various other chronic disorders. The etiology of obesity is manifold, but essentially there is commonly a disproportion between intake and consumption of calories.

The central role of the hypothalamus in the regulation of food intake has been known for decades, and obesity is a marker of certain hypothalamic syndromes, e.g. Fröhlich's syndrome. Several theories have been suggested to explain the hypothalamic regulation of food intake, e.g. the glucostatic, lipostatic, and thermostatic theories (Mogenson, 1976). The classical view was that the hunger center, located in the ventrolateral hypothalamus (VLH), and the satiety center in the ventromedial hypothalamus (VMH) would be mutually balanced in normal conditions. Therefore the damage to either center would be the immediate cause of the ensuing aphagia or hyperphagia, respectively. Keesey and Powley (1975) have proposed another interpretation for this hypothalamic function: the primary role of the ventrolateral and ventromedial hypothalamic centers would be to regulate jointly a "set point" for body weight and particularly for the amount of fat.

Regardless of the exact mechanism by which this hypothalamic balance operates, insulin has been implicated as a likely mediator in this sytem. Several experimental observations lend support to this hypothesis. Pancreatectomy (Young and Lin, 1965) or the destruction of the pancreatic beta-cells by streptozotocin (Ork and Bray, 1972) block the development of obesity in VMH-lesioned animals. The hyperinsulinemia of VMH-lesioned rats is a primary effect of the lesion (Martin *et al.*, 1974). Therefore a chronically elevated level of circulating insulin is probably a necessary condition for an elevated "set point" in a VMH-lesioned animal (Keesey and Powley, 1975). According to Keesey and Powley, this dual control model of weight regulation might not only account for the changes in weight following hypothalamic lesions but could also help to explain how individuals usually control their level of food intake.

External factors are also central in the regulation of food intake, and especially temperature is noteworthy in this respect.

As already indicated, insulin is important in the regulation of food intake. Insulin release is affected by many factors. Among them is the autonomous nervous system, parasympathetic nerve stimulation increasing and sympathetic nerve stimulation inhibiting insulin release (Woods and Porte, 1974). Humoral regulation of insulin release by the central nervous system may be a possibility as well. Yaksh and Myers (1972) described in cross-perfusion experiments in monkeys the release of neurohumoral substances from the hypothalamus, regulating food intake. A humoral factor has been found from the VLH, stimulating insulin release both *in vitro* and *in vivo* in several animal species (Idahl and Martin, 1971; Martin *et al.*, 1974; Lockhart-Ewart *et al.*, 1976). This humoral factor has been shown also in rat plasma (Martin *et al.*, 1973). In addition, hyperinsulinemia is found in obesity following stimulation of the VLH (Steffens, 1975). Recently further support for the hypothesis of hypothalamic participation in the regulation of endocrine pancreas was provided by the observation of decreased plasma insulin concentrations in rats injected with VMH medium (Moltz *et al.*, 1975).

Woods and Porte (1976) have suggested that insulin concentration in the cerebrospinal fluid may be the messenger informing the ventral hypothalamus about the amount of body fat.

But none of the above-mentioned hypotheses regarding the regulation of food intake and insulin release have been definitely proven. Furthermore, the possible pathogenetic role of a humoral VLH factor stimulating insulin release in some forms of human obesity is still unknown. Therefore, the present study was initiated to find out whether children with various types of obesity would have in their sera a factor, capable of stimulating *in vitro* insulin release.

I. SUBJECTS AND METHODS

A. *Subjects*

Obese children, aged 3 to 16 years, examined and treated at the Department of Pediatrics, University of Oulu and the Tahkokangas Institute for Mentally Retarded Children in Oulu were studied. Obesity was confirmed according to the weight and height standards for Finnish children. The etiology of obesity was various and in many cases unknown. Endocrinologically healthy non-obese children, aged 1½ to 14 years served as controls. Up to now we have studied the sera of 16 obese and 10 non-obese children.

B. *Methods*

Venous blood samples (15–20 ml) were collected during an oral glucose tolerance test (OGTT) at 0 and 30 min of the test for evaluating the presence of an islet-stimulating factor. In some cases, single fasting samples were taken. Serum was separated immediately after sampling and stored at −20°C until fractionation. Since previous observations (Martin *et al.*, 1973) have shown that the islet-stimulating factor in plasma is attached to albumin, we treated the serum samples with urea, 0.643 g/ml of serum, in an attempt to split the factor from albumin bonds. Samples were filtrated through Amicon membranes XM 50, UM 10, and UM 2*. The fraction on the top of the UM 2 membrane, of m.w. 1,000–10,000 was repeatedly washed with 0.9% NaCl until all the urea was removed as checked chemically. This washed fraction (approximately 5 ml) was immediately frozen and kept at −20°C until assayed.

The ability of the serum fraction to stimulate insulin release was tested *in vitro* using isolated islets of rat pancreas. Wistar rats of both sexes weighing 250–380 g were used. Islets were isolated (Lacy and Kostianovsky, 1967) and then preincubated in tissue culture medium (Parker's solution) for 2 hours before the final incubation period (Lockhart-Ewart *et al.*, 1976). The actual incubation was performed in Gey and Gey buffer containing a) 3.3 mmole glucose/litre (baseline), b) 16.5 mmole glucose/litre, and c) 3.3 mmole glucose/litre + 0.1 ml of the serum fraction in the atmosphere of 95% O_2 and 5% CO_2. The incubation medium contained $CaCl_2$ 2.0 mmole/litre and bovine serum albumin 1 mg/ml. Insulin released into the medium was measured radioimmunologically according to a modification of the method of Herbert *et al.* (1965). The amount of insulin released by islets incubated with the serum fractions (c) was compared to that of the islets incubated in baseline medium (a). Stimulation with high glucose (b) served as an internal control to assess the viability of the islets.

In addition, blood glucose and serum immunoreactive insulin (IRI) were measured on all specimens obtained during the OGTT. IRI was also measured in the serum fraction to be tested for islet-stimulating activity.

II. RESULTS

The classification of the cases according to the presence of an islet-stimulating factor in the serum is given in Table I.

Table I. Classification of the subjects according to the presence of an islet-stimulating factor (F +) in their serum.

	F + n	F − n
Obese children	4	12
Non-obese children	1	9
	5	21

The clinical data of the children positive for islet-stimulating activity in the fractionated serum as well as the results of the islet-incubation in each case are summarized in Table II.

Most of the serum fractions did not contain measurable amounts of IRI and in a few cases their insulin content was negligible (between 1 to 3 μU/ml). Despite

* Amicon Ultrafiltration Membranes, Amicon Corporation, Lexington, Mass., U.S.A.

Table II. Summary of the clinical data and the results of islet incubations in the cases with detectable islet-stimulating factor in the serum.

Case No.	Sex	Age yr	Excess weight SD	Clinical features	Insulin release during the incubation μU/islet/hour Mean ± SD Baseline	Serum fraction	p
1.	M	12	+ 3.5	Hypothalamic tumor, obesity	13.6 ± 6.1	28.1 ± 12.8	< 0.05
2.	F	9	+ 4.2	Obesity	6.6 ± 5.2	18.2 ± 4.4	< 0.005
3.	M	13	+ 5.5	Obesity	14.8 ± 3.3	20.6 ± 2.6	< 0.02
4.	F	2½	+ 2.0	Obesity	4.5 ± 1.4	7.1 ± 2.5	0.05<p<0.1
5.	F	1½	± 0	Urinary tract infection	7.1 ± 2.2	18.5 ± 2.1	< 0.001

their hyperinsulinemic response, there was no significant difference in the blood glucose and IRI values during the OGTT between obese children with and without islet-stimulating activity in their serum fractions. In all non-obese children blood glucose and IRI responses were normal.

III. DISCUSSION

In our study, various types of obese children were examined in respect of the presence of islet-stimulating activity in their sera. According to the results in animal experiments (Idahl and Martin, 1971; Martin *et al.*, 1973; Martin *et al.*, 1974; Lockhart-Ewart *et al.*, 1976) we have reason to believe that this activity is of hypothalamic origin. One of these obese children (Table II, Case No.1) is a boy who started to become obese about one year before the operation of angiosarcoma in the region of sella and hypothalamus. The other three obese children have no clear clinical signs of a hypothalamic syndrome. Surprisingly, we found islet-stimulating activity in the serum of one 1½ year old non-obese girl (Table II, Case No.5). The meaning of this finding needs more clarification. However, eleven months after the specimen was taken for the present study, the girl now has a slight overweight (excess weight + 1.5 SD).

The etiology of obesity is most likely multifactorial. In our study, the islet-stimulating activity was not found in the sera of all obese children studied. Our present hypothesis of the neurohormonal regulation of insulin release is that there might be a build-up system with different components for short- and long-term regulation: the acute effect on insulin release is mediated via the autonomous nervous system, whereas a slower starting and longer lasting effect could be mediated by humoral factor(s), the latter changing the threshold of the pancreatic beta-cells to various stimuli, for instance to glucose, amino acids, etc.. There is preliminary evidence that the humoral factor, which stimulates insulin release *in vitro* and *in vivo* and which in animal experiments has been shown to be of hypothalamic origin, also has a direct stimulatory effect on the metabolism of glucose in adipose tissue (Grimes *et al.*, 1976). Regardless of the mechanisms by which the food intake is steered, we assume that there should normally be a balance between factors increasing and decreasing the release of insulin. Therefore, to the VLH factor that increases insulin release there should be a counterpart which might be either somatostatin or the VMH material, described by Moltz *et al.* (1975), which decreases plasma insulin.

Our results, although preliminary, suggest that the islet-stimulating activity might have some role in the development of hyperinsulinemia in obesity and possibly also in the development of childhood obesity. Current investigations attempt to find out the possible role of the islet-stimulating factor in the pathogenesis of various types of obesity and its possible occurrence in children at various ages. Prospective studies are also needed, e.g. in cases with clinically recognized hypothalamic syndromes and in any type of childhood obesity, particularly during the first year(s) of obesity.

ACKNOWLEDGEMENTS

The financial support given by the Sigrid Juselius Foundation, including a travel grant given to Professor Julio M. Martin (Visiting Scientist, Department of Pediatrics, University of Oulu, 1975), and the Finnish Culture Foundation is gratefully acknowledged. We thank Novo Research Institute, Copenhagen, for providing us with the insulin radioimmunoassay kits.

ADDENDUM

Between the time of the presentation of this paper and the revision of the manuscript, we have additionally studied the sera of five obese and three non-obese children. In the first group, insulin stimulating activity was found in three cases and none in the second group.

REFERENCES

Grimes, L.J., Mok, C. and Martin, J.M. (1976). *Clin. Res.* **24** *(in press).*

Herbert, V., Lau, K-S, Gottlieb, C.W. and Bleicher, S.J. (1965). *J. clin. Endocr.* **25**, 1375-1384.

Idahl, L.-Å. and Martin, J.M. (1971). *J. Endocr.* **51**, 601-602.

Keesey, R.E. and Powley, T.L. (1975). *Am. Scient.* **63**, 558-565.

Lacy, P.E. and Kostianovsky, M. (1967). *Diabetes* **16**, 35-39.

Lockhart-Ewart, R.B., Mok, C. and Martin, J.M. (1976). *Diabetes* **25**, 96-100.

Martin, J.M., Mok, C.C., Penfold, J., Howard, N.J. and Crowne, D. (1973). *J. Endocr.* **58**, 681-682.

Martin, J.M., Konijnendijk, W. and Bouman, P.R. (1974). *Diabetes* **23**, 203-208.

Mogenson, G.J. (1976). *In* "Hunger: Basic Mechanisms and Clinical Implications" (D. Novin, W. Wyrwicka and G.A. Bray, eds) pp.473-485. Raven Press, New York.

Moltz, J.H., Fawcett, C.P., McCann, S.M., Dobbs, R.H. and Unger, R.H. (1975). *Endocr. Res. Commun.* **2**, 537-547.

Steffens, A.B. (1975). *Am. J. Physjol.* **228**, 1738-1744.

Woods, S.C. and Porte, D., Jr. (1974). *Physiol. Rev.* **54**, 596-619.

Woods, S.C. and Porte, D., Jr. (1976). *In* "Hunger: Basic Mechanisms and Clinical Implications" (D. Novin, W. Wyrwicka and G.A. Bray, eds) pp.273-280. Raven Press, New York.

Yaksh, T.L. and Myers, R.D. (1972). *Am. J. Phsyiol.* **222**, 503-515.

York, D.A. and Bray, G.A. (1972). *Endocrinology* **90**, 885-894.

Young, T.K. and Liu, A.C. (1965). *Chin. J. Physiol.* **19**, 247-253.

MONOAMINERGIC CONTROL OF GROWTH HORMONE SECRETION IN CHILDREN

F. Dammacco, N. Rigillo, G. Chetrì, C. Torelli, C. Mastrangelo
and A. Zuccaro

Department of Pediatrics, University of Bari, Italy

The mechanisms controlling the growth hormone (hGH) secretion in man, although extensively studied, remain not yet completely elucidated. Numerous reports have appeared indicating the existence of monoaminergic regulation of GH release, but the role played by single monoamines in the control of growth hormone secretion in man is still controversial.

Alpha-adrenergic receptors blockade with phentolamine reduces, while beta-andrenergic receptors blockade with propranolol enhances hGH responses to various stimuli in normal adults (Blackard and Heidingsfelder, 1968) and children (Parra *et al.*, 1970). These effects by central adrenergic mechanisms appear well-documented so that numerous GH-provocative stimuli have been devised with propranolol in combination with other pharmacologic agents in children (Collu *et al.*, 1975a; Maclaren *et al.*, 1975; Shanis and Moshang, 1976).

Uncertainty, however, persists about the dopaminergic and serotoninergic control of GH secretion in man. In this chapter we report the results obtained in children with drugs acting on central dopaminergic and serotoninergic mechanisms in order to elucidate further the role played by these systems in hGH secretion in children.

I. DOPAMINERGIC CONTROL OF hGH SECRETION

L-3,4-dihydroxyphenylanine (levodopa), a precursor of dopamine and noradrenaline, has been shown to increase hGH plasma concentrations in normal adults (Boyd *et al.*, 1970) and children (Chakmakjian *et al.*, 1973; Gomez-Sanchez and Kaplan, 1972; Laron *et al.*, 1973; Rigillo *et al.*, 1975; Root and Russ, 1972; Weldon *et al.*, 1973) after a single oral administration. The levodopa test is widely

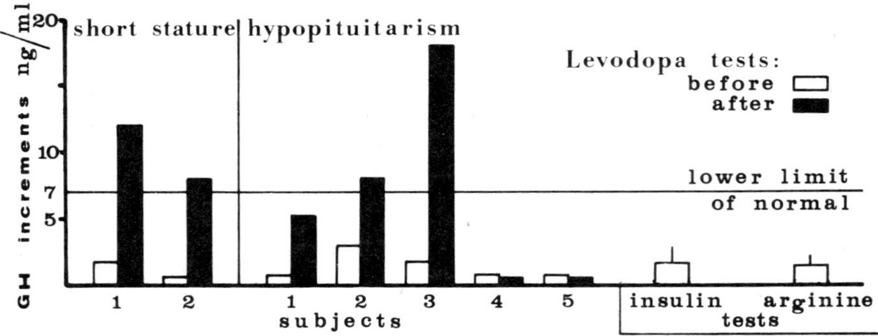

Fig.1 Plasma hGH peak increments after levodopa tests (250 mg po) before and after levodopa pretreatment in two children with non-endocrine short stature and in five hypopituitary subjects. Normal increment: > 7 ng/ml. Mean ± SEM of hGH responses to insulin and arginine tests in hypopituitary children.

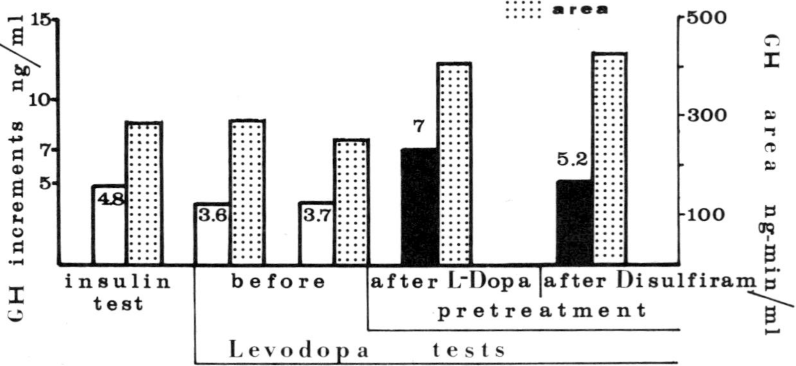

Fig.2 Plasma hGH peak increments and secretory areas to insulin test and to levodopa tests before and after levodopa or disulfiram pretreatment in a child with partial isolated GH deficiency.

employed in the identification of hypopituitary children, although associated with a variable percentage of false negative responses.

We have studied (Dammacco *et al.*, 1976b) the effect of an oral levodopa pretreatment (250 mg, twice a day, for five days) on the hGH release to levodopa test in children non "responders" to this drug. In two children with non-endocrine short stature the hGH response to levodopa became normal when the tests were performed after the pretreatment period (Fig.1). The same result was obtained in four of six hypopituitary dwarfs (three with total and one with partial isolated hGH deficiency) (Figs 1 and 2). The diagnosis of hGH deficiency in our hypopituitary children, aged 7—12 years, was made on the basis of clinical findings and absent hGH responses to insulin hypoglycemia (+1.52 ± 1.43 ng/ml), arginine infusion (+1.26 ± 0.82 ng/ml) and the first levodopa test (+1.32 ± 0.90 mean ± SEM ng/ml) (Fig.1). After the study reported here, these patients were treated with exogenous GH, showing the expected increase in growth velocity. These re-

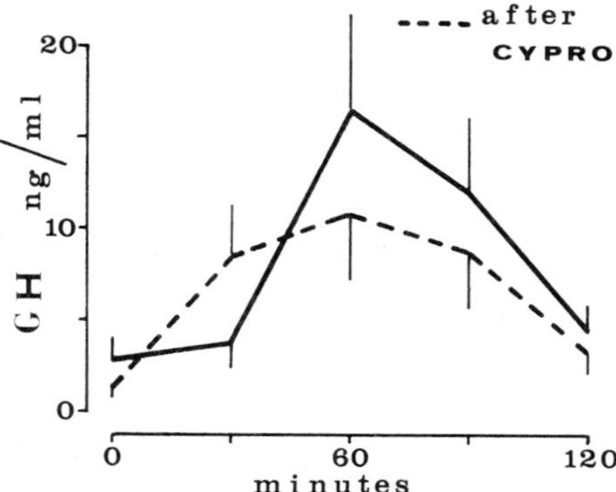

Fig.3 Plasma hGH levels during levodopa tests (250 mg po) before and after cyproheptadine in six constitutional short children.

sults confirmed the diagnosis of GH deficiency in our patients. As reported above, in four of these hypopituitary children the GH release induced by levodopa was found increased or normalized after five days of levodopa administration. A possible explanation for these results may be the existence of a defective hypothalamic monoaminergic control of hGH secretion at least in some of these patients. However, more GH deficient children have to be examined before conclusive pathogenetic information might be drawn from the levodopa priming diagnostic protocol.

It has been reported that levodopa, in addition to the expected increase in dopamine and noradrenaline levels, can induce a displacement of serotonin from nerve endings (Everett and Borcherding, 1970). Thus, it is possible that serotoninergic mechanisms may be involved in the GH response to levodopa administration.

In order to elucidate better the monoaminergic role in the hGH secretion induced by levodopa, we have employed two drugs: disulfiram, which increases dopamine concentrations blocking noradrenaline synthesis and cyproheptadine, a clinically used antiserotonin agent (Dammacco *et al.*, 1975).

In one child with isolated partial hGH deficiency, showing repeatedly intermediate hGH responses to levodopa tests, oral disulfiram administration (0.5 mg twice a day) significantly improved the response to levodopa tests (Fig.2). The same results were obtained in five adults by Giordano *et al.* (1973).

These findings suggest that dopaminergic mechanisms may play an important role in the hGH release observed after levodopa administration.

On the contrary, no significant modifications were observed in the hGH responses to levodopa after cyproheptadine administration in six constitutionally short children (Fig.3).

These results, suggesting no significant involvement of serotoninergic mechanisms in the levodopa induced hGH release, appear in contrast with those reported in adults with the same drug (Collu *et al.*, 1975b). A possible age-related difference in the control of growth hormone secretion may be invoked for this discrepancy.

A dopaminergic control of hGH secretion in man appears also to be suggested by our results (Dammacco *et al.*, 1976a) obtained with two other drugs:

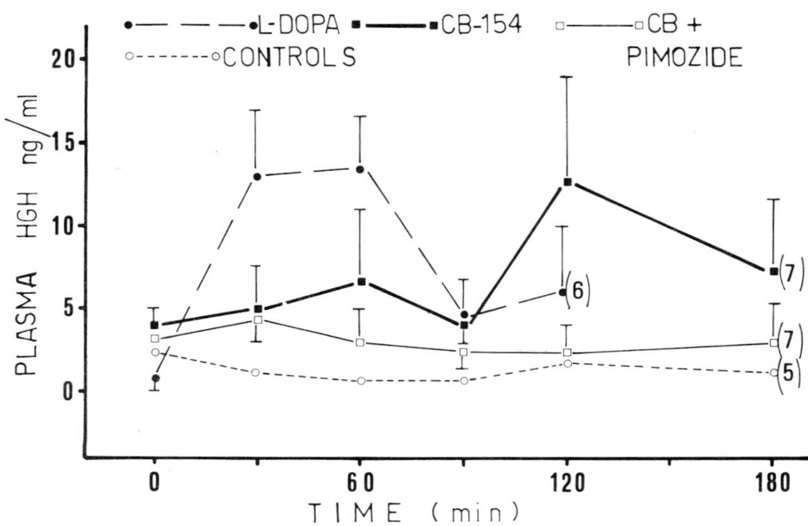

Fig.4 **Plasma hGH levels after administration of levodopa (6 children), CB-154 (2.5 mg po) and CB-154 following pimozide pretreatment (7 adult subjects) and placebo (5 normal adult subjects) (Mean ± SEM).**

2-bromo-α-ergocryptine (CB-154), a specific dopamine receptor agonist (Corrodi *et al.*, 1973), and pimozide, a specific long-acting dopaminergic receptor blocking agent (Anden *et al.*, 1970).

As shown in Fig.4, the oral administration of CB-154 significantly stimulated hGH secretion in normal volunteers, aged 17 to 21 years. In these subjects pimozide pretreatment (1 mg, orally, twice a day) abolished the hGH response to CB-154.

The same inhibitory effect of pimozide on plasma hGH levels was observed in one child, 12 years old, with Laron dwarfism (Laron, 1968). This child was given pimozide (0.5 mg orally, twice a day) for three days. On the third day of pimozide administration, several basal plasma hGH levels were found suppressed to less than 0.4 ng/ml. On the contrary, the fasting GH levels were in the acromegalic range before pimozide administration (7 determinations: 15.10 ± 6.80 ng/ml, mean ± SEM) and returned elevated three days after pimozide (Fig.5). Thus, pimozide showed its inhibitory effects on hGH secretion both in normal secretory states and in hGH hyperincretory diseases.

II. EFFECTS OF CYPROHEPTADINE ON hGH SECRETION

Cyproheptadine, a clinically used antiserotonin agent with antihistamine and anticholinergic effects (Stone *et al.*, 1961), has been shown to have inhibitory influences on GH secretion in animals (Smythe *et al.*, 1975) and man.

In adult subjects the growth hormone responses to insulin hypoglycemia (Bivens *et al.*, 1973; Smythe and Lazarus, 1974), arginine infusion (Nakai *et al.*, 1974), physical exercise (Smythe and Lazarus, 1974), levodopa (Collu *et al.*, 1975b) and 5-hydroxythriptophan (Nakai *et al.*, 1974) have been found reduced

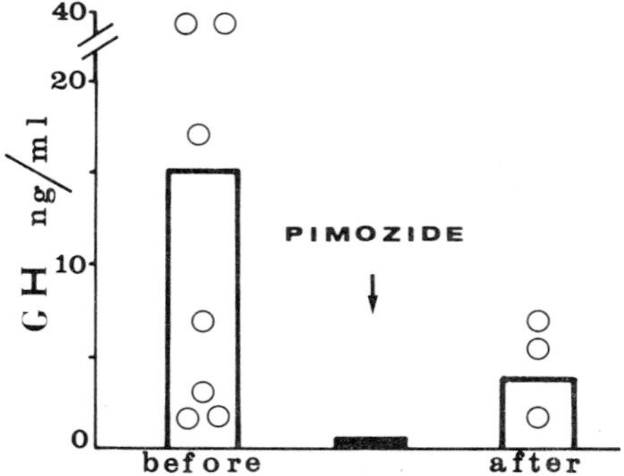

Fig.5 Basal hGH levels in a child with Laron dwarfism before, during and after pimozide administration.

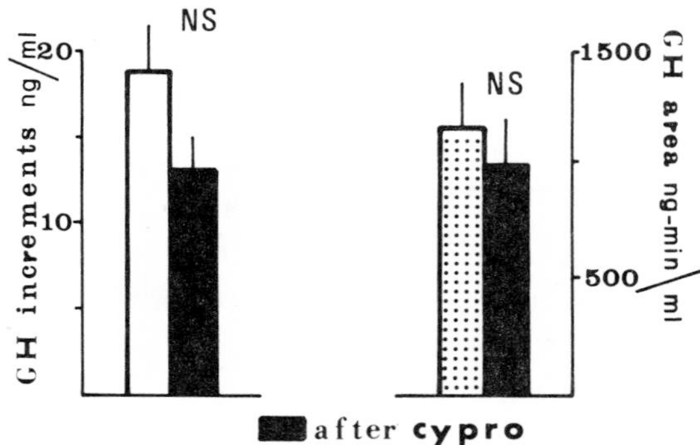

Fig.6 Mean ± SEM of hGH peak increments and secretory areas observed during insulin, arginine, physical exercise and levodopa tests in 18 children before and after cyproheptadine administration. NS: no statistical significance.

after cyproheptadine administration.

We have studied the effects of cyproheptadine on hGH secretion induced by different provocative stimuli in children. The subjects were eighteen non-endocrine growth-retarded children. Levodopa (250 mg in single oral dose) was administered to six subjects; insulin hypoglycemia (0.1 U/kg), arginine infusion (0.5 g/kg) and physical exercise were performed in groups of four children for a total of twelve subjects. After the baseline tests, the children were given cyproheptadine, 8 mg/day, for five days. On the morning of the sixth day, a final dose of cyproheptadine, 4 mg, was administered two hours before repeating the tests. Cyproheptadine did not significantly change the GH responses to different stimuli in each group of subjects. When the children were examiend all together, the means of plasma hGH increments and secretory areas were found reduced, 30% and 14% respectively, after cyproheptadine administration (Fig.6). However, this reduction did not reach statistical significance.

Furthermore, we have studied the effect of cyproheptadine administration on the sleep-related growth hormone secretion in three children and six adult

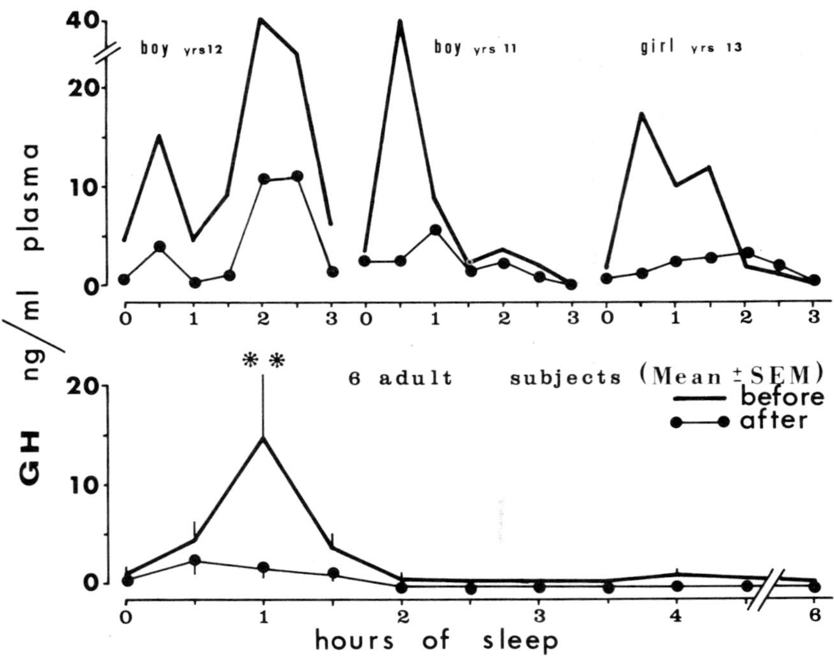

Fig. 7 Plasma hGH levels during sleep in 3 children and 6 adults before and after cyproheptadine administration. **: $p < 0.01$.

subjects, 8 and 12 mg/day for five days respectively (Dammacco *et al.*, 1976c). The subjects were studied before cyproheptadine and on the fifth night of cyproheptadine administration. All-night polygraphic recordings were carried out in the adult volunteers. As shown in Fig. 7, a significant reduction of hGH release was observed in children as well as in adults. Thus, cyproheptadine showed its inhibitory effect mainly on the physiologic GH secretion related to the onset of sleep.

If this drug acts at central levels, as an antiserotonin agent, our results would suggest that in children serotoninergic mechanisms play a major role in the physiologic sleep-related growth hormone secretion. However, other studies with more specific antiserotonin agents are needed to define better the serotoninergic role in the control of the growth hormone secretion in children.

REFERENCES

Anden, N.E., Butcher, S.G., Corrodi, H., Fuxe, K. and Ungerstedt, U. (1970). *Eur. J. Pharmac.* **11**, 303-314.

Bivens, C.H., Lebovitz, H.E. and Feldman, J.M. (1973). *New Engl. J. Med.* **289**, 236-240.

Blackard, W.G. and Heidingsfelder, S.A. (1968). *J. clin. Invest.* **47**, 1407-1414.

Boyd, A.E., Lebovitz, H.E. and Pfeiffer, G.B. (1970). *New Engl. J. Med.* **283**, 1425-1429.

Chakmakjian, Z.H., Marks, J.F. and Fink, C.W. (1973). *Pediatr. Res.* **7**, 71-75.

Collu, R., Leboeuf, G., Letarte, J. and Ducharme, J.R. (1975a). *Pediatrics* **56**, 262-267.

Collu, R., Jequier, J.C., Letarte, J., Leboeuf, G. and Ducharme, J.R. (1975b). *Horm. Metab. Res.* **7**, 96-97.

Corrodi, H., Fuxe, K., Hokfelt, T., Lidbrink, P. and Ungerstedt, U. (1973). *J. Pharm. Pharmac.* **25**, 409-410.

Dammacco, F., Rigillo, N., Zimbalatti, F., Brunetti, L., Scaramuzzi, O. and Dammacco, A. (1975). *In* "Atti Giornate Endocrinologiche Senesi" (E.E. Muller and S.E. Piazzi, eds) pp.351-356. Edizioni ISVT, Sclavo, Siena.

Dammacco, F., Rigillo, N., Tafaro, E., Gagiardi, F., Chetrì, G. and Dammacco, A. (1976a). *Horm. Metab. Res.* **8**, 247-248.

Dammacco, F., Rigillo, N., Chetrì, G., Tafaro, E. and Torelli, C. (1976b). *In* "Atti XVI Congresso Naz. Soc. I. Endocrinologia", p.39. Serono, Symposia.

Dammacco, F., Puca, F.M., Rigillo, N., Genco, S., Specchio, L.M., Chetrì, G., Torelli, C., Mastrangelo, C., Candeliere, C. and Galeone, D. (1976c). Presented at "Third European Congress of Sleep Research", Montpellier, France *(in press).*

Everett, G.M. and Borchoerdering, J.W. (1970). *Science* **168**, 849-850.

Giordano, G., Marugo, M., Minuto, F., Barreca, T. and Foppiani, E. (1973). *Folia Endocrinologica* **26**, 523-535.

Gomez-Sanchez, C. and Kaplan, N.M. (1972). *J. clin. Endocr. Metab.* **34**, 1105-1107.

Laron, Z., Josefsberg, Z. and Doron, M. (1973). *Clin. Endocrinol.* **2**, 1-7.

Laron, Z., Pertzelan, A. and Karp, M. (1968). *Isr. J. Med. Sci.* **4**, 883-897.

Maclaren, N.K., Taylor, G.E. and Raiti, S. (1975). *Pediatrics* **56**, 804-807.

Nakai, Y., Imura, H., Sakurai, H., Kurahachi, H. and Yoshimi, T. (1974). *J. clin. Endocr. Metab.* **38**, 446-449.

Parra, A., Schultz, R.B., Foley, T.P. and Blizzard, R.M. (1970). *J. clin. Endocr. Metab.* **30**, 134-137.

Rigillo, N., Dammacco, F., Pentasuglia, N. and Zimbalatti, F. (1975). *Minerva Pediatrica* **27**, 908-914.

Root, A.W. and Russ, R.D. (1972). *J. Pediatr.* **81**, 808-813.

Shanis, B.S. and Moshang, T. (1976). *Pediatrics* **57**, 712-714.

Smythe, G.A. and Lazarus, L. (1974). *J. clin. Invest.* **54**, 116-121.

Smythe, G.A., Brandstater, J.F. and Lazarus, L. (1975). *Neuroendocrinology* **17**, 245-257.

Stone, C.A., Wenger, H.C., Ludden, C.T., Stavorsky, J.M. and Ross, C.A. (1961). *J. Pharmac. exp. Ther.* **131**, 73-84.

Weldon, V.V., Gupta, S.K., Haymond, M.W., Pagliara, A.S., Jacobs, L.S. and Daughaday, W.H. (1973). *J. clin. Endocr. Metab.* **36**, 42-46.

AN UNIDENTIFIED ACTH STIMULABLE ADRENAL STEROID IN CHILDHOOD HYPERTENSION

M.I. New and L.S. Levine

Department of Pediatrics, The New York Hospital, Cornell Medical Center New York, USA

We would like to add to the body of data suggesting the existence of an unknown mineralocorticoid in low renin hypertension.

In the clinical studies about to be presented we have produced evidence that there is an ACTH stimulable steroidal hormone capable of raising blood pressure. Further, the data indicate that this steroidal hormone is not a *known* mineralocorticoid.

The first patient studied was an 18 year old boy with dexamethasone suppressible hyperaldosteronism and hypertension. He was first reported at the age of 12 years and subsequent studies indicated that the only steroid he oversecreted was aldosterone (New *et al.*, 1976; New *et al.*, 1973). At age 18, the slightly elevated levels of urinary aldosterone were still readily suppressed with 1 mg of dexamethasone though he rarely complied with medication at home (Fig.1, Panel E).

With dexamethasone suppression aldosterone excretion fell below 0.7 mcg/day within 24 h (Panel F). The initially low renin (normal values 0.5–5 ng/ml/h) rose as natriuresis occurred accompanied by a slight weight loss. Blood pressure returned to normal over 5 days. Urinary potassium decreased transiently. We reasoned that if aldosterone were causing the hypertension in the untreated state, then administration of aldosterone in the suppressed state should cause a rise in blood pressure.

With aldosterone excretion suppressed and while the patient was normotensive, aldosterone was administered 1 mg daily over 24 h intravenously for 5 days (Panel G). This administration is reflected in the increased urinary excretion of aldosterone. Marked sodium retention and weight gain occurred but there was no significant change in blood pressure. There was slight kaliuresis and,

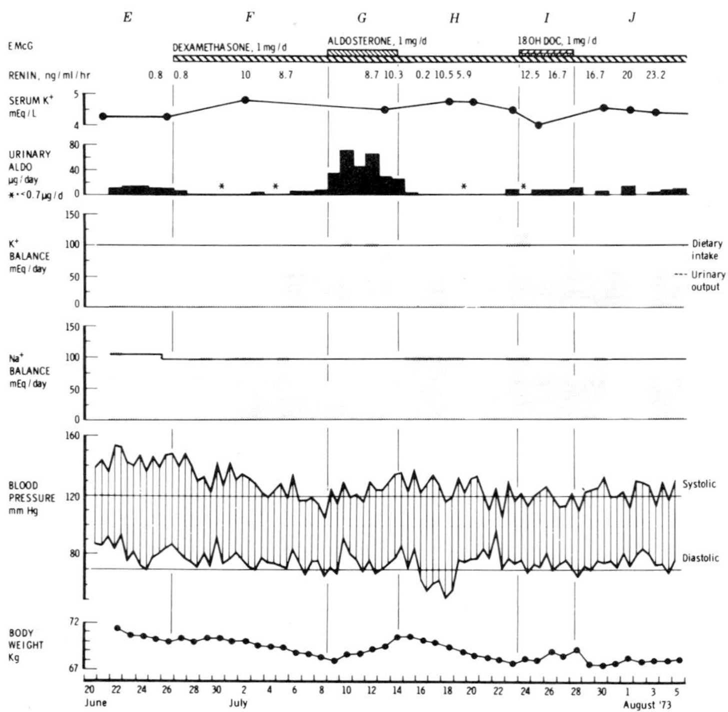

Fig.1 Metabolic balance of sodium and potassium correlated with blood pressure and various periods of therapy and hormonal measurements. In this figure as in others are depicted the medication, plasma renin activity, serum potassium, urinary aldosterone (pH1), potassium balance, sodium balance, blood pressure and weight. The blood pressure was taken 6 times during the day and 6 times during the night. The mean day and night time pressures are depicted.

inexplicably, plasma renin did not decrease, although 2 days later it was low. Thus it appeared that aldosterone administration in large quantities induced sodium retention but *not* hypertension in this patient within a 5 day period.

Aldosterone infusion was discontinued (Panel H). The aldosterone excretion fell and natriuresis occurred with loss of body weight and potassium retention. The patient remained normotensive.

18-OH-DOC was given, 1 mg intravenously over 24 h for 5 days (Panel I). Minimal changes in sodium and potassium balance occurred and no change in blood pressure. Low mineralocorticoid activity of 18-OH-DOC has been reported in bioassays (Melby *et al.*, 1972; Porter *et al.*, 1971). The unexplained high renin levels were observed repeatedly. The failure of administered aldosterone and 18-OH-DOC to suppress renin may be the result of continuous dexametha-

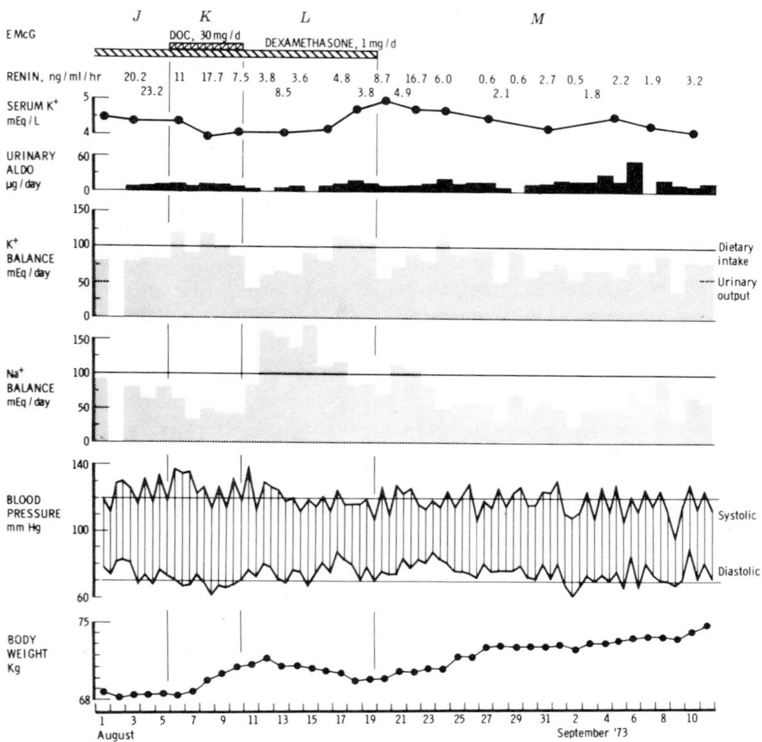

Fig.2 Metabolic balance of sodium and potassium correlated with blood pressure and various periods of therapy and hormonal measurements.

sone suppression. Dexamethasone suppresses the ACTH-regulated aldosterone secretion, allowing plasma renin to rise, which then stimulates renin mediated aldosterone secretion. This mechanism has been described in 17-hydroxylase deficiency (New, 1971; Biglieri *et al.*, 1966). No significant metabolic or blood pressure changes occurred when 18-OH-DOC administration ceased (Panel J).

With continued dexamethasone treatment, DOC was administered 30 mg daily intravenously for 5 days (Fig.2, Panel K). A slight fall in serum potassium and increased urinary excretion of potassium occurred. There was marked sodium retention and a weight gain of 2 kg. Again *no* increase in blood pressure was observed. Renin decreased somewhat but not to baseline levels. Failure of DOC to suppress plasma renin activity is unexplained. The effects of 30 mg of administered DOC are similar to the effects of 1 mg of administered aldosterone.

With discontinuation of DOC, natriuresis and potassium retention occurred accompanied by a rise in serum potassium (Panel L). The sodium retention, kaliuresis and weight gain resulting from the administered DOC is validated by reversal of the effect when DOC is discontinued. The lack of a DOC effect on blood pressure is also confirmed by the absence of change in blood pressure whether or not the DOC was being administered. As was suggested for Panel J, the continued excretion of small amounts of aldosterone suggests that the increased renin stimulates aldosterone despite ACTH suppression.

These studies of the effects of aldosterone, 18-OH-DOC, and DOC suggest that none of these hormones administered alone is capable of raising blood pressure after five days of continuous infusion at superphysiological doses despite a strong mineralocorticoid effect observed with aldosterone and DOC. The next series of studies was designed in order to determine whether the five-day period was too short to observe an effect of adrenal steroids on blood pressure.

After all treatment was discontinued, we wished to observe how long it would take for the patient's endogenous ACTH to reappear and produce hypertension and sodium retention (Panel M). Within five days of discontinuing dexamethasone treatment, sodium retention and weight gain occurred. After 14 days without dexamethasone, urinary aldosterone excretion increased and plasma renin activity decreased after seven days. However, hypertension did not recur even after three weeks without dexamethasone therapy, at a time when aldosterone excretion was high.

The dual regulation of aldosterone is again demonstrated in this period. After short-term dexamethasone suppression in this patient, aldosterone excretion decreased to below detectable levels, while renin remained suppressed indicating ACTH regulation of aldosterone. It was shown in a previous report of this patient (New *et al.*, 1973), that during dexamethasone treatment, a low salt diet provoked a rise in renin and aldosterone suggesting renin rather than ACTH was regulating aldosterone in the dexamethasone-suppressed state. This renin regulation is again suggested at the end of prolonged dexamethasone suppression (Panel L), when the renin remained elevated and aldosterone secretion was low but measurable. Two weeks following discontinuation of dexamethasone treatment, the urinary aldosterone excretion increased and the plasma renin activity decreased. This suggests that ACTH regulation of aldosterone resumed by the twelfth day after discontinuation of dexamethasone. Though aldosterone was being excreted in excess at the end of this period, hypertension did not recur, indicating that aldosterone did not raise blood pressure in this patient even after three weeks of excess aldosterone secretion, sodium retention and weight gain.

In order to evaluate whether infusion of ACTH was capable of producing an increase in blood pressure within the period of five days in which steroids were infused, ACTH (40 units intravenously over 24 h for six days; 80 units intravenously over 24 h for two days) was administered (Fig.3, Panel N). This was associated with increased aldosterone excretion, sodium retention, weight gain and a fall in serum potassium. The increased aldosterone excretion continued throughout the period of ACTH administration. The plasma renin activity did not decrease to pretreatment levels observed in panel E (Fig.1).

The infusion of ACTH produced a rise in blood pressure within five days whereas infusion of aldosterone, 18-OH-DOC or DOC administration were without effect on blood pressure in this period of time (Panels G, I, K) (Figs 1 and 2). This suggests that ACTH stimulated the adrenal secretion of a steroid other than those infused which was capable of causing a rise in blood pressure within

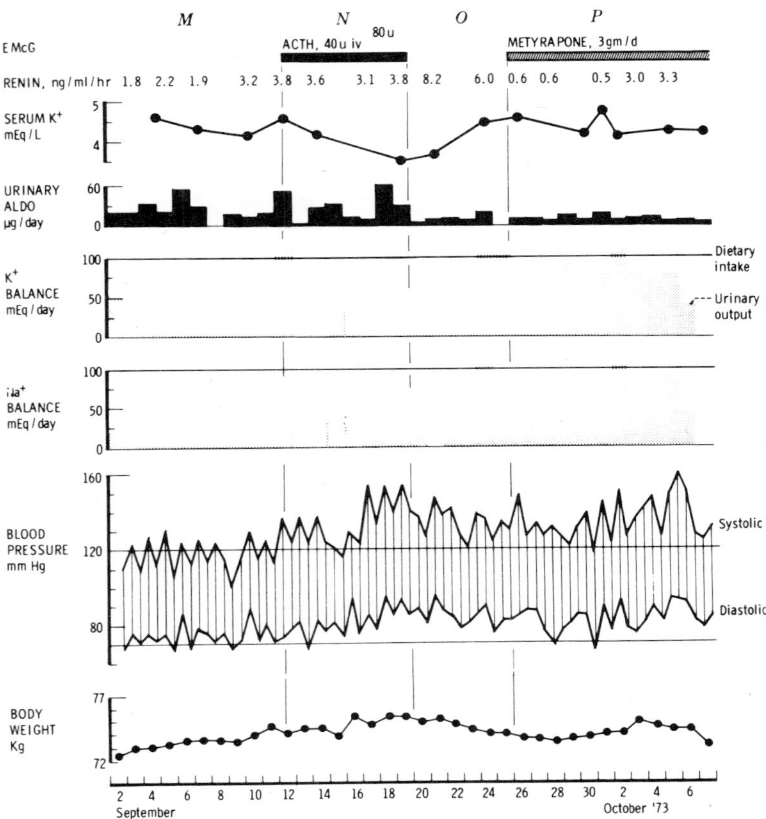

Fig.3 **Metabolic balance of sodium and potassium correlated with blood pressure and various periods of therapy and hormonal measurements.**

5 days. Quantitatively the amount of aldosterone administered was far greater than that stimulated by the ACTH. Blood pressure, however, rose only during ACTH administration, further supporting the hypothesis that the blood pressure effect of ACTH was mediated through a hormone other than aldosterone. The failure of aldosterone to decrease during continuous ACTH administration was unexpected. Continuous ACTH administration has been reported to cause an initial increase in aldosterone excretion followed by a decrease within five days. The decrease is interpreted as "escape" from ACTH (Newton *et al.*, 1968; Biglieri *et al.*, 1969). Although sodium retention and weight gain were observed during ACTH, aldosterone, or DOC administration, plasma renin activity failed to decrease to pretreatment levels observed in Panel E. The failure of ACTH to induce regularly a fall in renin has been reported by others (Newton *et al.*, 1968; Scoggins *et al.*,

1974). In addition, it has been demonstrated that DOC administration does not cause a plasma renin activity in subjects with various forms of hypertension (Biglieri *et al.*, 1972), in contrast to the prompt decline observed in normal subjects when DOC is administered (Shade *et al.*, 1975). This failure of DOC to suppress renin in hypertensive states has been attributed to the reduced cumulative sodium retention and weight gain in hypertensives as compared to normals (Biglieri *et al.*, 1970). In this patient, however, renin suppression with mineralocorticoid administration failed to occur even in the presence of sodium retention and weight gain. The response of renin to the administration of mineralocorticoids in hypertensives has not been studied extensively. Thus, the renin data in this patient as well as in other hypertensives remains to be clarified.

After ACTH was discontinued, aldosterone excretion decreased. Within five days the patient returned to potassium and sodium balance (Panel O). The patient lost 2 kg of weight so that his weight was the same as that before the ACTH administration. Blood pressure decreased slightly. Plasma renin activity increased and serum potassium rose to 4.5 mEq/L. Thus, with discontinuation of ACTH a rapid reversal of the mineralocorticoid effects was seen although blood pressure changes were minimal.

Blood pressure had not returned to baseline levels at the start of metyrapone treatment. Administration of metyrapone produced a transient sodium retention and a marked fall in plasma renin activity (Fig.4, Panel P). As sodium retention subsided, blood pressure and plasma renin activity increased. Aldosterone excretion remained low but detectable throughout the period of metyrapone treatment.

In this patient blood pressure was maintained at an elevated level with metyrapone. It has been demonstrated that metyrapone interferes with the formation of cortisol by inhibiting the initial cleavage of cholesterol into pregnenolone in addition to inhibiting the 11β-hydroxylation of 11-desoxycortisol (Carballeira *et al.*, 1976). However, a compensatory ACTH increase can overcome the metyrapone inhibition of cholesterol side-chain cleavage activity (Carballeira *et al.*, 1976). The rise in ACTH secretion in the presence of the 11β-hydroxylase inhibition results in a rise in DOC secretion. The elevation of blood pressure during metyrapone is probably not due to increased DOC secretion since it was demonstrated (Panel K) that five days of continuous infusion of DOC in large amounts did not produce hypertension. The effects of metyrapone are probably secondary to increased secretion of ACTH. This is supported by the similar changes in weight, blood pressure, sodium and potassium balance and plasma renin activity observed at the end of the ACTH and metyrapone treatment periods. The major difference between the ACTH (Panel N) and metyrapone (Panel P) treatment is in the quantity of aldosterone excretion. During metyrapone administration aldosterone excretion was not elevated. These studies further suggest that endogenous or exogenous ACTH can induce the adrenal secretion of an unidentified steroid capable of raising blood pressure. This unidentified hormone is not completely dependent on sodium retention for its capacity to raise blood pressure.

In order to determine whether ACTH mediates its effect on blood pressure via secretion of a steroid hormone, or is in itself the blood pressure raising agent, metyrapone was continued and aminoglutethimide was added. The elevated blood pressure returned to normal, aldosterone excretion was markedly reduced, and a sodium diuresis and a rise in serum potassium ensued. Body weight de-

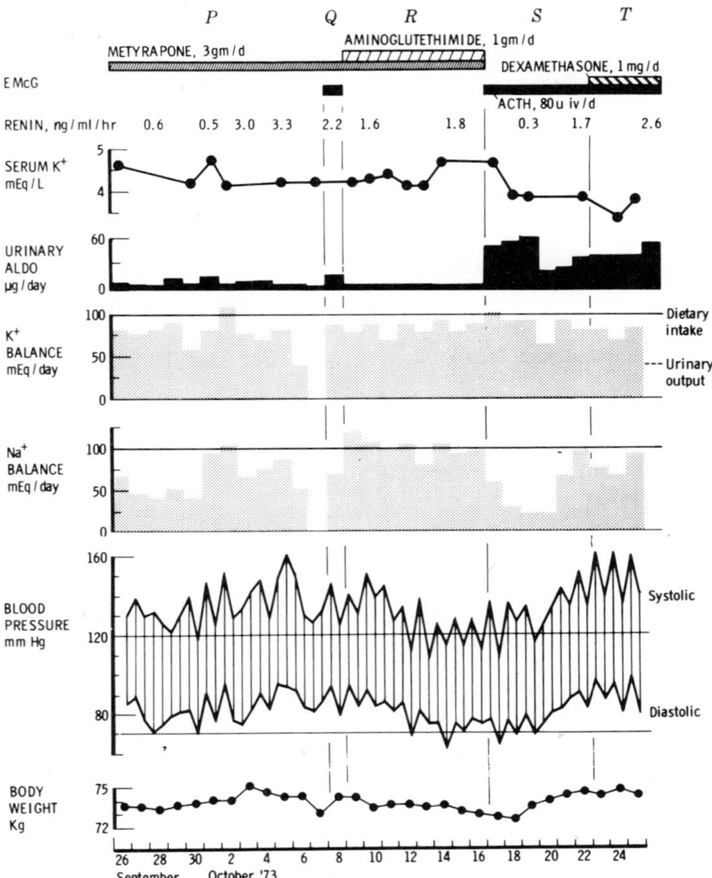

Fig.4 **Metabolic balance of sodium and potassium correlated with blood pressure and various periods of therapy and hormonal measurements.**

creased slightly. Plasma renin activity remained at low normal levels. Aminoglutethimide inhibits steroid synthesis by blocking the conversion of cholesterol at C_{21} steroids. Via the negative feedback, adrenal-pituitary mechanism, ACTH secretion rises during aminoglutethimide treatment. The rapid fall in blood pressure to normal levels during this period is strong evidence that the hypertension observed during the periods of metyrapone (Panel P) and ACTH administration (Panel N) is due to adrenal secretion of an unidentified steroid and is not due to a direct pressor action of ACTH.

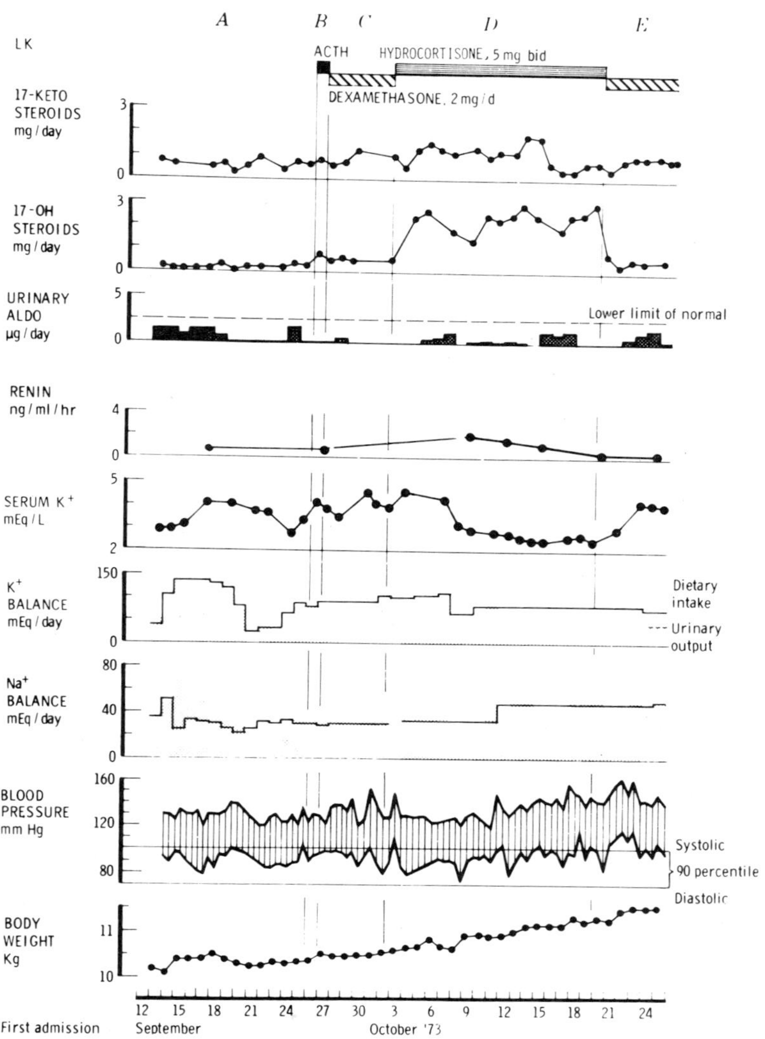

Fig.5 Metabolic balance of sodium and potassium correlated with blood pressure and various periods of therapy and hormonal measurements. The mean daytime and nighttime blood pressures are presented. The 90th percentile blood pressure for a child her age is indicated in each panel (McCammon, 1970).

Finally, ACTH was administered again as before with an even more dramatic rise in blood pressure, rise in urinary aldosterone and sodium retention (Panel S). The hypertension was persistent while the sodium retention was transient. Thus the hypertensive effect of ACTH was reproducible (Panels N and S) and was not dependent on sodium retention. In both periods of ACTH administration aldosterone excretion increased and remained elevated.

This failure of "escape" of aldosterone secretion from ACTH regulation is abnormal, and has been observed in hyperaldosteronism associated with adrenal hyperplasia (Miura *et al.*, 1968). It has also been demonstrated in another kindred with dexamethasone-suppressible hyperaldosteronism (Grim *et al.*, 1975).

The effect of ACTH was not diminished by concurrent administration of dexamethasone, demonstrating that dexamethasone treatment lowers blood pressure and aldosterone by suppressing ACTH and not by a peripheral action on the adrenals as suggested by Ruse *et al.* (1972) (Panel T).

We concluded from these studies that an ACTH stimulable steroid other than aldosterone, 18-OH-DOC, or DOC may be the cause of hypertension in this patient. The metyrapone and aminoglutethimide studies further suggest it is an adrenal steroid.

This hypothesis was strengthened by the study of a 3-year-old Zuni Indian girl with a 46/XX karyotype. She presented with hypertension and hypokalemia. She had been hospitalized many times for gastroenteritis and survived without steroid treatment. The following studies were carried out on the Pediatric Clinical Research Center of New York Hospital-Cornell Medical Center.

Urinary excretion of 17-ketosteroids, 17-hydroxysteroids, aldosterone and morning plasma cortisol (4.9 μg/dl) were low (Fig.5, Panel A). Hypokalemia was present and persisted despite potassium supplementation of 150 mEq/d. Plasma renin activity was decreased (normal values, 0.5–5 ng/ml/h). Blood pressure was markedly elevated. Low potassium intake at the end of this period resulted in decreased sodium wasting. Potassium has been shown to cause sodium wasting experimentally (Brandis *et al.*, 1972).

Thus, this 3-year-old child demonstrated hypertension and hypokalemia in the absence of excessive aldosterone excretion. A standard ACTH test, 40 U intravenously over six hours caused an increase in plasma cortisol to 23 μg/dl (Panel B). Urinary 17-hydroxysteroid excretion increased slightly when measured by the Porter-Silber chromogen method. Plasma renin activity remained low.

These findings suggest that the patient's capacity to secrete cortisol was impaired both in the baseline period and in response to ACTH. The low plasma renin activity in the presence of low urinary aldosterone, hypokalemia and hypertension suggest the presence of a mineralocorticoid other than aldosterone.

Dexamethasone and hydrocortisone were administered sequentially (Panel C, D, E). The blood pressure did not decrease and indeed appeared to increase. The child became quite cushingoid and weight increased progressively. The 17-hydroxysteroids reflected the administration of hydrocortisone. Aldosterone excretion and plasma renin activity remained low. While dexamethasone administration was continued, dietary sodium was reduced to 10 mEq/day (Fig.6, Panel F). This resulted in a negative sodium balance, and a prompt decrease in blood pressure. No change in weight or urinary aldosterone was observed. When potassium intake was reduced from 60 mEq/day to 30 mEq/day, a marked decrease in urinary sodium occurred.

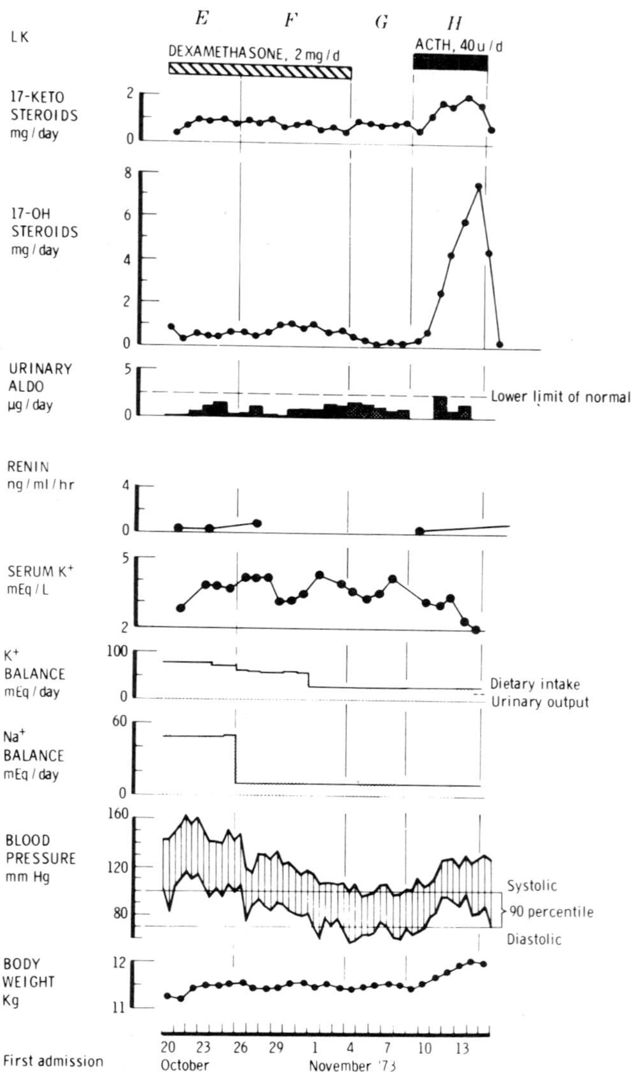

Fig.6 Metabolic balance of sodium and potassium correlated with blood pressure and various periods of therapy and hormonal measurements.

Despite the decreased potassium intake she remained in positive potassium balance and serum potassium rose. The fall in blood pressure upon restriction of dietary sodium demonstrates the dependence of blood pressure on sodium intake. This decrease in blood pressure occurred despite the continuation of dexamethasone treatment which had previously caused elevation of blood pressure. The ability to conserve sodium in the absence of an elevation of urinary aldosterone suggests the presence of another mineralocorticoid. Her capacity to conserve sodium as well as potassium indicated good renal function.

The fall in blood pressure observed in the absence of weight loss suggests there was no net fluid loss. Blood pressure and serum potassium remained in the normal range when dexamethasone was discontinued (Panel G). Plasma renin activity as well as urinary aldosterone excretion remained low at the end of this period and after 15 days of dietary sodium restriction (10 mEq/day). We interpreted these results to mean that the important element in the fall in blood pressure was the sodium restriction; dexamethasone did not contribute to the fall in blood pressure.

The absence of weight loss when blood pressure was reduced indicates that the sodium effect was not mediated through a measurable loss of body water. The persistent suppression of plasma renin activity despite dietary sodium restriction suggests that a mineralocorticoid was present. The effect of the unknown mineralocorticoid on blood pressure, however, was not apparent in the sodium restricted state.

While the low sodium diet was maintained, ACTH was administered intravenously (40 U/day) continuously for five days (Panel H). Urinary 17-ketosteroids and 17-hydroxycorticoids rose to 2 and 7 mg/d respectively, but aldosterone excretion never increased above 2 μg/d. Plasma cortisol rose to a maximum of 32 μg/dl. Serum potassium concentration fell to less than 2 mEq/L. Blood pressure increased significantly and there was 0.5 kg gain in weight. Urinary sodium and potassium excretion did not change from the pre-ACTH period.

Thus, an increase in blood pressure was produced by ACTH without a concomitant increase in aldosterone excretion. This suggests that ACTH stimulated a factor other than aldosterone capable of raising blood pressure. This factor appears to be a mineralocorticoid as is evident by the precipitous fall in serum potassium concentration. The fall in serum potassium was apparently not the result of kaliuresis as no increase in urinary potassium was observed. The weight gain suggests fluid retention despite the low sodium intake. The ability of ACTH to increase blood pressure was sufficient to override the hypotensive effect of a low sodium diet. Blood pressure was restored to hypertensive levels observed on a normal sodium diet. Thus, the factor stimulated by ACTH which raises blood pressure is only partly dependent on sodium intake. The rise in 17-hydroxycorticoid excretion and plasma cortisol suggests that the adrenal is capable of secreting glucocorticoids but not to a normal degree. Children of similar size and age increase urinary 17-hydroxycorticoids to 60 mg/day and plasma cortisol to 70 μg/100 ml after five days of ACTH (unpublished data). Thus it seems likely that ACTH was stimulating a hormone which is a mineralocorticoid capable of raising blood pressure and that this hormone may be the same hormone causing hypertension, hypokalemia and hyporeninemia in the untreated state. The failure of ACTH to stimulate aldosterone even transiently shows a defect in aldosterone secretion which is marked. The subnormal increase in urinary 17-hydroxycorti-

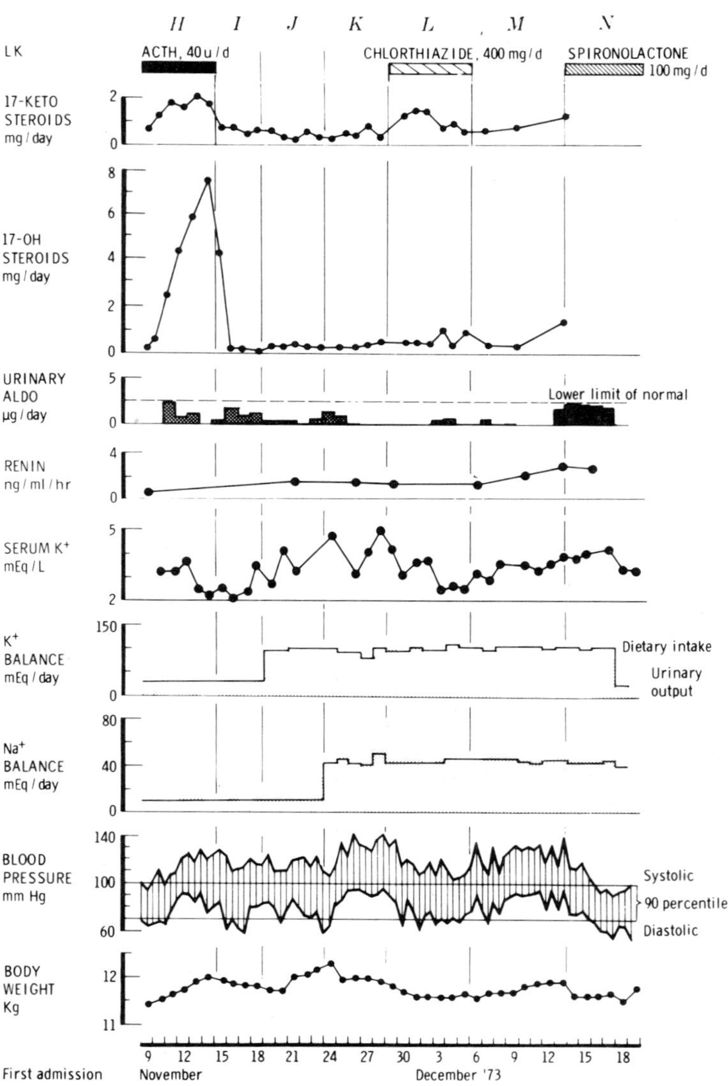

Fig. 7 Metabolic balance of sodium and potassium correlated with blood pressure and various periods of therapy and hormonal measurements.

coids and plasma cortisol with prolonged ACTH treatment indicates that glucocorticoid secretion is also impaired but to a lesser extent than aldosterone.

With discontinuation of ACTH, blood pressure decreased within 48 h (Fig. 7, Panel I). Urinary 17-hydroxycorticoids and 17-ketosteroids fell promptly to low pretreatment levels. Weight declined slightly. Serum potassium rose after ACTH had been discontinued for five days. Aldosterone excretion did not change significantly.

Throughout the whole study, aldosterone excretion and plasma renin activity remained low and fairly fixed. The rise in 17-hydroxysteroids and plasma cortisol with ACTH and the rapid fall when ACTH was discontinued raises the possibility that in the untreated state ACTH is suppressed by an unidentified steroid resulting in a very low glucocorticoid secretion. (See plasma ACTH concentration below.)

When potassium intake was increased to 100 mEq/d, blood pressure did not change significantly (Panel J). There was net potassium retention and a rise in serum potassium to 4.5 mEq/L. Aldosterone excretion and plasma renin activity remained at low levels. There was a slight weight gain and natriuresis occurred. Although administration of large amounts of potassium is recognized as a potent stimulator of aldosterone secretion in normal subjects and subjects with hyperaldosteronism, in this patient the stimulus did not produce any increase in aldosterone. Renin was also not stimulated despite a natriuresis in association with a high potassium intake. The effect of dietary sodium restriction in lowering the blood pressure persisted.

With an increase in dietary sodium to normal amounts for age (40 mEq/d) (Panel K), the blood pressure rose to the hypertensive levels observed prior to institution of the low sodium diet. Serum potassium fluctuated. Urinary excretion of 17-hydroxysteroids, aldosterone and plasma renin activity did not change significantly. It appears, therefore, that in this child blood pressure is responsive to both ACTH and sodium.

Administration of chlorothiazide (400 mg/d) produced a transient natriuresis, a fall in blood pressure to normal limits, and a weight loss of 0.5 kg (Panel L). A decrease in serum potassium ensued without kaliuresis. Urinary excretion of aldosterone and 17-hydroxysteroids and plasma renin activity remained low. The effect of chlorothiazide to decrease blood pressure is probably mediated via the natriuretic effect. Although natriuresis is usually a stimulus to renin and aldosterone, the failure of these parameters to increase under provocative conditions was again demonstrated.

Discontinuation of chlorothiazide resulted in a rise in blood pressure and a weight increase of 0.5 kg (Panel M). A rise in serum potassium concentration to 3.6 mEq/L was associated with potassium retention. The capacity of normal dietary sodium to raise blood pressure was again demonstrated. That the decrease in blood pressure produced by chlorothiazide was mediated by the natriuresis is supported by the rise in blood pressure when natriuresis ended. The changes in weight were not as marked as changes in blood pressure. The known kaliuretic and hypokalemic effect of chlorothiazide makes it an unlikely therapeutic modality in this child.

Spironolactone administration produced a prompt fall in blood pressure without significant change in urinary aldosterone (Panel N). Serum potassium concentration rose. Plasma renin activity was slightly higher but appeared to have risen before spironolactone was administered. There was a slight natriuresis and a weight gain of 0.5 kg. Since spironolactone blocks mineralocorticoid action in the kidney, the fall in blood pressure and the normalization of serum potassium concentration with spironolactone strongly suggests that this patient secretes a mineralocorticoid capable of raising blood pressure and capable of causing hypokalemia. This mineralocorticoid is not aldosterone since aldosterone is not secreted in significant quantities in this patient. The capacity of spironolactone to lower blood pressure distinguishes this patient from those described by Liddle *et al.* (1963) who responded to triamterene and not to spironolactone. Spironolactone is a good therapeutic drug in this patient, since it lowered blood pressure and corrected the hypokalemia.

The secretion rates of desoxycortisol, cortisol, desoxycorticosterone, corticosterone and aldosterone were low in the baseline period. This patient had a surface area of 0.5 m^2 and the normal data is given for comparison (Table I) (New *et al.*, 1970). With ACTH stimulation, there was a slight increase to still subnormal levels in the patient. With dexamethasone the secretion rates of both normal subjects and those of the patient were extremely low.

Table I. Adrenal hormone secretion rates (mg/day).

Baseline	B	S	F	DOC	Aldosterone
Normal adult	3.8	0.38	11.5	0.085	0.18
Normal adult/m^2	2.0	0.26	7.5	0.055	0.13
Normal child/0.5 m^2	1.2	0.13	3.8	0.025	0.02–1.6
LK	0.057	0.06	0.04	0.026	0.02
ACTH - 1 day					
Normal child/0.5 m^2	5.0	10.0	12.0	0.2	0.100
LK	0.21	0.22	1.4	0.068	0.013
Dexamethasone					
Normal adult/0.5 m^2	<1	<1	<1	<1	0.04
LK	0.03	0.05	0.04	0.027	0.005

The ACTH level on the morning of her seventh day of admission (Fig.1, Panel A, 9/18/73) was less than 50 pg/ml as measured by Dr. Roslyn Yalow (Berson *et al.*, 1968). At this level, low and normal values cannot be distinguished but it is clear that the level is not elevated in this patient. The absence of elevated ACTH levels in the presence of low cortisol secretion rate, low 17-hydroxycorticoid excretion and low plasma cortisol suggests some factor other than cortisol suppresses ACTH. If the ACTH level were low it would explain the low secretion of all the steroids measured. Since the patient does respond to administered ACTH, albeit sluggishly, it is apparent that the adrenal has the capacity to secrete these hormones. Indeed, with prolonged ACTH administration (Panel H, Fig.2) there is a significant rise in the excretion of 17-hydroxycorticoids which suggests a significant increase in the secretion rate of adrenal hormones at this time. A steroid recently suggested to be important in low-renin hypertension, 16-hydroxydehydroepiandrosterone (16-OH-DHEA) (Liddle *et al.*, 1975), was very low in this patient's urine (Table II). Other steroids of interest in low renin hypertension were also low (Jänne *et al.*, 1969; Ulick, 1976).

Table II. Excretion of steroid metabolites of interest in low-renin hypertension.

Urinary steroids (μg/day)	LK	Normal adult	Normal child	Reference to normal range
16β-hydroxydehydroepiandrosterone	7.8	19–116	–	25
3β,17β-dihydroxy-5-androstene-16-one	83.0	60–360	–	25
18-OH-tetrahydro-DOC	<4	15	–	57
18-OH-tetrahydro-A	<4	122±35	39±21	27
Tetrahydroaldosterone	<4	53±20	19±9	27

DISCUSSION

The evidence for secretion of an unknown adrenocortical steroid in low renin hypertension has been recently summarized by Liddle *et al.* (1973). Various mineralocorticoids have been implicated in low renin hypertension. A role for DOC in the etiology of low renin hypertension may be speculated upon since DOC is secreted in excess in certain hypertensive states (New, 1971; Biglieri *et al.*, 1966; New *et al.*, 1970). DOC administration has produced hypertension (Biglieri *et al.*, 1970, Luft *et al.*, 1954; Soffer *et al.*, 1940) and elevated plasma DOC concentrations have been found in some patients with low renin hypertension (Brown *et al.*, 1972). The role of aldosterone in the production of hypertension is less clear, although hyperaldosteronism is associated with certain hypertensive disorders (Ross, 1975). Administration of aldosterone to humans has produced strong mineralocorticoid effects, but variable effects on blood pressure (Rosemberg *et al.*, 1962; Dawborn, 1969). Two studies showed no change in blood pressure (Rosemberg *et al.*, 1962; Dawborn, 1969); one did not mention blood pressure (Ross *et al.*, 1965) and the two studies carried out by August *et al.* (1958, 1959) showed a rise in blood pressure at the end of 26 days of aldosterone administration when maximal weight gain occurred. The other studies cited here (Rosemberg *et al.*, 1962; Ross *et al.*, 1965; Dawborn, 1969) administered aldosterone for a maximum of ten days. Thus the variable effects on blood pressure may be influenced by the duration of aldosterone administration. The role of 18-OH-DOC in hypertension remains controversial (Ulick, 1973; Messerli *et al.*, 1976).

In the first patient, EMG, in whom the only steroid known to be oversecreted is aldosterone, remission of hypertension occurs when aldosterone is suppressed by dexamethasone. We have documented, however, that aldosterone is not the ACTH stimulable hormone which produced hypertension within five days. ACTH when given to either normal individuals or patients with hyperaldosteronism has been shown to produce a transient increase in aldosterone secretion or excretion but no change in plasma renin (Newton *et al.*, 1968). In patients, including those with hyperaldosteronism, aldosterone excretion returns to unstimulated levels by the third day of ACTH administration. The same phenomenon of transient ACTH effect on aldosterone excretion has been observed by others (Biglieri *et al.*, 1969; Dluhy *et al.*, 1969; Slaton *et al.*, 1969) which is in contrast to the persistent stimulation of aldosterone by ACTH in this patient.

Although hypertension is common in Cushing's syndrome (Plotz *et al.*, 1952), and is frequently associated with steroid administration (Ragan, 1953), the role of hypercortisolemia in the etiology of hypertension is obscure. Of interest is the greater incidence of hypertension with chronically administered ACTH compared to treatment with corticosteroids (Savage *et al.*, 1962) suggesting that a steroid other than cortisol may be responsible for the hypertension. The effect of ACTH administration on blood pressure in man has not received great attention.

In the first patient, EMG, the data suggest that a patient with dexamethasone-suppressible hyperaldosteronism secretes an adrenal steroid, induced by ACTH, which is not a known mineralocorticoid. Though we have not identified the steroid, we have demonstrated that neither aldosterone nor 18-OH-DOC nor DOC administered alone produces hypertension within five days, in contrast to the rapid hypertensive effect of ACTH administration. We did not, however, administer steroids in combination as was done in sheep (Fan *et al.*, 1975). The pressor effect of five days of metyrapone and the absence of pressor effect of five days of DOC administration in this patient suggests that the ACTH-induced hypertensive steroid is an 11-desoxysteroid other than DOC. Further studies using blood and urine collected under ACTH and metyrapone stimulation may provide a source from which we may characterize this steroid.

The second patient, LK, provides the most persuasive evidence for the presence of an unidentified ACTH stimulable hormone which has both mineralocorticoid and glucocorticoid activity and is capable of raising blood pressure. This patient manifests strong mineralocorticoid effects and hypertension in the absence of excessive secretion of any known sodium retaining steroid. The mineralocorticoid activity of this hormone is reflected in the hypokalemia and suppressed renin in the untreated state and the aggravation of the hypokalemia with ACTH administration.

The glucocorticoid effect is suggested by the lack of elevation of plasma ACTH in the presence of low 17-hydroxycorticoid excretion, plasma cortisol and cortisol secretion. Further evidence for glucocorticoid activity is provided by the ability of the patient to survive repeated episodes of severe gastroenteritis, including salmonella sepsis, without glucocorticoid replacement despite low secretion and excretion of cortisol.

The pressor effect of this unknown hormone is evident in the hypertension in the untreated state which increased with ACTH administration. Although the pressor effect of the ACTH stimulable hormone showed sodium dependence, administration of ACTH apparently overrode the hypotensive effect of low sodium diet.

Hypertension produced in sheep following administration of ACTH (Scoggins *et al.*, 1974; Fan *et al.*, 1975) is in some ways similar to that observed in the patient, L.K. Both are hypokalemic, hypertensive states which persist even on a low sodium intake and can occur without changes in weight and external electrolyte balance. In both, the hypertensive effect of ACTH can be observed on a low sodium intake. The known components of the sheep's adrenocorticol effluent, including 18-OH-DOC when reinfused, did not reproduce the hypertension within 24 hours as did the administration of ACTH (Fan *et al.*, 1975).

In a recent preliminary report, Scoggins *et al.* (1976) indicate that the steroid in the sheep's adrenal vein blood that is capable of reproducing the rapid hypertensive effect of ACTH when administered along with the known adrenal secretory components is 17a,20a-dihydroxy-4-pregnene-3-one. Several cases of apparent mineralocorticoid excess have been described in which the patients are hypertensive and hypokalemic but aldosterone secretion is very low. The first study was that of Liddle *et al.* (1963) who described eight patients in a kindred who had severe hypertension and hypokalemia which was resistant to treatment with spironolactone or low sodium diet. Treatment with triamterene reduced blood pressure and caused a rise in serum potassium when dietary sodium was decreased.

Other cases with similar findings have been described (Aarskog *et al.*, 1967; Milora *et al.*, 1967). One of these cases responded to spironolactone (Ross, 1975) while another required triamterene (Milora *et al.*, 1967).

The patient whose disorder is most like that of patient L.K. is that of Werder *et al.* (1973). Like our patient, Werder's patient was a 3-year-old female with low excretion of glucocorticoids and mineralocorticoids. The most important difference appears to be the rise in renin and aldosterone with salt restriction and spironolactone in Werder's case. These authors also propose an unknown steroid with mineralocorticoid activity as the best explanation for all the features, including a low normal ACTH level.

In summary, we have presented a case of apparent mineralocorticoid excess in a 3-year-old girl. The features are hypertension, hypokalemia, hyporeninemia and reduced-to-absent secretion of mineralocorticoids and glucocorticoids. The data suggest the presence of an as yet unidentified hormone which is stimulated by ACTH and which has both mineralocorticoid and glucocorticoid activity. The pressor effect of the hormone is partly dependent on sodium. The hypertension and hypokalemia are improved with spironolactone treatment.

These patients, L.K. and E.M.G., provide strong evidence for an unidentified ACTH stimulable adrenal steroid having an important role in certain forms of low-renin hypertension. It would seem important to characterize this steroid and investigate its role in other forms of hypertension.

ACKNOWLEDGEMENTS

This investigation was supported in part by USPHS, NIH Grants HL 177749 and HD 00072; USPHS, NIH Division of Research Facilities and Resources, Clinical Research Centers RR 47; and the National Foundation March of Dimes Award CRBS-278.

REFERENCES

Aarskog, D., Støa, K.F., Thorsen, T. and Wefring, K.W. (1967). *Pediatrics* **39**, 884.
August, J.T., Nelson, D.H. and Thorn, G.W. (1958). *J. clin. Invest.* **37**, 1549.
August, J.T. and Nelson, D.H. (1959). *J. clin. Invest.* **38**, 1964.
Berson, S.P. and Yallow, R.S. (1968). *J. clin. Invest.* **47**, 2725.
Biglieri, E.G., Herron, M.A. and Brust, N. (1966). *J. clin. Invest.* **45**, 1946.
Biglieri, E.G., Schambelan, M. and Slaton, P.E., Jr. (1969). *J. clin. Endocr. Metab.* **29**, 1090.
Biglieri, E.G., Schambelan, M., Slaton, P.E. and Stockigt, J.R. (1970). *Circ. Res.* **26, 27** **(Suppl.I)**, 1-195.

Biglieri, E.G., Schambelan, M. and Stockigt, J.R. (1972). *Proceedings of the IV Intnl. Congress Endocrinology*, Washington, D.C., p.109, (**Abstract No.271**).
Brandis, M., Keyes, J. and Windhager, E.E. (1972). *Am. J. Physiol.* **222**, 421.
Brown, J.J., Fraser, R., Love, D.R. *et al.* (1972). *Lancet* **ii**, 243.
Carballeira, A., Fishman, L.M. and Jacobi, J.D. (1976). *J. clin. Endocr. Metab.* **42**, 687.
Dawborn, J.K. (1969). *Med. J. Australia* **1**, 1079.
Dluhy, R.G. and Williams, G.H. (1969). *J. clin. Endocr. Metab.* **29**, 1319.
Fan, J.S.K., Coghlan, J.P., Kenton, D.A., Oddie, C.J., Scoggins, B.A. and Shulkes, A.A. (1975). *Am. J. Physiol.* **228**, 1695.
Ferrebee, J.W., Ragan, C., Atchley, D.W. and Loeb, R.F. (1939). *JAMA* **113**, 1725.
Genest, J., Nowacyznski, W., Kuchel, O. and Sasaki, C. (1972). *In* "Hypertension '72" (J. Genest and E. Koiw, eds) p.293. Springer-Verlag, New York.
Gotshall, R.W. and Davis, J.O. (1973). *Am. J. Physiol.* **224**, 1116.
Grim, C.E., Weinberger, M.H., Anand, S.K. and Northway, J.D. (1975). *Proceedings of VI Intnl. Congr. Nephrology*, Florence, Italy. (**Abstract No.605**).
Jänne, O. and Vihko, R. (1969). *Steroids* **14**, 235.
Kagawa, C.M. and Pappo, R. (1962). *Proc. Soc. exp. Biol. Med.* **109**, 982.
Liddle, G.W. and Sennet, J.A. (1975). *J. Steroid. Biochem.* **6**, 751.
Liddle, G.W., Bledsoe, T. and Coppage, W.S. (1963). *Trans. Assoc. Am. Phys.* **76**, 199.
Liddle, G.W., Carey, R.M. and Douglas, J.G. (1973). Intnl. Congr. Series **273**, pp.752-756. Excerpta Medica.
Luft, R., Sjøgren, B., Ikkos, D. *et al.* (1954). *Recent Prog. Horm. Res.* **10**, 425.
McCammon, R.W. (1970). "Human Growth and Development", pp.49-59. C.C. Thomas, Springfield, Ill.
Melby, J.C., Dale, S.L., Greikin, R.J., Gaunt, R. and Wilson, T.E. (1972). *Recent Progr. Horm. Res.* **28**, 287.
Melby, J.C., Dale, S.L., Grekin, R.J., Gaunt, R. and Wilson, T.E. (1972). *In* "Hypertension '72" (J. Genest and E. Koiw, eds), p.350. Springer-Verlag, Berlin.
Messerli, F.H., Kuchel, O., Nowaczynski, W. *et al.* (1976). *Circulation* **53**, 406.
Milora, R., Vagnucci, A. and Goodman, A.D. (1967). *Clin. Res.* **15**, 482.
Miura, K., Yoshinaga, K., Goto, K., Katsushima, I., Maebashi, M., Demura, H., Iino, M., Demura, T. and Toriki, T. (1968). *J. clin. Endocr. Metab.* **28**, 1807.
New, M.I. (1971). *J. clin. Invest.* **49**, 1930.
New, M.I. and Peterson, R.E. (1967). *J. clin. Endocr. Metab.* **27**, 300.
New, M.I. and Seaman, M.P. (1970). *J. clin. Endocr. Metab.* **30**, 361.
New, M.I., Siegal, E. and Peterson, R.E. (1973). *J. clin. Endocr. Metab.* **37**, 93.
Newton, M.A. and Laragh, J.H. (1968). *J. clin. Endocr. Metab.* **28**, 1006.
Perera, G.A. (1948). *Proc. Soc. exp. Biol. Med.* **68**, 48.
Perera, G.A., Knowlton, A.I., Lowell, A. and Loeb, R.F. (1944). *JAMA* **125**, 1030.
Plotz, C.M., Knowlton, A.I. and Ragan, C. (1952). *Am. J. Med.* **13**, 597.
Porter, G.A. and Kimsey, J. (1971). *Endocrinology* **89**, 353.
Ragan, C. (1953). *Bull. N.Y. Acad. Med.* **29**, 355.
Rosemberg, E., Demany, M., Budnitz, E. *et al.* (1962). *J. clin. Endocr. Metab.* **22**, 465.
Ross, E.J. (1959). *Proc. Roy. Soc. Med.* **52**, 1086.
Ross, E.J. (1975). "Aldosterone and Aldosteronism", p.306. Lloyd-Luke Ltd., London.
Ross, E.J. and Hurst, P.E. (1965). *Clin. Sci.* **28**, 91.
Ruse, J.L., Price, C., Stiefel, M. and Laidlaw, J.C. (1972). *In* "Hypertension '72" (J. Genest and E. Koiw, eds) pp.326-333. Springer-Verlag, Berlin.
Savage, O., Copeman, W.S;, Chapman, L., Wells, M.V. and Treadwell, B.L. (1962). *Lancet* **1**, 232.
Scoggins, B.A., Coughlan, C.P., Denton, D.A., Fan, J.S.K., McDougall, J.G., Oddie, C.J. and Shulkes, A.A. (1974). *Am. J. Physiol.* **226**, 198.
Scoggins, B.A., Coghlan, J.P., Denton, D.A., Fan, J.S. and McDougall, J.G. (1976). *Program and Abstracts – 58th Annual Meeting, The Endocrine Society*, San Francisco (**Abstract No.211**).
Shade, R.E. and Grim, C.E. (1975). *J. clin. Endocr. Metab.* **40**, 652.
Slaton, P.E., Jr., Schambelan, M. and Biglieri, E.G. (1969). *J. clin. Endocr. Metab.* **29**, 239.
Soffer, L.J., Engle, F.L. and Oppenheimer, B.S. (1940). *JAMA* **115**, 1860.
Ulick, S. (1973). Intnl. Congr. Series **273**, pp.761-767. Excerpta Medica.

Ulick, S. (1976). *J. clin. Endocr. Metab.* **43**, 92.
Ulick, S. (1976). *Am. J. Med. (in press).*
Vagnucci, A.H. and Shaprio, A.P. (1974). *Metabolism* **23**, 273.
Werder, E., Zachmann, M., Vollman, J.A., Veyrat, R. and Prader, A. (1973). *Intnl. Study Group for Steroid Hormones*, Rome. (Abstract).

RELATIONSHIP BETWEEN PRA PLASMA LEVELS AND SODIUM DIETARY INTAKE IN NORMAL CHILDREN, IN THE SUPINE AND UPRIGHT POSITIONS

G. Giovannelli, G. Banchini, A. Ammenti and S. Bernasconi
Department of Pediatrics, University of Parma, Italy

While the interest of pediatricians in hypertension increasingly grows, there still remains a lack of information on the behaviour of Plasma Renin Activity (PRA) in children. For instance, plasma levels of PRA have been reported to be inversely related to age up to puberty (Kotchen *et al.*, 1972; Krause *et al.*, 1972; Marshall *et al.*, 1976; Sassard *et al.*, 1975), but in this research PRA values were not normalized versus sodium intake; whereas it is well known from adult research that in normal subjects (i.e. in normotensive, normovolemic subjects) PRA values are greatly modified by sodium and potassium intake on the one hand and by the sympathetic nervous system activity on the other (the latter, active mainly in the upright position).

As a matter of fact, pediatric literature is lacking in a significant reference point constituted by the PRA behaviour in normal children of various ages, at different dietary sodium intakes, determined both in the supine and upright positions.

In order to fill in this gap we measured plasma levels of PRA in a group of normal children (38 to present), ages from 2 months to 14 years, maintaining a constant dietary potassium (50 $mEq/m^2/24$ h) and different sodium intakes (from 10 to 160 $mEq/m^2/24$ h), both in the supine and upright positions, at equilibrium of sodium balance. The attainment of balance was checked by daily controls of the prescribed dietary intake and the 24 h urinary excretion of sodium; satisfactory equilibrium (i.e. a difference between intake and output within ±20%) was reached after approximately 3 days in most cases. The same process and standard of judgment was applied to potassium.

PRA was determined by radioimmunoassay (RIA) using BAL-IC as an inhibitor, with plasma pH ajdusted to 5.5, in the early morning, after several hours of fasting,

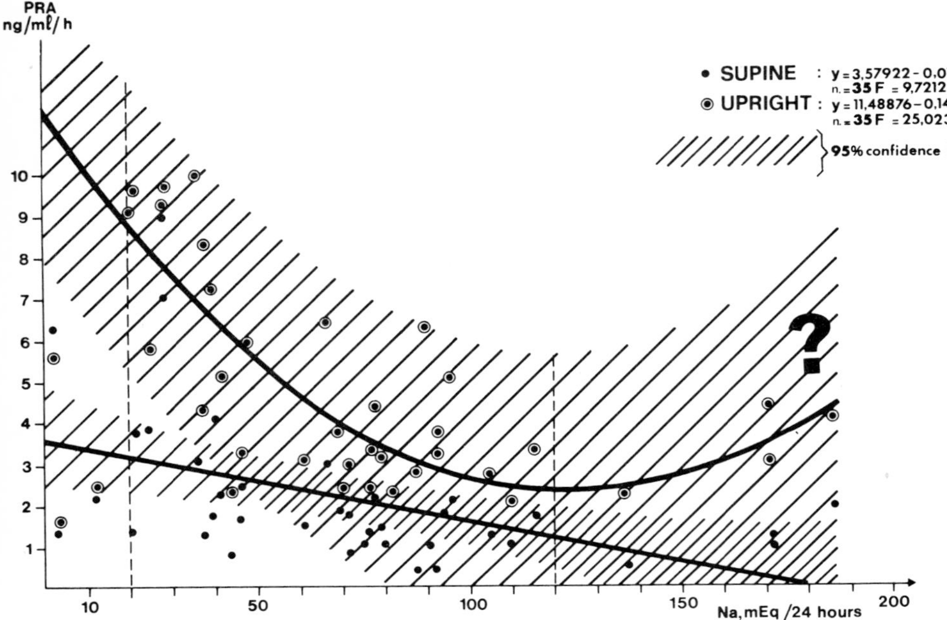

Fig. 1 PRA plasma levels *v.* urinary sodium excretion in 38 normal children in the supine and upright positions.

first in the supine position after overnight rest and then after 1 h in the upright position with unrestricted physical activity.

PRA values were plotted against the daily rate of urinary sodium excretion and statistically analyzed; rectilinear and parabolic regression equations for PRA versus sodium excretion were calculated and compared in terms of reduction of the variance (on the basis of Fisher's test). A third regression equation, the hyperbolic, was not tested; it was considered practically equivalent to the parabolic on the basis of similar research in adults (Salvetti *et al.*, 1974).

The end result of our investigations is a nomogram (Fig. 1) which deserves brief comment:

1) PRA levels increase in the upright position.

The 3 sucklings examined (cases with the lowest sodium intakes in Fig. 1) seem to be an exception to the rule (prevalence of the sympathetic nervous system?); therefore they were not considered in our calculations.

2) PRA decreases by increasing dietary sodium intake, both in the supine and upright positions. However, at the highest intakes, a tendency to inversion is observed for PRA response in the upright position; in fact, values rise again and give the regression line a true parabolic form. If confirmed by wider research (see the question mark in Fig. 1), this paradoxical behaviour merits our attention.

3) In the supine position only about 25% of the total variance of PRA values is accounted for by the correlation with sodium excretion. This finding, while supporting the claimed influence of the parameter "age" in prepuberal subjects, points out the limited value of isolated supine PRA levels for clinical pur-

poses, even after normalization for sodium excretion. In the upright position, more than 60% of the total variance of PRA values is accounted for by the parabolic correlation with sodium excretion. These percentages are likely to improve by increasing the number of examined cases.

Altogether, this nomogram affords a rational interpretation of PRA plasma levels in single cases, in different physiopathological conditions, provided sodium excretion and changes in the upright position are known, as should always be the case.

In our opinion, two points are worthy of future investigation:

1) behaviour of PRA in sucklings, where relevant; unexplained variations may be encountered from one case to the other;

2) PRA pattern at very high sodium dietary intake.

ACKNOWLEDGEMENT

This work was supported by a grant from the C.N.R.

REFERENCES

Kotchen, T.A., Strickland, A.L., Rice, T.W. and Walters, D.R. (1972). *J. Pediatr.* **80**, 938.
Krause, D.K., Schillmoeller, U. and Hayduk, K. (1972). *German Medical Monthly* **2**, 103.
Marshall, R., Bartlett, C., Sheehan, M., Maurer, M., Ellenberger, D. and Blumberg, A. (1976). *Pediatr. Res.* **10**, 326 (Abstr.).
Salvetti, A., Sassano, P., Arzilli, F. and Gazzetti, P. (1974). *J. Nucl. Biol. Med.* **18**, 119.
Sassard, J., Sann, L., Vincent, M., Francois, R. and Cier, J.F. (1975). *J. clin. Endocr. Metab.* **40**, 524.

EARLY DIAGNOSIS OF CONGENITAL ADRENAL HYPERPLASIA BY MEASUREMENT OF PLASMA 17 OH PROGESTERONE, TESTOSTERONE, CORTISOL, ALDOSTERONE AND RENIN ACTIVITY

G. Natoli, P. De Luca, C. Ossicini, R. Berardinelli, F. Sciarra*, C. Piro*, F. Sparano* and M.V. Adamo*

**Department of Child Health and Medicine, University of Rome, Italy*

SUMMARY

Plasma 17 OHP, T, F, PAC and PRA were measured by radioimmunoassay at 8--9 a.m. in 18 patients, aged 16 hours – 23 years affected by congenital adrenal hyperplasia.

In 7 patients with 21 OH deficiency, when therapy was discontinued for 20 days, high levels of 17 OHP (29.6 – > 100 ng/100 ml), T (140–800 ng/100 ml), PAC (30–38 ng/100 ml) and PRA (4–6 ng/ml/h) were found.

In 8 patients with salt losing 21 OH deficiency, high levels of 17 OHP (5.9–58.6 ng/ml) and T (95–800 ng/100 ml) were detected. In one case PRA was high (11 ng/ml/h), whilst PAC and F were decreased (3 ng/100 ml and 0.6 μg/100 ml respectively).

In 3 patients with 11 OH deficiency 17 OHP was slightly increased (3–4 ng/ml), T was high (560–950 ng/100 ml) and PAC and PRA low (2–2.5 ng/100 ml and 0.13–0.25 ng/ml/h respectively).

These results, therefore, suggest that early diagnosis of congenital adrenal hyperplasia can be established by measurement of these steroids in plasma.
17 OHP and T decreased significantly during dexamethasone treatment (single dose late in the evening) and levels not higher than 20 ng/ml and 30 ng/100 ml respectively in prepubertal children, are generally associated with a normal linear growth rate.

The diagnosis of congenital adrenal hyperplasia (CAH) is usually etablished on the basis of the clinical findings and the results of urinary 17-ketosteroids (17KS) and pregnanetriol (PT) determinations (Wilkins, 1952; Natoli, 1961; Newns, 1974). Various difficulties, however, are encountered in infancy and especially in the newborn since (a) 24 h urine collection is not accurate (b) pregnanetriol may be within the normal range during the first weeks of life on account of a low hepatic steroid glucuronyl transferase activity (Migeon, 1961; Shackleton *et al.*, 1972), and (c) 17-ketosteroids are often elevated even in normal newborns during the first days of life as an index of the foetal zone hyperactivity, and may be also within the normal range or slightly elevated in CAH (Wilkins, 1965).

The monitoring of treatment also presents difficulties since, while criteria such as growth rate, skeletal age, 17KS and PT determinations can be followed, growth disorders, virilization and other complications are frequently encountered (Bongiovanni *et al.*, 1973; Rappaport *et al.*, 1973).

Recently plasma levels of steroids such as 17 OH progesterone (17 OHP) and testosterone (T) have been found elevated and taken into consideration for the diagnosis of CAH (Strott *et al.*, 1969; Loras *et al.*, 1974; Chaussain *et al.*, 1974; Loriaux *et al.*, 1974; Lippe *et al.*, 1974; Franks, 1974; Hami *et al.*, 1975; Solomon and Schoen, 1975; Youssefnezadian and David, 1975). The aim of the present investigation therefore was to assess the usefulness of these two parameters and of cortisol (F), aldosterone (PAC) and plasma renin activity (PRA) measurements in the management of CAH.

MATERIALS AND METHODS

Studies were carried out on 18 patients (aged between 1 day and 25 years) affected by CAH (7 due to 21 hydroxylase (21 OH) deficiency, 8 with the salt-losing form and 3 due to 11 β-hydroxylase (11 OH) deficiency).

Patients were treated with dexamethasone, 0.125–0.750 mg *pro die* according to age, given as a single dose at 10 p.m. (Malaguzzi Valeri and Natoli, 1963; Natoli and Schwarzenberg, 1976). In salt-losing form, dietary supplementation with salt and 12.5–25 mg DOCA (Cortiron Depot, Schering) was administered every two weeks.

The parameters used to monitor the efficacy of treatment, based on monthly physical examinations, included growth rate, skeletal age, urinary 17 KS and PT determinations. More recent examinations have also included plasma 17 OHP and T assays. F, PAC and PRA were also measured in a few cases.

Blood samples for steroid determinations were collected at 8–9 a.m. in basal condition (treatment was interrupted for at least 20 days prior to collection) and 3 months after recommencement of therapy. Only 2 cases (14 and 15) had not received any form of treatment at the time of the investigation.

Plasma 17 OHP was determined using the RIA technique proposed by Abraham *et al.* (1971). Normal values:

Newborns (1st week)	0.7–2.25 ng/ml
Prepubertal children	0.20–0.58 ng/ml
Men	0.60–1 ng/ml
Women (follicular phase)	0.34–0.96 ng/ml
(luteal phase)	1.4–2.5 ng/ml.

Plasma T was measured with the RIA technique of Sciarra *et al.* (1974). Normal values in male and female newborns (1st week) are 35–200 ng/100 ml and 15–60 ng/100 ml respectively, in prepubertal children 15–30 ng/100 ml and in female and male adults 15–70 ng/100 ml and 300–1000 ng/100 ml respectively.

Plasma aldosterone was determined in clinostatism with the RIA technique of Sparano *et al.* (1974). Normal values in adults are 3–12 ng/100 ml. PRA was evaluated using the RIA technique of Haber *et al.* (1969). Normal values in adults are 0.3–1.3 ng/ml/h.

Plasma cortisol was assayed with RIA after chromatographic separation on a Sephadex LH 20 column (cm 8.5 × 0.8). Normal values in adults are 5–20 μg/100 ml (Murphy, 1967).

Urinary 17 KS were evaluated according to the method of Moxam and Nabarro (1956) (normal values in newbowns mg 0.28–1.3/24 h), prepubertal children (2–10 years old) mg 0.5–3/24 h and in male adults 8–20 mg/24 h, and urinary pregnanetriol with the method of Bongiovanni and Eberlein (1958) (normal values < 1 mg/24 h).

RESULTS

Data from the 7 patients (aged between 2 and 23 years) affected by CAH due to 21 OH deficiency are reported in Table I.

Table I. Plasma 17α-hydroxy-progesterone (17 OHP) urinary pregnanetriol, plasma testosterone and urinary 17 ketosteroids (17 KS) in C.A.H. patients with 21 hydroxylase (21 OH) deficiency.

CASE	SEX	C.A.H. DEFICIT OF.....	AGE (years) present	AGE (years) at first observation	AGE (years) duration of observation	HEIGHT (cm) present if completed	HEIGHT (cm) at last observation	BONE AGE (years)	STEROIDS PLASMA 17 OHP ng/ml	STEROIDS URINARY PREGNANETRIOL mg/24h	STEROIDS PLASMA TESTOSTERONE ng/100ml	STEROIDS URINARY 17 KS mg/24h
1	♀	21 OH	23	4 4/12	18 8/12	143.5		A	> 100	50.4	150	20
2	♀	21 OH	16 2/12	1 6/12	14 8/12	150		18	95.24	40.50	188	16.56
3	♀	21 OH	12 9/12	3 7/12	9 2/12		147.5	12	55.5	23	243	25
4	♀	21 OH	8 5/12	2 3/12	6 2/12		125	9	29.6		140	6.3
5	♂	21 OH	6 2/12	2	4 2/12		116	8 7/12	60	22.7	400	9.3
6	♀	21 OH	8 9/12	1 1/12	7 8/12		122	9	35	14.5	155	9.2
7	♀	21 OH	2 3/12	mo. 1	2 2/12		78	1 2/12	> 100		800	

At the time of the last examination height was normal in patients 3–7 and below normal in patients 1 and 2. Bone age was correlated with the chronological age in all cases.

Plasma 17 OHP was elevated in all patients with values ranging between 29.6 ng and > 100/ml. The increase in plasma 17 OHP was correlated with the high urinary levels of PT (14.5–50.4 mg/24 h).

Plasma T was also elevated in all cases with values ranging between 140–800 ng/100 ml, whilst urinary 17 KS were significantly high only in case 3, slightly elevated in cases 1, 2, 5 and 6 and within the normal range in case 4.

Results in the 8 patients (aged between 16 hours – 15 years) with the salt-losing form of CAH are shown in Table II. At the time of the last examination height and bone age were normal in cases 8, 9, 10 and 13, and below normal in cases 11 and 12.

Table II. Plasma 17α-hydroxy-progesterone (17 OHP), urinary pregnanetriol, plasma testosterone and urinary 17 ketosteroids (17 KS) in CAH patients with sodium-losing variant (21 OH S.L.).

CASE	SEX	C.A.H. DEFICIT OF.....	AGE (years) present	AGE (years) at first observation	duration of observation	HEIGHT (cm) present if completed	HEIGHT (cm) at last observation	BONE AGE (years)	STEROIDS PLASMA 17 OHP ng/ml	URINARY PREGNANETRIOL mg/24 h	PLASMA TESTOSTERONE ng/100ml	URINARY 17 KS mg/24 h
8	♀	21 OH s. l.	15 2/12	mo. 6	14 8/12		150	15 9/12	37.1	15.1	140	14.25
9	♂	21 OH s. l.	5	d. 4	5		105	4	58.6		450	10.2
10	♀	21 OH s. l.	6 10/12	d. 5	6 10/12		110	7	37.1	13	112	13.1
11	♀	21 OH s. l.	5 10/12	d. 1	5 10/12		100	5	32.1	11.3	160	4.6
12	♂	21 OH s. l.	1 7/12	d. 2	1 7/12		71	1	14.4	4	150	10
13	♀	21 OH s. l.	12 11/12	mo. 1	12 10/12		150	14	40	22.4	220	18.19
14	♀	21 OH s. l.	mo. 5	d. 5	mo. 5		62	mo. 3	20	n.d.	800	1.21
15	♀	21 OH s. l.	†	h. 16	d. 35				5.9		95	

Plasma 17 OHP was high in all patients with values ranging between 5.9 ng (16 h newborn) and 58.6/ml. PT was also elevated with values ranging between 4 and 22.4 mg/24 h, in cases 8–13 and not detectable in case 14 (5 days old). Urinary steroids were not determined in case 15 (16 hours old) because of the difficulty in collecting 24 h urine samples. Plasma T was high with values ranging between 95 and 800 ng/100 ml and urinary 17 KS significantly elevated in cases 9, 10, 12 and 13 (mg 10–18.19/24 h), slightly elevated in cases 8 and 11 (mg 14.25 and 4.6/24 h) and normal in case 14.

Data from the 3 patients (aged 23, 25 and 10) affected by CAH due to 11 OH deficiency are reported in Table III. Patients 16 and 18 are brothers.

Height was normal in cases 17 and 18 and below normal in case 16. Plasma 17 OHP was slightly elevated with values of 3.33, 4 and 3 ng/ml, respectively,

Table III. Plasma 17α-hydroxy-progesterone (17 OHP), urinary pregnanetriol, plasma testosterone and urinary 17 ketosteroids (17 KS) in CAH patients with 11 hydroxylase (11 OH) deficiency.

CASE	SEX	C.A.H. DEFICIT OF	AGE (years) present	AGE (years) at first observation	duration of observation	HEIGHT (cm) present if completed	HEIGHT (cm) at last observation	BONE AGE (years)	STEROIDS PLASMA 17 OHP ng/ml	STEROIDS URINARY PREGNANETRIOL mg/24h	STEROIDS PLASMA TESTOSTERONE ng/100ml	STEROIDS URINARY 17 KS mg/24h
16	♂	11 OH	23	2	21	144.5		A	3.33	1	800	18.1
17	♂	11 OH	25 8/12	8 9/12	4-1	165		A	4.0	1.2	950	24
18	♂	11 OH	10 3/12	1 7/12	8 8/12		133.5	9 6/12	3.0	1.1	560	14.6

Table IV. Plasma aldosterone (PAC), plasma renin activity (PRA) and plasma cortisol (F) in CAH.

Cases N°	Sex	C.A.H. deficit of	age years	Plasma steroids F μg/100ml	Plasma steroids PAC ng/100 ml	Plasma steroids PRA ng/ml/h
16	♂	11 OH	23	4.0	2	0.13
18	♂	11 OH	10 3/12	5.2	2.5	0.25
1	♀	21 OH	23	1.5	30	4
4	♀	21 OH	8 5/12	1.5	34	6
6	♀	21 OH	8 9/12	2.5	38	4
13	♀	21 OH s.l.	12 11/12	0.6	3	11

whereas urinary PT was almost within the normal range (1, 1.2 and 1.1 mg/24 h respectively). Plasma T and urinary 17 KS were normal in the 2 adult males (cases 16 and 17) and high in case 18 (T = 560 ng/100 ml, 17 KS = 14.6 mg/24 h).

The results of plasma aldosterone (PAC), plasma renin activity (PRA) and cortisol (F), evaluated in 6 patients, are reported in Table IV. PAC was low (2 and 2.5 ng/100 ml) in cases 16 and 18 with 11 OH deficiency, high in cases 1.4 and 6 with 21 OH deficiency (30, 34 and 38 ng/100 ml respectively) and within low normal limits in case 13 with the salt-losing form (3 ng/100 ml).

PRA was low in cases 16 and 18 (0.13 and 0.25 ng/ml/h) and high (4–11 mg/ml/h) in the remaining cases, F was below normal or decreased (0.6–5.2 μg/100 ml) particularly in the patient with the salt-losing CAH (0.6 μg/100 ml).

Plasma 17 OHP and T, urinary PT and 17 KS concentrations before and after dexamethasone treatment are shown in Table V.

Table V. Plasma 17α-hydroxy-progesterone (17 OHP), urinary pregnanetriol, plasma testosterone and urinary 17 ketosteroids (17 KS) before and during dexamethasone treatment in CAH.

CASE Nº	SEX	C.A.H. DEFICIT OF	AGE (years)	STEROIDS: PLASMA 17 OH P ng/ml		URINARY PREGNANETRIOL mg/24h		PLASMA TESTOSTERONE ng/100 ml		URINARY 17 Ks mg/24 h	
				TREATMENT: BEFORE	during	BEFORE	during	BEFORE	during	BEFORE	during
1	♀	21 OH	23	>100	12.4	50.4	3.8	150	80	20	5.5
2	♀	21 OH	16 2/12	95.24	18.3	40.5	2.5	188	30	16.56	3
3	♀	21 OH	12 9/12	55.5	20	23	4.6	243	78	25	5.83
4	♀	21 OH	8 5/12	29.6	20			140	84	6.3	4.4
5	♂	21 OH	6 2/12	60	14	22.7	2.3	400	60	9.3	2.8
6	♀	21 OH	8 9/12	35	12	14.5	1.8	155	39	9.2	2
8	♀	21 OH s.l.	15 2/12	37.1	4.8	15.1	1.9	140	24	14.25	2.44
9	♂	21 OH s.l.	5	58.6	10			450	80	10.3	1.66
10	♀	21 OH s.l.	6 10/12	37.1	9.2	13	1.4	112	2	13.1	1.7
11	♀	21OH	5 10/12	32.1	7.4	11.3	1	160	5	4.6	0.24
12	♂	21OH	1 7/12	14.4	5.51	4	0.9	150	5	10	0.36
13	♀	21OH s.l.	12 11/12	40	30	22.4	8.3	220	93	16.19	8.76
14	♀	21OH s.l.	d 5	20				800	50		
15	♀	21 OH s.l.	1st day †	5.9				95	50		
16	♂	11 OH	23	3.33	1.33	1	0.4	800	580	18.1	7
17	♂	11 OH	25 8/12	4.0	0.9	1.2	0.6	950	430	24	7.8
18	♂	11 OH	10 3/12	3.0	0.9	1.1	0.7	560	30	14.6	2.7

17 OHP decreased significantly (0.9 and 18.3 ng/ml) during treatment in 12 cases (1, 2, 5, 6, 8–12 and 16–18) and decreased slightly (20, 20 and 30 ng/ml) in case 3, 4 and 13.

Urinary levels of PT were also significantly decreased (0.4–4.6 mg/24 h) with the exception of case 13 (8.3 mg/24 h) in whom 17 OHP was also high.

Plasma T and urinary 17 KS decreased under treatment in all cases (15–580 ng/100 ml and 0.24–8.76 mg/24 h respectively).

Figures 1, 2 and 3 represent the growth charts of some of the patients affected by the three forms of CAH, studied sequentially during childhood. The height and corresponding bone age are given.

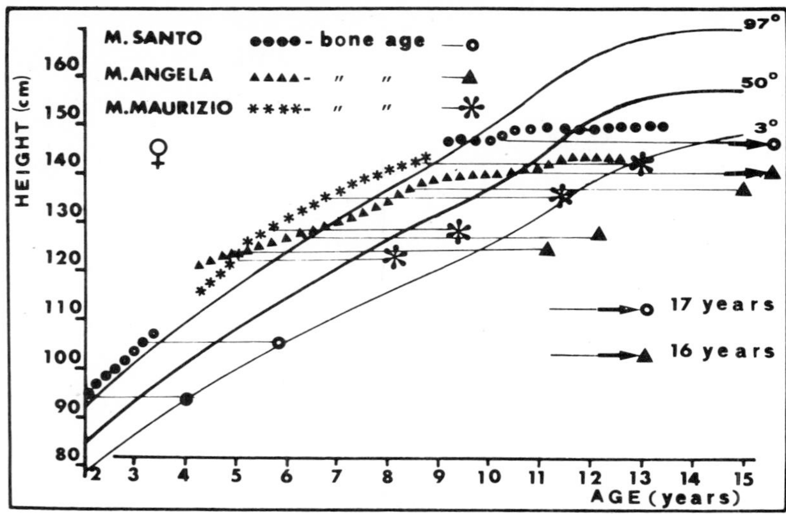

Fig. 1 Abnormal linear growth rate in 3 patients (M. Santo, case 2; M. Angelo, case 1; M. Maurizio, not shown in the tables) affected by CAH with 21 OH deficiency. Treatment interrupted or delayed.

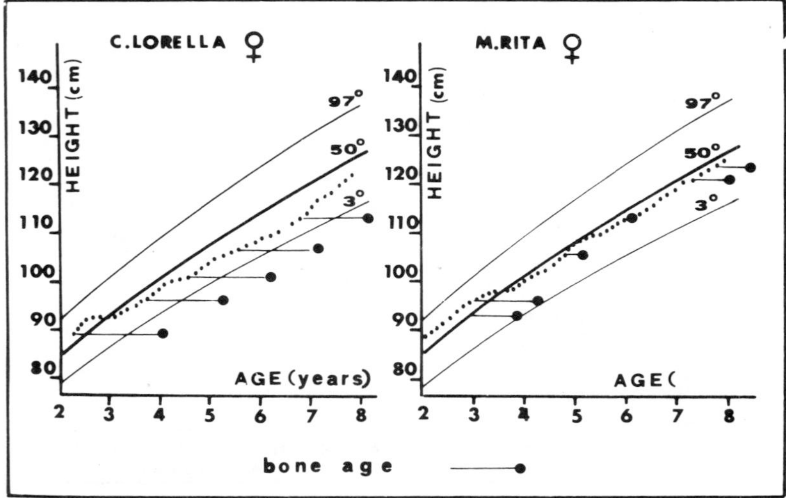

Fig. 2 Normal linear growth rate in 2 patients (C. Lorella, case 4 and M. Rita, case 6) affected by CAH with 21 OH deficiency. Regular treatment.

The abnormal linear growth rates of 3 patients with 21 OH deficiency are shown in Fig. 1: treatment was interrupted in M. Santo (case 2) by the parents, whilst in M. Angelo (case 1) and M. Maurizio (not shown in the tables) dexamethasone treatment was commenced with considerable delay. The normal linear growth rates observed in 2 patients (C. Lorella, case 4 and M. Rita, case 6) with

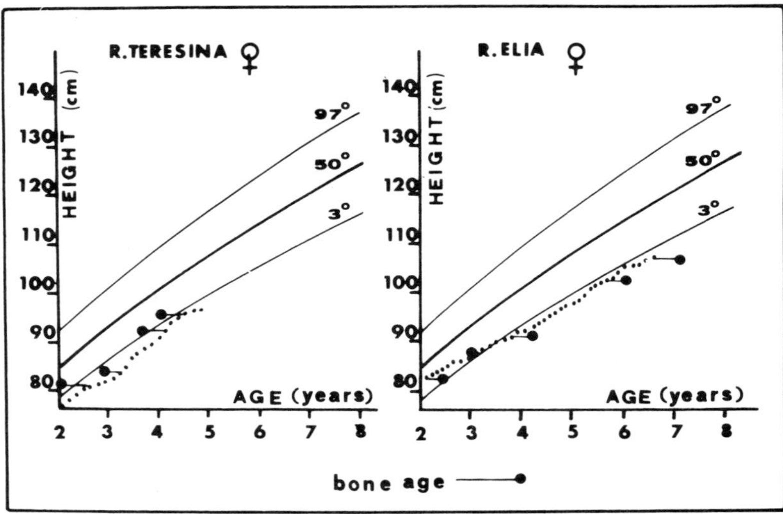

Fig.3 Abnormal linear growth rate in 2 sisters (R. Teresina, case 11 and R. Elia, case 10) affected by salt-losing CAH. Regular treatment from birth.

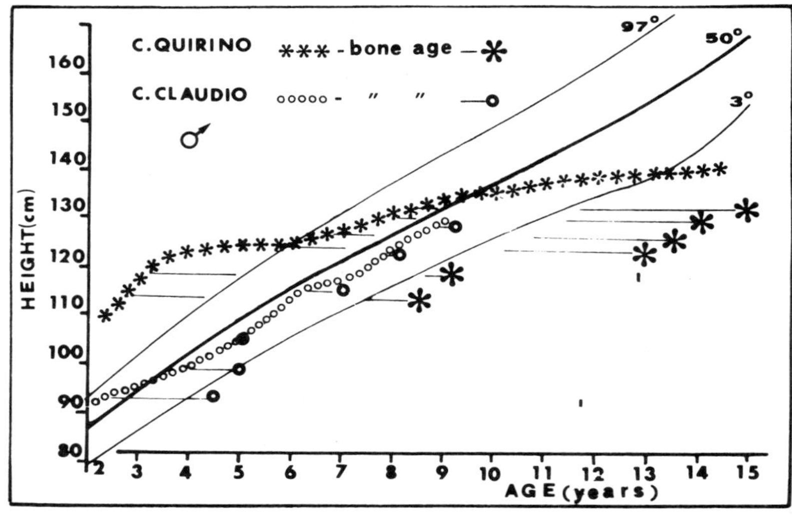

Fig.4 Abnormal linear growth rate in a patient (C. Quirini, case 1) treated with high doses of prednisone, in comparison with the normal growth of the brother (C. Caludio, case 7). Treated with low doses of dexamethasone. Both cases are affected by CAH with 11 OH deficiency.

21 OH deficiency treated regularly from an early age with dexamethasone are shown in Fig.2.

Furthermore, an abnormal growth rate was observed in 2 patients with the salt-losing form (R. Teresina, case 11 and R. Elia, case 10) of CAH (Fig.3), althoug[h] regularly treated from an early age.

Finally, data from 2 patients with 11 OH deficiency are shown in Fig.4. C. Quirino (case 16) in whom treatment was both delayed and insufficient shows an abnormal linear growth rate, whereas the brother C. Claudio (case 18) who received early and adequate treatment presents a normal linear growth rate.

DISCUSSION

The results of the present investigation performed on 18 patients affected by various forms of CAH demonstrate that plasma levels of 17 OHP and T are increased and that this increase may precede, at birth, that of urinary pregnanetriol, as observed by other authors (Strott *et al.*, 1969; Loras *et al.*, 1974; Chaussain *et al.*, 1974; Loriaux *et al.*, 1974; Lippe *et al.*, 1974; Franks *et al.*, 1974; Hami *et al.*, 1975; Solomon and Schoen, 1975; Youssefenejadian and David, 1975).

It is therefore confirmed that RIA determination of these steroids has a significant advantage, in the early diagnosis of CAH, over the classical tests based on the evaluation of their urinary catabolites (Youssefenejadian and David, 1975).

Plasma 17 OHP is significantly elevated in CAH due to 21 OH deficiency, with or without salt-losing, whilst it is only slightly increased in the form with 11 OH deficiency.

Urinary pregnanetriol is in the upper limits of the normal range in the 11 OH deficiency and elevated in the other forms.

Plasma T, on the contrary, is significantly increased in all cases, with no differences between the three forms of CAH. Urinary 17 KS are not always elevated and in some patients are slightly modified.

As far as concerns the other steroids taken into consideration, plasma cortisol is below normal or decreased, especially in the salt-losing form, whereas the behaviour of PRA and PAC differs according to the type of enzymatic defect, as found by others (Franks, 1974; Loras, 1970; Bartter, 1968; Dahl, 1972).

In fact in the 11 OH deficient form, PRA and PAC are low, probably on account of the increased production of DOC, whilst in the 21 OH deficiency PAC and PRA are elevated, suggesting an attempt to compensate for the sodium loss resulting from the overproduction of sodium-losing steroids such as progesterone. PAC, on the other hand, is in the low limits of the normal range in the salt-losing form of 21 OH deficiency, due to the more severe enzymatic block, which does not permit the 21 hydroxylation of progesterone necessary for the aldosterone biosynthesis, in spite of PRA elevation.

As far as the treatment of CAH is concerned, it has been demonstrated that a single low dose of dexamethasone late in the evening is sufficient to decrease the pituitary production of ACTH and consequently to depress adrenal hyperactivity, thereby permitting a normal growth rate and preventing or reversing virilization (Hayek *et al.*, 1971; Jacobs *et al.*, 1972; Natoli and Schwarzenberg, 1976).

The longitudinal follow-up shows that the linear growth rate was normal in those cases in which treatment was commenced immediately after birth and given without interruption. This observation, however, is not related to a normalization of plasma 17 OHP which remains higher than normal although its levels do not rise above 20 ng/ml. In some cases, moreover, urinary pregnanetriol is slightly above the normal range.

The present results are in agreement with those of Lippe *et al.* (1974) and particularly of Loras *et al.* (1974) who demonstrated that the normalization of plasma 17 OHP levels is obtained only with high doses of glucocorticoids which alter, thereafter, the regular growth.

Plasma T, on the contrary, in the majority of children under 12 years remains below 30 ng/100 ml, whilst urinary 17 KS are low, with the exception of patients 4, 5 and 9 aged 5, 6 and 8 years respectively, who although presenting a normal linear growth rate and higher T concentrations (60, 80 and 84 ng/100 ml).

Patient 14 on the other hand had high values of 17 OHP and T and an abnormal linear growth rate as a consequence of discontinuous treatment.

On account of the limited time of observation it is not possible from the present data to draw any definite conclusions on the evaluation of the efficacy of glucocorticoid therapy in the management of CAH by means of plasma 17 OHP and T determinations. In prepubertal children, however, plasma levels of 17 OHP below 20 ng/ml and T around 30 ng/100 ml seem to be acceptable for a normal linear growth rate. The possible repercussion that this hormonal situation may have on the future development of these patients, particularly on pituitary gonadal function, has to be verified.

REFERENCES

Abraham, G.E., Hopper, K., Tulchinsky, D., Swerdloff, R.S. and Odell, W.D. (1971). *Anal. Lett.* **4**, 325.

Bartter, F.C., Harkin, R.I., and Bryan, G.T. (1968). *J. clin. Invest.* **47**, 1742-1752.

Bongiovanni, A.M. and Eberlein, W.R. (1958). *Analyt. Chem.* **30**, 388-393.

Bongiovanni, A.M., Moshang, T.H., Jr. and Parks, T.S. (1973). *Helv. Paedit. Acta* **28**, 127-134.

Chaussain, J.L., Estrada, Y., Roger, M., Tea, N.T., Scholler, R., Canlorbe, P. and Job, J.C. (1947). *Nouv. Presse Méd.* **3**, 2621-2624.

Dahl, V., Rivarola, M.A. and Bergada, C. (1972). *J. clin. Endocr. Metab.* **34**, 661-665.

Franks, R.C. (1974). *J. clin. Endocr. Metab.* **39**, 1099-1102.

Haber, E., Koerner, T., Page, L.B., Klinan, B. and Purnode, A. (1969). *J. clin. Endocr. Metab.* **29**, 1349-1355.

Hami, M., Rosler, A. and Rabinowitz, D. (1975). *J. clin. Endocr. Metab.* **40**, 863-867.

Hayek, A., Crawford, J.D. and Bode, H.H. (1971). *Metabolism* **20**, 897-901.

Jacobs, H.S., Abraham, G.E., Glasser, E.J., Hopper, K. and Kondon, J. (1972). *J. Endocrinol.* **53**, XXXVI-XXXVII.

Lippe, B.M., La Franchi, S.H., Lavin, N., Parlow, A., Coyotupa, J. and Kaplan, S.A. (1974). *J. Paediat.* **85**, 782-787.

Loras, B., Haour, F. and Bertrand, J. (1970). *Paediat. Res.* **4**, 145-146.

Loras, B., Roux, H., Audi-Parera, L., David, M. and Bertrand, J. (1974). *Biomedicine* **21**, 317-322.

Loriaux, D.L., Ruder, H.J. and Lipsett, M.B. (1974). *J. clin. Endocr. Metab.* **39**, 627-630.

Malaguzzi Valeri, O. and Natoli, G. (1963). Scritti in onore del Prof. Gaetano Salvioli in occasione del XXX anno d'insegnamento, pp.607-616. Scuola Tipografica Benedettina, Parma.

Migeon, G.J. (1961). *In* "Ciba Foundation Symposium" (G.E.W. Wostenholme and M. O'Connor, eds), p.226. Churchill, London.

Moxam, A. and Nabarro, J.D.M. (1956). *J. clin. Path.* **9**, 351-356.

Murphy, B.E.P. (1967). *J. clin. Endocr. Metab.* **27**, 973-990.

Natoli, G. and Schwarzenberg, L. (1976). *Mon. Ped.* **28**, 1418-1436.

Newns, G.H. (1974). *Arch. Dis. Child.* **49**, 1-3.

Rappaport, R., Bouthereuil, R., Basmaciogullari, A. and Marti-Henneberg, C. (1973). *Acta Pediat. Scand.* **62**, 513-519.

Sciarra, F., Toscano, V., Concolino, G., Piro, C. and Sorcini, G. (1974). *Folia Endocrinol.* **27**, 657-662.

Shackleton, C.H., Mitchell, F.L. and Farquhar, J.W. (1972). *Pediatrics* **49**, 198-205.

Solomon, I.L. and Schoen, E.J. (1975). *J. clin. Endocr. Metab.* **40**, 355-362.

Sparano, F., Tosti Croce, C. and Sciarra, F. (1974). *Folia Endocrinol.* **27**, 423-431.

Strott, C.A., Yoshimi, T. and Lipsett, M.B. (1969). *J. clin. Invest.* **48**, 930-939.
Wilkins, L. (1952). *J. Pediat.* **41**, 860-874.
Wilkins, L. (1965). *In* "The Diagnosis and Treatment of Endocrine Disorders in Childhood and Adolescence", p.412, 3rd Ed. Thomas Springfield, Illinois.
Youssefenejadian, E. and David, R. (1975). *Clin. Endocrinol.* **4**, 451-454.

17α-HYDROXYLASE DEFICIENCY IN THREE SIBLINGS

F. Mantero, M. Contri* and D. Armanini

Department of Medicine, University of Padova
General Hospital, Vicenza, Italy

INTRODUCTION

The 17α-hydroxylase deficiency syndrome was described for the first time in a genetically female individual by Biglieri *et al.* (1966) and is characterized by hypertension, hypokalemia and signs of hypoestrogenism (absent pubic and axially hairs, lack of breast development, primary amenorrhea) (Mills *et al.*, 1967; Goldsmith *et al.*, 1967; Mallin, 1969; Linquette *et al.*, 1971; Tranchetti *et al.*, 1973; de Lange *et al.*, 1973). Later it was found to be present also in genotypically male subjects who presented with pseudohermaphroditism (New, 1970; Mantero *et al.*, 1971; Bricaire *et al.*, 1972; Hammerstein *et al.*, 1973; Kershnar *et al.*, 1973; Alvarez *et al.*, 1973). The syndrome may have a familial character having been described in members of the same family (two genetically male brothers and two female). Recently, we have had the opportunity to study for the first time in a family three affected members, two female and one male, all of whom, however, were phenotypically female and grew up as such. Two other sisters in the family died in early infancy for unknown reasons. The parents are blood related as in other cases already described in the literature.

CASE REPORTS

Case 1

Graziella, D., 14 years old, tenth of thirteen children. The patient was brought to us for observation complaining of severe headaches, episodes of vomiting and presented recently with periods of hypertension. On physical examination (Fig.1), the patient appeared to be phenotypically female, hyposomic (1.40 m tall), without secondary sexual characteristics; she had not menstruated. Her

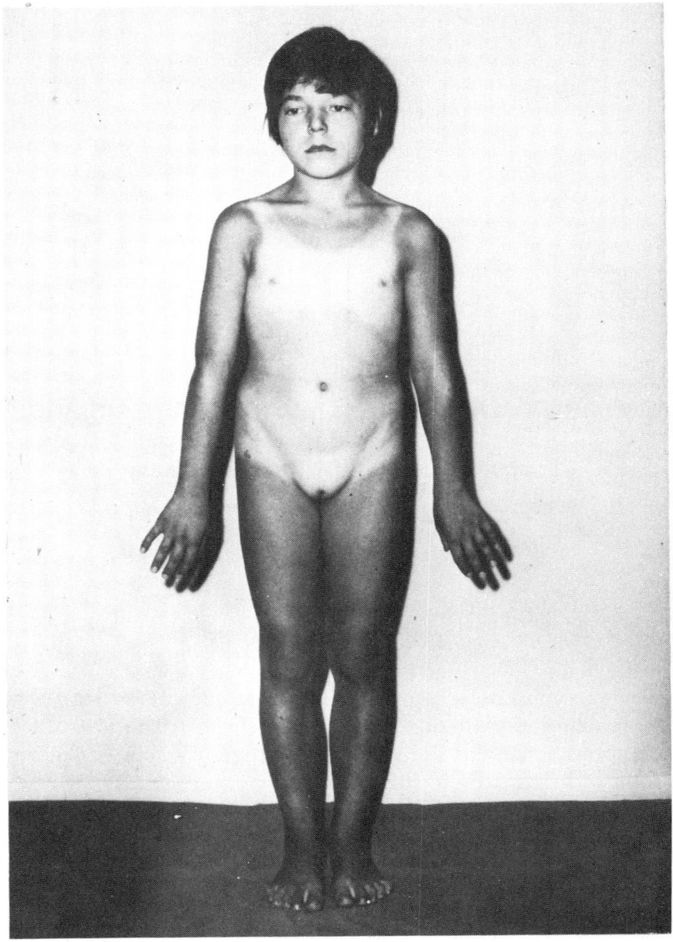

Fig.1 Patient G.D. (46/YY), at age 14. Note the female prepubertal aspect.

arterial blood pressure was 190/130 in both positions. Her external genitalia were female but hypotrophic, with no signs of clitoromegaly. The vagina was small and 2.8 cm long. On rectal examination neither the uterus nor its adnexa were palpable. Chromosomal analysis showed a normal male karyotype (46/XY). On laparotomy no structures referable to the uterus or to the fallopian tubes were evident. At the level of both the right and the left internal inguinal rings a small nut-sized whitish colored spongy mass was found (referable to the gonads). The masses protruded into the abdominal cavity and were held in position by a peduncle which inserted into the inguinal canal itself. The histologic examination showed fragments of testicular structure (Fig.2). The tubules appeared atrophic and were covered more or less exclusively by Sertoli cells. The interstitial tissue was well represented and enclosed several Leydig cells.

Case 2

Augusta, D. (Fig.3), 19 years old, 7th offspring, was first seen when she was 13 years old at a Pediatric Department for delayed growth and amenorrhea. On

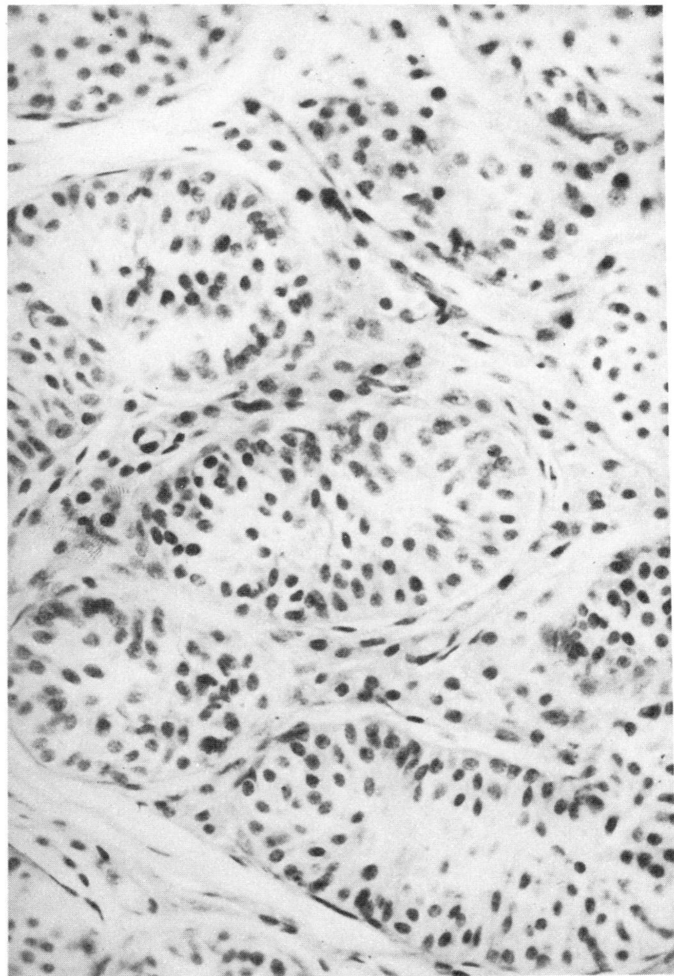

Fig. 2 Testicular biopsy of patient G.D.; the tubules contain only Sertoli cells. Leydig cells are present in the interstitial tissue.

laparoscopic examination she was found to have fibrocystic ovaries and underwent laparotomy, which revealed a uterus which seemed to be a medial thickening of the broad ligaments, and multiple ovarian cysts which appeared as orange-sized, smooth and multilocular masses containing a serous fluid. Histological examination of ovaries showed numerous cysts with hyperplasia and luteinization of the theca (Fig.4). A bilateral ovarian resection and reconstruction was performed. We are not aware of her blood pressure at that time. When we first saw the patient she presented with severe hypertension having a systolic of 180 over a diastolic of 130, with short stature and poorly developed sexual characteristics. Her karyotype was that of a normal female, 46/XX. She still accused primary amenorrhea. Her routine admission laboratory data were normal, except for a blood potassium of 2.9 mEq/l.

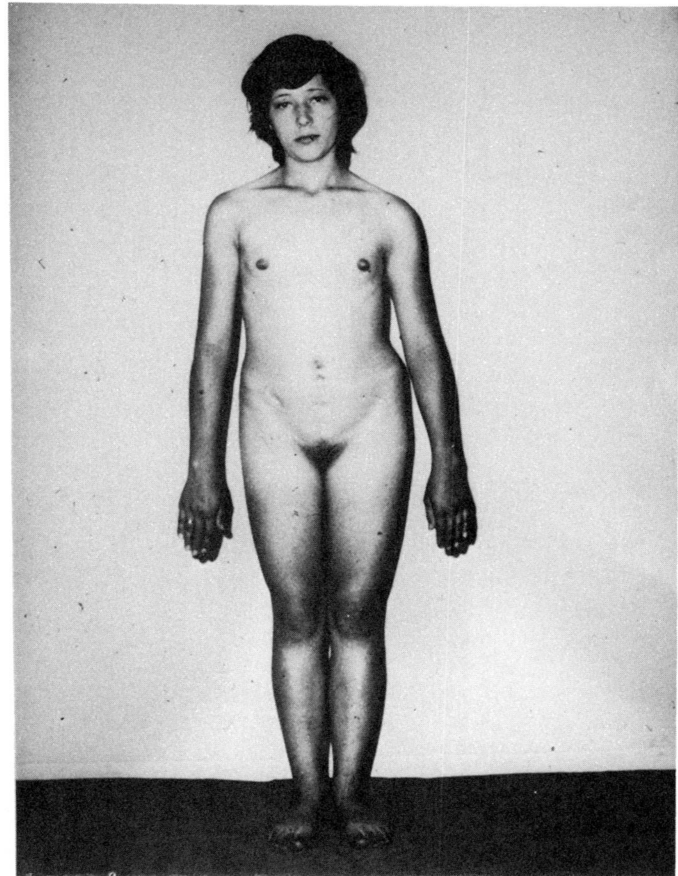

Fig.3 Patient A.D. at age 19. Previous estrogens treatment has developed a minimal degree of secondary sexual characteristics.

Case 3

Marilisa, D., 23 years old, third offspring. In her case history there is an attack of glomerulonephritis when she was six years old which apparently healed. Her menarche was induced by estrogen administration at 16 years old but was amenorrheic without therapy. She was admitted one year prior to our observation in a Gynecology Clinic for investigation for absent axially and pubic hairs and for underdeveloped breasts. Her external genitalia appeared to be normal. On rectal gynecologic examination her uterus was felt displaced to the left, on the right being felt an orange-sized movable mass. On laparotomy, the uterus presented with pubertal characteristics, the tubes were thin, tortuous but opened. The ovaries were egg-sized with a covering albuginea mother-of-pearl like and had many microcystic follicles. A bilateral ovarian resection was performed. When we first observed the patient she presented with arterial hypertension of 180/130. Her blood and urine studies were normal except for notable hypokalemia 1.95 mEq/l. Blood sodium was 145 mEq/l. Fundoscopic examination revealed a grade II retinopathy. Renal function studies were all within normal limits. The karyotype was 46/XX.

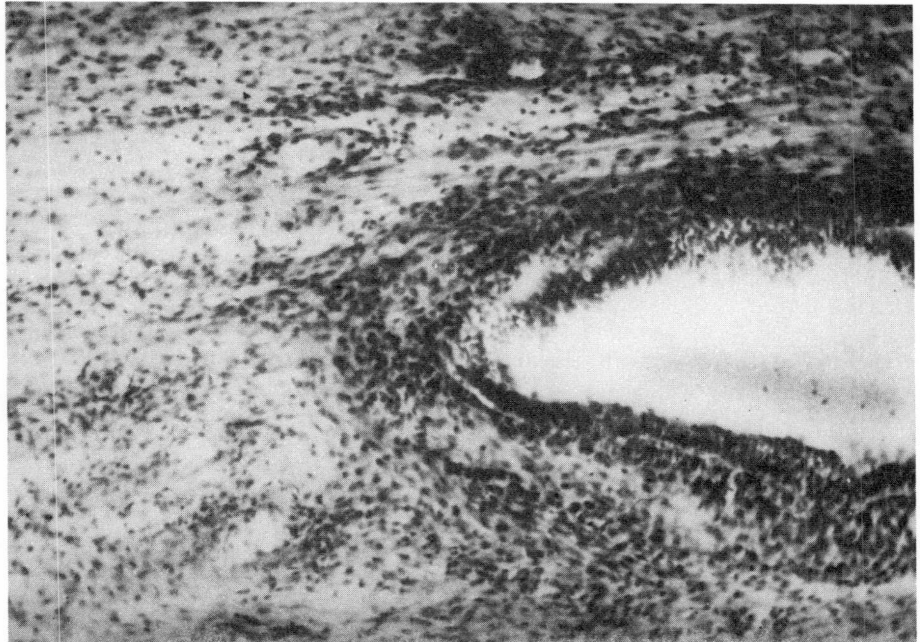

Fig.4 A follicle cyst from ovarian biopsy of patient A.D.

HORMONAL STUDIES

The results of hormone levels found in each case are shown in Table I, as well as the methods used and the normal values (sex hormones, for females in follicular phase). The diagnosis of 17α-hydroxylase deficiency in all three cases seems evident by the high progesterone, deoxycorticosterone and corticosterone levels (steroids not hydroxylated in the C17 position) and by the low or undeterminable levels of 17-OH-progesterone, deoxycortisol and cortisol (secretion rate) as well as androgens and estrogens. Consequently, the plasma ACTH, FSH and LH levels are elevated. The PRA is suppressed in all three cases, the aldosteronuria is also very low. The apparently high levels of plasma "cortisol" and "aldosterone" seem due to the cross-reacting high levels of corticosterone.

THERAPY

Once we suspected the diagnosis of a 17α-hydroxylase deficiency we carried out in all three patients an acute dexamethasone therapy test (2 mg per day for seven days). The variations in arterial blood pressure, electrolyte and equilibrium and hormonal parameters are recorded in Table II. In two cases (Graziella and Augusta) the blood potassium levels returned to normal with a marked reduction in arterial blood pressure, while in the third case (Marilisa, the eldest of the three) only an improvement in blood potassium without any change in arterial B.P. occurred. In all three patients, the plasma deoxycosterone and corticosterone levels fell to within normal limits. The PRA rose also to within normal limits while

Table I. Hormonal studies in 17 OHDS.

Steroid Assayed	Graziella XY	Augusta XX	Marilisa XX	Method & N.V.
17OH Steroids				
Pl. 17OH-Progesterone (ng%)	16.9	6.8	3.7	RIA: 25-200
Pl. 11-Deoxycortisol (ng%)	22	22	27	RIA: 50-100
Pl. "Cortisol" (μg%)	16.9	20.6	18.8	RIA: 5-20
Ur. 17OH-Steroids (mg/24 h)	1.6	5.2	3.9	P.S.: 5-15
Cortisol secretion rate (mg/24 h)	undetectable	undetectable	0.4	IS.DIL.: 8-20
Sterpids Derived From 17OH Steroids				
Ur. 17Ketosteroids (mg/24 h)	1.6	1.5	4.3	ZIMM.: 4-10
Pl. Dehydroepiandrosterone (ng%)	7	11	21	RIA: 200-250
Pl. Androstenedione (ng%)	—	53	19.5	RIA: 80-200
Pl. Testosterone (ng%)	34.7	33.6	25.9	RIA: 10-50
Ur. Estrogens (μg/24 h)	43.5	18	60	JAYL.: 20-90
Non 17OH Steroids				
Pl. Progesterone (ng%)	255	460	160	RIA: 20-80
Ur. Pregnandiol (mg/24 h)	2.3	—	12.8	SOMM: 0.5-1.5
Pl. Deoxycorticosterone (ng%)	251	251	134	RIA: 3-12
Pl. Corticosterone (μg%)	20.5	28.2	33.0	RIA: 0.2-1.5
Pl. Aldosterone (ng%)	55.2	9.0	29.6	RIA: 3-12
Ur. Aldosterone (μg/24 h)	2.0	1.6	undetectable	RIA: 5-15
Related Hormones				
Pl. Renin activity (ng/ml/3 h)	0.2	0.6	0.2	RIA: 1-4
Pl. ACTH (pg%)	171	216	246	RIA: 40-120
Pl. FSH (ng%)	20	6.6	20	RIA: 1.8-3
Pl. LH (ng%)	5.5	4.2	10	RIA: 1.6-2

the aldosteronuria remained unchanged.

Chronic treatment: all three patients were placed on continuous dexamethasone treatment of 0.5 mg per day to be taken in the evening and have undergone periodic monitoring of their blood pressures and electrolytes. After one year of therapy the blood pressures are more or less normal in the first two cases and only slightly reduced in the third, whereas the electrolyte values in all three cases have remained within normal limits. Conjugated estrogens are also being given to the three patients, with some development of their secondary sexual characteristics.

DISCUSSION

Further proof of the familial nature of the 17α-hydroxylase deficiency syndrome is provided by the simultaneous occurrence of the deficiency in these three siblings. The fact that the parents are blood related is also very interesting since the same was true in three other cases previous reported. It is also possible that the two offspring who died in early childhood for unknown reasons had a defect in their steroid synthetic mechanism. Evidently, the disease may exist in

Table II. Dexamethasone suppression test (2 mg/day for 1 week).

	Graziella		Augusta		Marilisa	
	before	after	before	after	before	after
Na_S (mEq/l)	142	141	139	134	145	139
K_S (mEq/l)	3.3	4.3	2.9	3.7	1.9	2.5
B.P. (mm Hg)	160/110	130/90	180/130	145/110	180/130	180/130
P1. Corticosterone (ng/100 ml)	20.5	0.75	28.2	0.72	33.0	0.98
P1. Deoxycorticosterone (ng/100 ml)	251	1.3	251	17	134	9
P1. Renin activity (ng/ml/3 h)	0.20	3.80	0.62	1.84	0.29	1.72
Ur. Aldosterone (μg/24 h)	2.04	undet.	1.69	0.15	undet.	undet.

the same family in genotypically dissimilar subjects but invariably the complete form of the disease presents in phenotypical females who are reared as such. From the literature, the diagnosis of the syndrome seems to be limited to the post-pubertal period when primary amenorrhea and lack of secondary sexual characteristics brings the patient to the doctor's attention. Although surely present during early childhood, hypertension does not seem to contribute to the early diagnosis of the disease, a fact which might be due to the unattentive blood pressure control by the primary care physician during infancy, or also to the fact that this disease was still to be described when at least part of the cases reported were children. Only when there have been important disturbances secondary to the hypertension in early childhood (headache, vomiting) or to the hypopotassiemia (paresthesia, paresis, myalgia) as in the youngest of the three patients reported here, an early diagnosis of the syndrome was made. We expect that more cases in the pediatric age group will be reported in the future; with early ACTH suppressive therapy, the damage caused by chronic hypertension could in fact be avoided and by early estrogen substitution therapy an improvement in the abnormalities of the secondary sexual characteristics might be achieved.

The problem of a patient with a chromosomal XY pattern and therefore possessing testicles is more complex. The testicles remain undescended and present as bilateral inguinal hernias which may be removed during surgical intervention to correct such a problem. The case presented in this study had testicles retained totally within the abdominal cavity. We recommend that they be removed in all cases, not merely because of the probability of malignant degeneration but they might also prove to be embarrassing to a patient reared as a female and convinced to be such. It is interesting that polycystic ovaries were found also in our two cases with a female genotype. It is very probable that they are the consequence of chronic overstimulation by FSH. The risk of an erroneous interpretation in the subject who presents with an associated amenorrhea is obvious. In fact, our two cases had been previously considered by a Gynecological Department to be affected by the Stein-Leventhal syndrome.

These three cases presented with the classical endocrine abnormalities for the complete form of the syndrome. They have almost total lack of cortisol secretion; also cortisol precursors, as 11-deoxycortisol and 17 OH progesterone, are found to be very low in the blood, as are their metabolites in the urine. Corresponding with these levels is a rather elevated plasma ACTH even though it is not as high as expected given that the cortisol secretion is so low. Evidently, some other adrenal steroid in high concentration (corticosterone?) may possess some negative feedback effectiveness on ACTH.

As would be expected, gonadotropin levels are high, since the sex hormones both estrogenic and androgenic, being hydroxylated in the C17 position, are extremely reduced in a deficiency of the 17α-hydroxylase enzyme, which is common to both the gonads and the adrenals.

A specific aspect of this syndrome is represented by the low aldosterone levels, which have been found also in our three new cases. This finding is commonly considered to be due to an ACTH-dependent increased production of DOC and B, which, through sodium retention and volume expansion, would reduce renin and thus the angiotensin-dependent aldosterone secretion. The exact mechanism may not be so simple, as pointed out by Biglierie and Mantero (1973); however, it seems likely that the impairment of aldosterone secretion is due only to a functional block, since it may be reproduced in normal subjects under chronic ACTH stimulation (Biglieri *et al.*, 1969). In our patients, short-term ACTH suppression with dexamethasone has induced only a normalization of the PRA, whereas urinary aldosterone remained unchanged: the return of the aldosterone reaction to angiotensin stimulation may take some more time, as shown in some of the previously-reported patients, including our own (Busnardo *et al.*, 1973), but invariably occurs.

REFERENCES

Alvarez, M.N., Cloutier, M.D. and Hayles, A.R. (1971). *Pediat. Res.* 7, 325.

Biglieri, E.G., Herron, M.A. and Brust, N. (1966). *J. clin. Invest.* **45**, 1946-1954.

Biglieri, E.G., Shambelan, M. and Slaton, P.E. (1969). *J. clin. Endocr. Metab.* **29**, 1090-1095.

Biglieri, E.G. and Mantero, F. (1973). "Research on Steroids", **Vol.V**, pp.385-399. S.E.U. Ed., Rome.

Bricaire, H., Luton, J.P., Laudat, P., Legrand, J.C., Turpin, G., Corvol, P. and Lemmer, M. (1972). *J. clin. Endocr. Metab.* **35**, 67-72.

Busnardo, B., Mantero, F., Riondel, A.M., Vayrat, R. and Austoni, M. (1973). "Research on Steroids", **Vol.V**, pp.499-503. S.E.U. Ed., Rome.

De Lange, W.E., Weeke, A., Artz, W., Jansen, W. and Doorenbos, H. (1973). *Acta Med. Scand.* **193**, 565-571.

Goldsmith, O., Solomon, D.H. and Horton, R. (1967). *New Engl. J. Med.* **277**, 673-677.

Hammerstein, J., Zielske, F., Distler, A. and Wolff, H.P. (1973). *Acta endocr. (Copenh.)* **176**, 76.

Kershnar, A.K., Borut, D. and Kogut, M.D. (1973). *Pediat. Res.* 7, 329.

Linquette, M., Dupont, A., Racadot, A., Lefebre, J., May, J.P. and Coppoen, J.P. (1971). *Ann. d'Endocrinol.* **32**, 574-582.

Mellin, S.R. (1969). *Ann. int. Med.* **79**, 69-75.

Mantero, F., Busnardo, B., Riondel, A.M., Veyrat, R. and Austoni, M. (1971). *Schweiz. Med. Wochenschr.* **101**, 38-43.

Mills, L.H., Wilson, R.J., Tait, A.D. and Cooper, A.R. (1967). *J. Endocrinol.* **38**, XIX-XX.

New, M. (1970). *J. clin. Invest.* **49**, 1930-1940.

Tronchetti, P., Matterazzi, F., Franchi, P. and Luisi, M. (1973). "Actualités Endocrinologiques" 13eme série, pp.78-88. L'expansion Editions, Paris.

HLA SYSTEM AND ISLET CELL ANTIBODIES IN DIABETES MELLITUS

M.T. Illeni, G. Pellegris, M.J. del Guercio, A. Tarantino, F. Busetto, C. Di Pietro, E. Clerici, G. Garotta and G. Chiumello

Department of Pediatrics, Department of Immunology, Department of Urology of the University of Milan
and
Istituto Nazionale per lo Studio e la Cura dei Tumori, Milan, Italy

Hereditary factors play an important role in the aetiology of maturity-onset type of diabetes mellitus of childhood (Tattersal *et al.*, 1975). The importance of these factors in the most frequent type of diabetes in childhood, the insulin-dependent disease, is not clear (Rimoin, 1967; Tattersal *et al.*, 1972).

Some authors have observed a statistically significant increase in frequency of the antigens HLA-B8 and HLA-BW15 in patients with insulin-dependent juvenile diabetes (Singal *et al.*, 1973; Nerup *et al.*, 1974; Cudworth *et al.*, 1975), thus suggesting the presence of predisposing genes near HLA loci. In susceptible children, viral infactions could initiate beta-cell damage and bring about clinical diabetes within a few weeks or months from the infection (Rolles *et al.*, 1975).

In our study, 90 insulin-dependent diabetics (46 males and 44 females) aged 2-20 years were HLA typed. All had acute onset of the disease between 11 months and 16 years of age, and its duration varied from a few days to 10½ years. Fifty-two percent of the children had the onset of clinical diabetes between October and January (Fig. 1). The control population was made up of 488 blood donors from the same geographic area of the diabetic patients.

The significantly different frequencies of HLA antigens in diabetic children and controls, and the relative risks (R.R.) are reported in Table I, which shows a statistically significant increase in the frequency of HLA-AW30 and HLA-B8, and decrease of HLA-A11 and HLA-BW35 in diabetics as compared to controls. As regards the negative association of HLA-A11 and HLA-BW35 antigens, a similar finding has been reported (Ludwig *et al.*, 1976) for HLA-B7 and the maturity-onset type of diabetes, suggesting that also the decreased frequency of some antigens may increase the risk of contracting the disease. The importance, if any, of

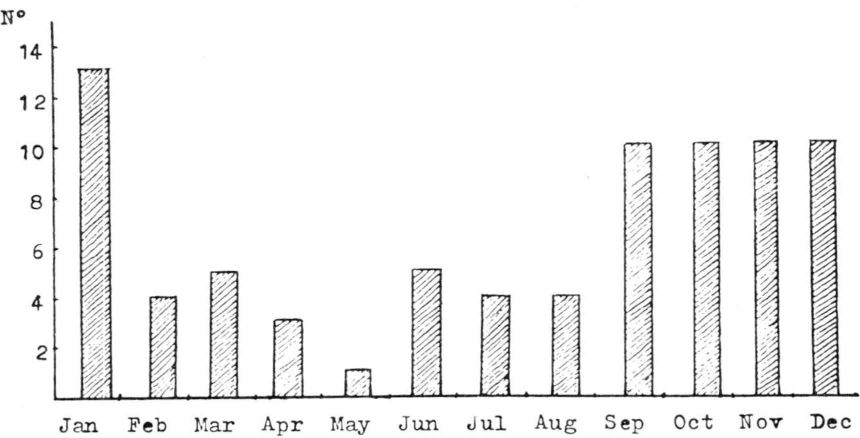

Fig.1 Month at onset of diabetes in 75 diabetic children.

Table I. Significantly different frequencies of HLA antigens in diabetic children and controls.

	Diabetic Children		Controls
Locus A		R.R.	
A11	3.3%*	0.28	11%
AW30	17.8%***	2.89	7%
Locus B			
B8	23.3%***	2.13	12.5%
BW35	16.7%***	0.38	34.7%

* $p < 0.05$; *** $p < 0.01$.

these antigens as protective factors against insulin-dependent diabetes could be evaluated by studying families with high incidence of the disease.

In Table I the relative risks are also indicated: for example the R.R. of 2.13 for HLA-B8 means that for an individual carrying this antigen the risk of developing diabetes is more than double as compared to individuals lacking HLA-B8.

In Table II the age at onset of diabetes is considered. The incidence of HLA-AW30 and HLA-B8 is significantly increased and the incidence of HLA-BW35 decreased as compared to controls when the disease occurs before the age of 5 years. In the group of 5–10 years onset, the frequency of HLA-A2, HLA-AW30, HLA-B18 is increased, and the frequency of HLA-BW35 decreased. As regards the group with onset of diabetes between 10 and 16 years, there are no significant differences.

When the seasonal beginning of the symptoms is considered (Table III), in the group in which the clinical onset was between October and January, the frequency of the antigens HLA-A2, HLA-AW30 and HLA-B8 is significantly increased,

Table II. Frequency of HLA antigens in diabetic children in relation to age at onset of the disease and controls.

	Diabetic Children Age at onset (years) 0–5	5–10	Controls
Locus A			
A2	53.6%	67.6%***	44%
AW30	21.4%***	17.6%*	7%
Locus B			
B8	35.7%***	11.8%	12.5%
BW35	7.1%***	17.6%*	34.7%
B18	17.9%	26.5%*	12.6%

* $p < 0.05$; *** $p < 0.01$.

Table III. Frequency of HLA antigens in diabetic children in relation to season at onset of the disease and controls.

	Diabetic Children Month at onset Oct–Jan	Feb–Sept	Controls
Locus A			
A2	61.9%*	52.6%	44%
A11	0*	7.9%	11%
A29	2.4%	13.2%*	4.9%
AW30	19%***	13.2%	7%
Locus B			
B8	26.2%**	23.7%	12.5%
B12	11.9%	31.6%*	17%
BW35	14.3%**	15.8%*	34.7%

* $p < 0.05$; ** $p < 0.02$; *** $p < 0.01$.

and that of HLA-A11 decreased. In the February–September group the frequency of of antigens HLA-A29 and HLA-B12 is increased; in both groups that of HLA-BW35 is significantly decreased.

The present data support the findings that HLA-B8, the antigen most commonly associated with insulin-dependent diabetes, occurs in most children who had the onset of clinical diabetes before 5 years of age (Rolles *et al.*, 1975).

It is possible that the association between diabetes and HLA antigens reflects a high degree of linkage disequilibrium between *HLA* genes and other unknown genes which may be directly involved in the pathogenesis, by means of specific responses against various antigens. The fact that siblings of the patients with the same HLA haplotype are not diabetics suggests that other genes may be necessary, by interacting with the HLA-linked gene, in order to reach the threshold of susceptibility, and that other environmental factors may be necessary in order to develop the disease in predisposed individuals. The HLA region contains about 2000 cistrons between loci A and B, and as many between loci C and D: some of them govern specific immune response towards various antigens. Although the pathogenesis of insulin-dependent diabetes is not completely known, autoimmune phenomena have been frequently demonstrated.

A lymphocytic infiltration of the Langerhans islet seems to be a common finding in diabetics under 30 years of age studied less than six months after the clinical onset of the disease; but insulitis is a transitory injury that was never found in young diabetics whose clinical symptoms lasted more than one year.

Even recently some authors reported the presence of antibeta cell antibodies in insulin-dependent diabetics (the antibodies were complement fixing IgG). The frequent association with autoimmune disease, the lymphocytic infiltration of the islets, the presence of lymphocytes sensitized towards human and animal pancreatic antigens, the high incidence of histocompatibility antigens like HLA-B8, frequently found also in autoimmune diseases like thyrotoxicosis, Hashimoto's thyroiditis, Addison's disease, all lead to the hypothesis that insulin-dependent diabetes mellitus, or at least in some cases, is an autoimmune disease. A viral infection by Coxsackie B4, rubella, mumps, may affect the carriers of particular antigens, and may trigger an autoimmune response leading to destruction of beta cells and to the development of clinical diabetes (Fig.2). While HLA-B8 negative diabetic children did not show evident seasonal variations, 81% of HLA-B8 positive children had the beginning of clinical symptoms of the disease within the months of October through February, and this is the period with the peak incidence of Coxsackie virus infections (Rolles *et al.*, 1975).

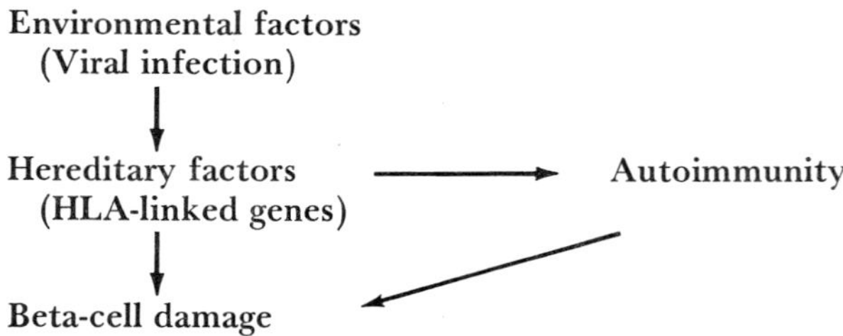

Fig.2 Possible aetiopathogenetic hypothesis for diabetes mellitus.

In our study the research of antibeta cells antibodies was performed by the technique of indirect immunofluorescence using fresh human pancreas frozen soon after surgical removal. The sera of children who had fluorescent antibodies directed against pancreatic structures were tested with fluorescent anti-IgG, -IgA and -IgM sera. In six cases antibodies against islet cells were found; they were of the IgA class and in two cases they were also of the IgG class. In eight children we found antibodies towards ductular cells of exocrine pancreas. In one case the

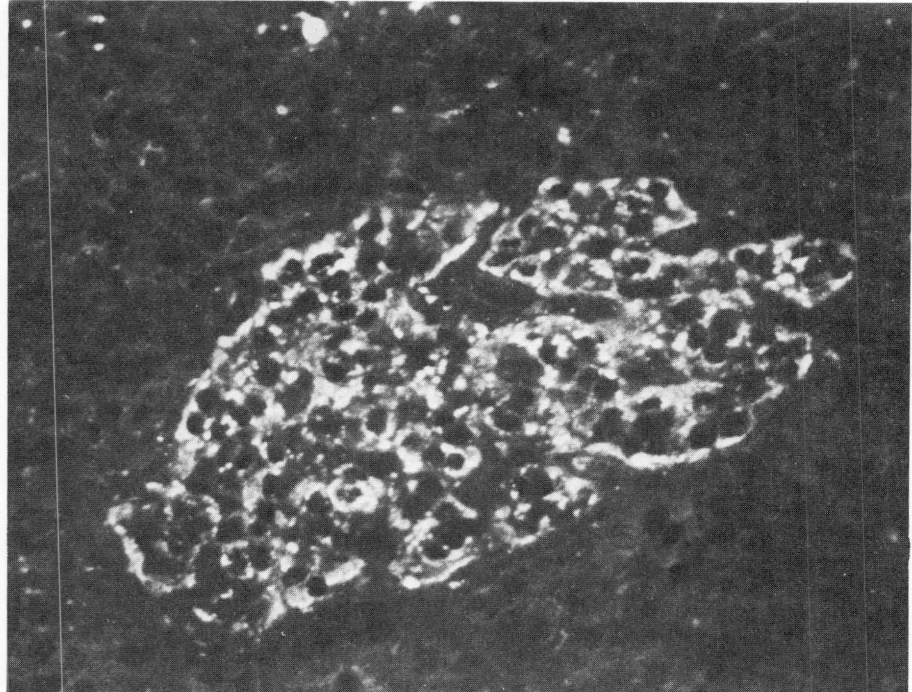

Fig.3 Immunofluorescent antibodies against pancreatic islet-cells.

diabetic symptoms began a few weeks and in the remaining cases more than one year before the identification of anti-islet cells antibodies.

The small number of positive cases makes it impossible to find a correlation between any histocompatibility antigens and the presence of anti-pancreas antibodies, even if most of them were HLA-B8 positive. The production of anti-islet cells antibodies may be under the control of an *Ir* gene within the HLA region, closely linked to HLA-B8 and, probably, to other genes. We could speculate that genetically predisposed children are easily affected by Coxsackie or other pancreas damaging viruses which may prime the production of autoantibodies. The fact that *HLA* system genes, on chromosome No.6, are very close to immune response genes, suggests that some *Ir* genes may be responsible for an altered immune response.

HLA antigens may interact or may be themselves membrane receptor sites for viruses or other pathogenic agents which may initiate an inflammatory process and damage the beta cells, so that hidden antigens may become manifest and initiate the immune response. HLA antigens may be similar to viral antigens, so that they may induce immune tolerance for some viral antigens. In this manner, the immune mechanism could fail to eliminate a virus which, after the acute phase, could persist for a long time in the organism and destroy beta cells directly or indirectly.

It is premature to speculate on the role of autoantibodies, in the positive cases, in the aetiology of diabetes, although it is possible that they may be associated with the insulitis observed in some juvenile insulin-dependent diabetics.

In conclusion, the present data demonstrate that in insulin-dependent diabetic children the frequency of some HLA antigens, as HLA-B8 and HLA-AW30, is significantly increased, while the frequency of other antigens is decreased. A great part of HLA-B8 positive children had the onset of clinical disease within the months of October through February, when the incidence of Coxsackie infections is higher. In a few cases anti-islet cells antibodies were found; it is most likely that the incidence of positive cases is higher when the patients are examined soon after the diagnosis or in the months before the clinical manifestations of the disease. These still fragmentary data shed new light on the aetiopathogenesis of diabetes and may also be useful in preventing insulin-dependent diabetes in childhood.

REFERENCES

Cudworth, A.G. and Woodrow, J.C. (1975). *Br. med. J.* **3**, 133-135.

Ludwig, H., Scherntlaner, G. and Mayr, W.R. (1976). *New Engl. J. Med.* **294**, 1066.

Nerup, J., Platz, P., Ortved-Andersen, O., Christy, M., Lyngse, J., Poulsen, S.E., Ryderr, L.P., Staub-Nielsen, L., Thomsen, M. and Svejgaard, A. (1974). *Lancet* **II**, 864-866.

Rimoin, D.L. (1967). *Diabetes* **16**, 346-351.

Rolles, C.J., Rayner, P.H.W. and Mackintosh, P. (1975). *Lancet* **II**, 230.

Singal, D.P. and Blajchman, M.A. (1973). *Diabetes* 22, 429-432.

Tattersal, R.B. and Pyke, D.A. (1972). *Lancet* **II**, 1120-1125.

Tattersal, R.B., Fajan, S.S. and Arbor, A. (1975). *Diabetes* **24**, 44-53.

THICKNESS OF MUSCLE CAPILLARY BASEMENT MEMBRANES IN NORMAL CHILDREN AND CHILDREN WITH DIABETES MELLITUS

R.L. Jackson, J.A. Esterly, R.A. Guthrie and N. Bilginturan

Department of Child Health, University of Missouri, School of Medicine Columbia, USA

Children with overt diabetes have hypoinsulinism so severe that for survival they invariably require exogenous insulin. The insulin requirement will vary depending on the weight of the child, how early the diagnosis is made, and how soon insulin therapy is initiated. The earlier the diagnosis is made and insulin is given the lower the insulin requirement and the easier it will be to attain and maintain a high degree of control with little risk of hypoglycemia.

Replacement therapy should be designed to maintain a state as physiological as possible, both to permit normal growth and development and to delay or prevent the insidious development of vascular complications. To attain that objective, the parents and, ultimately, the child must learn how to adjust insulin dosage and food intake to control the child's glycosuria yet allow him to participate fully in all activities of his peer group without fear of an insulin reaction. The task is not easy. It requires understanding, judgement, self discipline, and acceptance of the concept of maintaining optimum health. The parents have to teach these basic principles to their child by example.

Children with overt diabetes should be admitted to a hospital, as soon as possible, preferably to a pediatric unit, not only for the treatment of acute complications such as ketoacidosis but also to re-establish a good nutritional state, to determine the maintenance insulin requirement, to explore and identify difficult psychosocial areas, and to educate both the parents and the child. To attain these goals, the undernourished diabetic child with recent onset of diabetes requires hospital care for three to five weeks. The pediatric unit should have a school and recreational facilities so the child can continue his education and have normal physical activity.

It is an established fact but not fully appreciated that with prompt insulin treatment the exogenous insulin requirement of most children with recent onset of diabetes decreases rapidly to a relatively low level (0.05 to 0.40 units/kg/day). Jackson *et al.* in 1971 found the insulin requirement of children with very early diagnosis and treatment was as low as 0.05 to 0.10 units/kg/day and, if the parents were able to continue the treatment plan at home, this state of partial remission persisted for as long as four years. When the onset of overt diabetes was after puberty, the period of remission was found to extend for even a longer period of time. The insulin requirement is low because the patient's pancreas is still able to produce some endogenous insulin. During this period of partial remission, glycosuria can be controlled completely with two small doses of insulin daily and with little likelihood of even a mild insulin reaction. In contrast to the child with recent onset of diabetes who receives prompt and optimal treatment, the child with diabetes who receives delayed and suboptimal treatment usually requires 0.7 to 1.0 units/kg/day within a period of months and then becomes a so-called total or 'brittle' diabetic. We also recommend a period of hospital care for the child with total diabetes to attain a higher degree of control and to re-educate the child and his parents. To avoid hypoglycemia in a total diabetic, however, it becomes necessary to permit short periods of transient glycosuria with varying degrees of hyperglycemia. After a period of management in which the child with total diabetes has received only once-daily doses of insulin and relatively lax supervision of his meal plan, it becomes more difficult to establish a plan of treatment that requires more self discipline. Because these children have a much lower threshold of safety for hypoglycemia than do recently diagnosed children in partial remission, special attention must be given to teaching them and their parents how to adjust food intake with varying degrees of physical activity.

In our experience, at least two daily injections of insulins are needed for optimal treatment for all children with diabetes. As described in detail in their recent book "The Child with Diabetes", Jackson and Guthrie advise the use of a mixture of 2 parts NPH insulin and 1 part neutral regular insulin. Two-thirds of the total dose is given one-half hour before breakfast and the remaining 1/3 is given one-half hour before the evening meal.

The maintenance nutritional needs for the child with diabetes are the same as that for normal children. For that reason, we generally avoid the word 'diet' in talking to patients and their parents. 'Diet' has a connotation of fasting and denial; 'meal plan' does not.

We agree with the nutritional care plan for the diabetic child published in 1974 by Monroe *et al.* for the Diet Therapy Section of the American Dietetic Association. The meal plan for the child with diabetes should be based on the nutritional needs of healthy, nondiabetic children of similar age, height, and weight and should be compatible with his family's income and food habits. The essential difference is that food intake for the diabetic child is adjusted to the type and dose of insulin given and to his pattern of physical activity.

In addition to expert medical care, the child and family need to receive intensive education from a nurse and a dietitian experienced in management of children with diabetes. Detailed social information is essential to determine the family and community resources. The combined efforts of the health team also are needed to evaluate and prepare the family to continue the regimen after the child returns home.

An ever increasing number of patients with onset of diabetes in childhood are finding themselves handicapped by progressive vascular disease in early life. In 1956, Jackson and Hardin reported their findings on a group of 140 juvenile diabetic patients observed at the University of Iowa with a duration of their disease ranging from 10 to 29 years. They found that the degree of control of the diabetes was the only identifiable factor bearing a constantly significant relationship to the incidence and severity of vascular complications.

Recent biochemical studies are revealing the relationship between the duration and degree of hyperglycemia and hypoinsulinism and the rate of development of various complications of diabetes. Morrison and Winegrad (1972) and Rosio *et al.* (1972) have demonstrated an alternate pathway for glucose, namely the polyol pathway, to be operative during relatively short periods of more severe hyperglycemia. Gabbay (1973) and Bilginturan *et al.* (1976) have indicated that the polyol pathway is implicated in the production of cataracts, atherosclerosis, cerebral edema in some cases of ketoacidosis, and to the development of peripheral neuropathy.

Spiro has studied extensively the metabolism of the glycoprotein. In 1971 he found that the basement membranes of capillaries are glycoproteins consisting primarily of tightly bound chains of lysine molecules. In the diabetic with longstanding hyperglycemia and hypoinsulinemia as often as every third lysine molecule is substituted with galactose and glucose units resulting in thickening of the capillary basement membrane. The enzymes, transferases, responsible for the transfer of the galactose and glucose units to the lysine molecules are suppressed by insulin as reviewed by Spiro (1976) in his Claude Bernard lecture. Thus hyperglycemia increases the substrates for the basement membrane reaction and a low tissue insulin level allows the enzymes responsible for transfer of glucose to lysine to become activated. In 1971 Cahill presented evidence that there must be detectable serum levels of insulin during the entire 24 hours of each day in order to prevent the biochemical reactions described by Spiro.

Bloodworth and Engerman in 1973 studied dogs made diabetic with growth hormone or alloxan and showed conclusively that hereditary is not necessary for the development of microangiopathy and that the degree of diabetic control determines the rate of development of the microangiopathy. Osterby also in 1973 reported her extensive studies of the thickness of the capillary basement membranes of the glomerulus in non-diabetic and diabetic children. She found normal thickness of the capillary basement membranes (CBM) in children with diabetes at the time of onset of overt diabetes. Children with diabetes who received one dose of an intermediate acting insulin and who had varying degrees of glycosuria developed progressive thickening of their glomerular basement membranes over a 2 to 5 year period of time after the onset of the disease. In 1976, Maurer *et al.* reported their studies in animals and demonstrated that diabetic microvascularopathy is reversible.

Kilo *et al.* reported in 1972 that thickening of the capillary basement membranes in patients with adult-onset diabetes does not precede the onset of carbohydrate intolerance, but is related to the duration and severity of the diabetes. Their findings are confirmed by our studies at the University of Missouri, where Dr. Esterly using Williamson's method has measured the capillary basement membrane thickness (CBMT) in a large group of healthy adolescent children with no family history of diabetes and with normal oral glucose tolerance tests (OGTT's);

a large group of healthy older siblings of children with overt diabetes with one or more normal OGTT's including both blood sugar and serum insulin determinations; in a few older children with chemical diabetes; and in over 200 children with diabetes in varying degrees of control.

All measurements were done as unknowns and diabetic control was rated prior to any knowledge of CBMT's. Many of the diabetics were observed sequentially from onset. Patients were classified according to (a) age (prepubescent, pubescent, and postpubescent), (b) duration of the disease (0 to 5, 5 to 10, 10 to 15, and over 15 years), (c) overall control rating [(good), (fair to good), (fair to poor), and (poor to fair)]. For details of the criteria used to classify the overall degree of control of patients with insulin dependent diabetes, see Addendum A.

At present there are no reliable objective laboratory methods which reflect the overall degree of control of a diabetic patient over an extended period of time. The 1976 observations of Gabbay *et al.* and Koening *et al.* give hope that determination of A_{1c} hemoglobin may prove helpful in this regard. In our experience it is easy to identify and classify with confidence those patients who attain and maintain higher degrees of control. These patients are from stable, resourceful and well-disciplined families and keep reliable home records. In the early years after onset, the partial remission persists and during this period they establish good eating habits, learn how to increase gradually their insulin dosage and food intake with growth and also how to adjust their food intake and insulin dosage during periods of stress so as to keep their urine sugar-free except for minimal glycosuria over very short periods of time. Few, if any other clinics have a large group of children with diabetes in good control by our standards.

In 1946 Jackson and Kelly found that only children with (fair to poor) control by our criteria have a decreased growth rate. Therefore a decreased growth rate provides objective evidence of poorer degrees of control. However, there is a relatively large group of children whose level of control varies from time to time from (fair to good) to from (fair to poor). An overall classification for these patients is open to question as it has to be made on history of questionable reliability and interpretation of limited clinical and laboratory data.

In the recent past, a number of morphometric techniques have been introduced for determining capillary basement membrane width in normal subjects and patients with chemical and overt diabetes mellitus. Various fixatives, dehydrating agents and plastics have been used for processing the muscle tissues so that data from different laboratories are rarely comparable. We elected to use Williamson's method as we believe it is superior to and more reliable than other methods as verified by Dr. Williamson's recent study reported in July 1976. The only minor differences in our procedure as compared to Williamson's is that our laboratory uses a slightly different buffer system and a different plastic embedding media to process the tissues. To determine comparability of data from our laboratory with Dr. Williamson's muscle tissue obtained by needle biopsy from many normal and diabetic subjects was divided into two portions, one of which was fixed and processed in Dr. Williamson's laboratory and the others in our laboratory. Measurements in our laboratory have been found to be consistently slightly higher than measurements from Dr. Williamson's laboratory as exemplified in Fig.1.

Measurements of muscle capillary basement membrane thickness have been made from electron photomicrographs of 39 normal children (age 9 to 18, 22

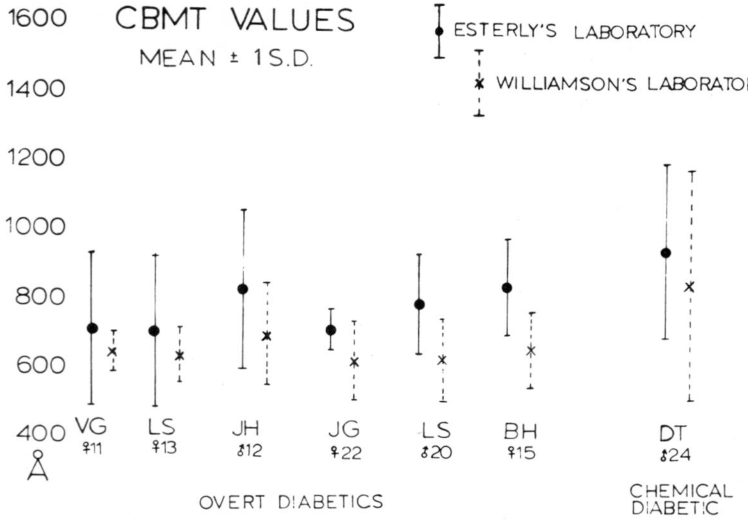

Fig. 1 **Comparative thickness of CBM of muscle tissue which was divided into two portions, one of which was fixed and processed in Williamson's laboratory and the other in Esterly's laboratory. All measurements were done by Dr. Esterly.**

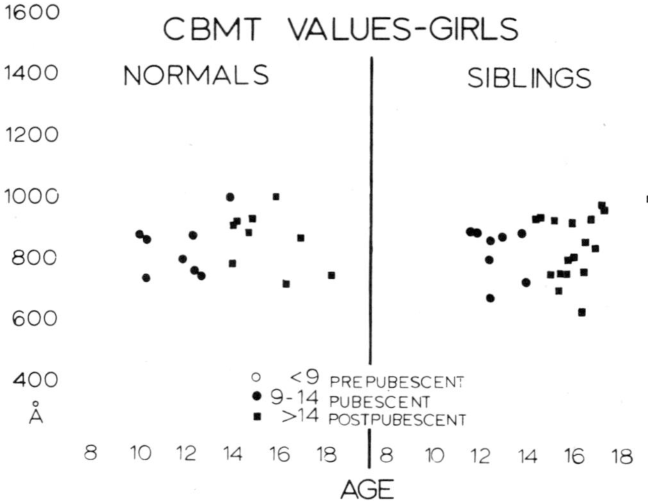

Fig. 2 **CBMT of healthy adolescent girls with no family history of diabetes and with normal OGTT's as compared to CBMT of healthy female siblings of children with overt diabetes with one or more normal OGTT's.**

boys and 17 girls) with no family history of diabetes and in 41 healthy siblings of diabetics (age 13 to 21; 17 boys and 22 girls) with one or more normal glucose tolerance tests (OGGTT's) including both blood sugar and serum insulin

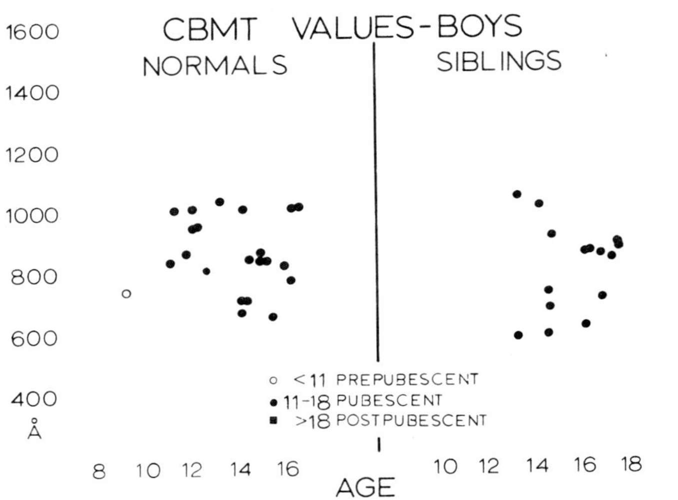

Fig.3 CBMT of healthy adolescent boys with no family history of diabetes and with normal OGTT's as compared to CBMT of healthy male siblings of children with overt diabetes with one or more normal OGTT's.

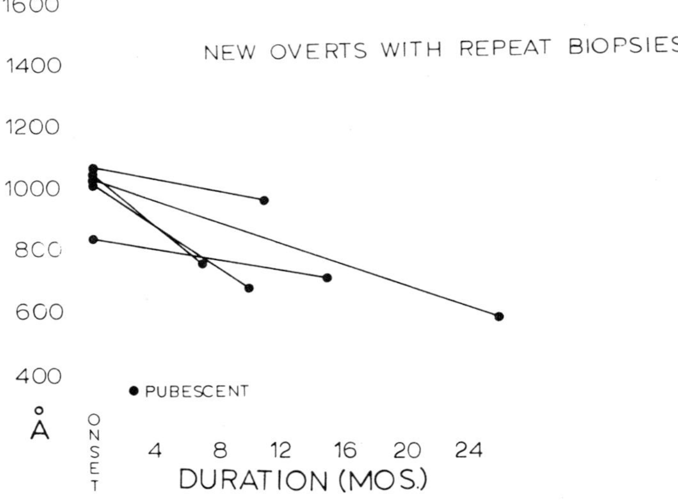

Fig.4 CBMT in 5 adolescent boys near time of onset and 7 to 24 months later during which time each boy had maintained excellent control.

determinations. Our data indicate that physiological thickening possibly accelerates during the prepubertal growth spurt but no definite increase in thickness was observed in the normal children or siblings with normal OGTT's during adolescence, i.e. girls 12 to 21 years and boys 14 to 21 years of age. No differences in CBMT were found between normal children and the siblings of children with overt diabetes with normal OGTT's (Figs 2 and 3).

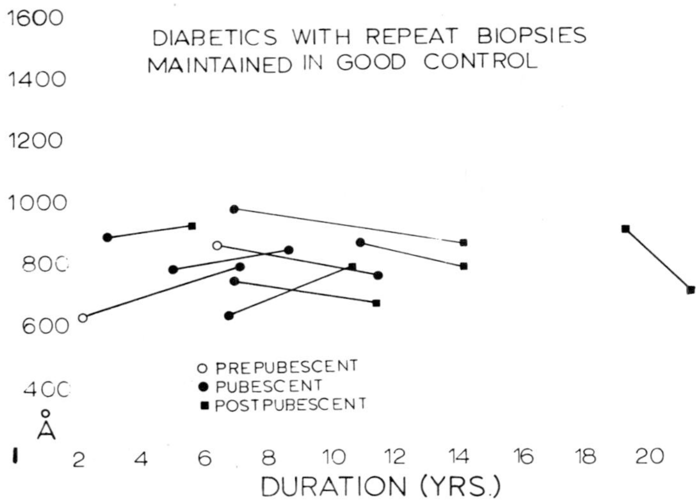

Fig.5 **Serial observation on eight children with diabetes maintained in good control. All values remained well within the expected range of normal children of comparable age.**

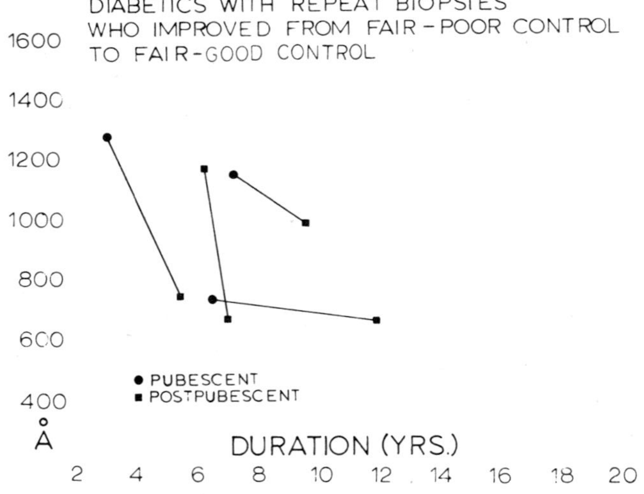

Fig.6 **Serial measurements of CBMT in 4 diabetics maintained in a higher degree of control over a period of years.**

Definite increase in CBMT was not observed in younger children with chemical diabetes but was increased in some young adults with more advanced chemical diabetes of longer duration. In 1973 Fajans and Williamson reported that young adult patients with documented chemical diabetes of many years duration had minimal but statistically significant increased CBMT of the muscle. Fajans and Williamson's data are important as they make it understandable why adult diabetic

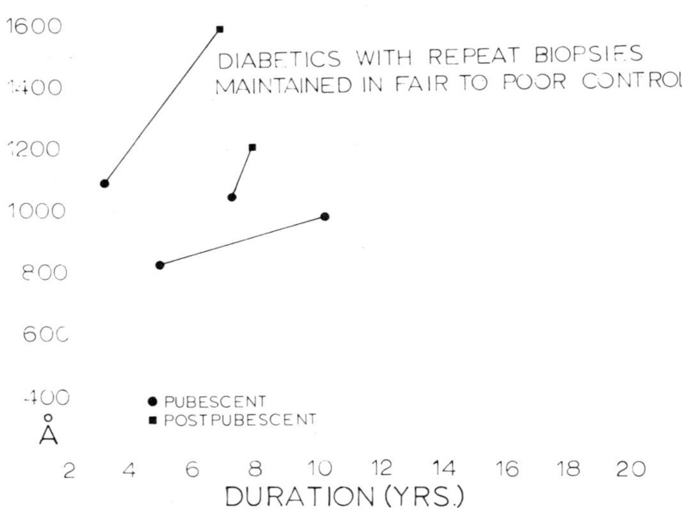

Fig. 7 **Progressive thickening of CBM in 3 diabetics maintained in fair to poor control.**

patients may have definite thickening of their capillary basement membrane at the time the diagnosis of overt diabetes is made.

Children with overt diabetes shortly after time of onset had normal or high normal CBMT (5 boys with high values at onset maintained in good control had decreased CBMT in less than 18 months) (Fig.4).

All 35 patients with diabetes classified to be in good control for as long as 15 years after onset had no increased CBMT. Sixty-three of the 67 patients classified to be in (fair to good) control for as long as 21 years after onset also had no increase in CBMT. Twenty-two of 46 patients classified to be in (fair to poor) control for 3 to 22 years after onset had increased CBMT. Most of the postpubescent girls in (fair to poor) control for more than 3 years and all of the postpubescent boys in (fair to poor) control, for more than 9 years, had increased CBMT. All 8 patients in (poor to fair) control had increased CBMT in less than 10 years.

Increase in CBMT was segmental, preceded retinopathy and was not observed before carbohydrate intolerance. No more than segmental thickening was observed in children with diabetes prior to puberty regardless of control rating.

Our longitudinal data are limited but the results to date are very consistent and indicate that the microvascular changes may not only progress during periods of poor control but also may regress during periods of improved control (Figs 5, 6 and 7). Additional studies including serial observations are in progress.

ADDENDUM A

Good Overall Control Rating

1. Most patients – under continuous observation in our clinic from time of onset of overt diabetes.

2. Early insulin treatment with 24 h insulin coverage. Using 2 injections with combination of regular and intermediate insulins.
3. Many patients – prolonged period of partial remission even up to 4 years (total insulin requirement less than 0.5 u/kg per day).
4. Good understanding and execution of meal planning.
5. Daily home records – reliable and relatively complete.
6. Essentially aglycosuric during entire period of partial remission, subsequently minimal transient glycosuria in no more than one of three or four daily urine specimens; no known ketonuria and very infrequent mild insulin reactions.
7. Postprandial blood sugar values at periodic clinic visits (3-5 times a year) usually normal or only slightly elevated.
8. Accurate growth record, excellent nutritional status, growth and maturation – normal.
9. Good psychosocial adjustment of child and family.
10. Responsible, stable family, good understanding, consistent compliance to regimen.

Fair to Good Overall Control Rating

1. Most patients – under continuous observation in our clinic at time or shortly after time of onset of overt diabetes.
2. Usually delayed insulin therapy but 24 h insulin coverage after treatment in our clinic. Using 2 injections with combination of regular and intermediate insulins.
3. Partial remission period usually 4 to 18 months, i.e., insulin requirement less than 0.5 u/kg/day.
4. Relatively good understanding and execution of meal planning.
5. Home records – reliable but less frequent testing.
6. Minimal transient glycosuria (less than one of 3 or 4 daily urine specimens). Transient ketonuria at times during infections. Occasional mild insulin reactions with very infrequent reactions of moderate severity.
7. Postprandial blood sugars at periodic clinic visits (3-5 times a year) variable but often normal or only moderately elevated.
8. Accurate growth record, excellent nutritional status, growth and maturation – normal.
9. Fair to good psychosocial adjustment of child and family.
10. Concerned, relatively stable family, good compliance to regimen most of the time.

Fair to Poor Overall Control Rating

1. Children usually total diabetics at time of admission to our clinic and insulin requirement is greater than 1.0 u/kg/day.
2. Usually delayed insulin therapy but 24 h insulin coverage after treatment in our clinic. Using 2 injections with combination of regular and intermediate insulins.
3. Variable dietary compliance.
4. Daily home records – often incomplete and somewhat questionable as to reliability.
5. Varying amounts of sugar in many urine specimens tested. Ketonuria known or suspected at times. More prone to insulin reactions of varying severity.
6. Postprandial blood sugars at clinic visits are usually high (300 ± 150 mg%) but sometimes normal or at hypoglycemic levels.

7. Accurate growth record, good nutritional status most of the time but maturation possibly delayed.
8. Increased incidence of psychosocial problems.
9. Relatively unstable family situation, erratic and less frequent clinic visits.

Poor to Fair Overall Control Rating

1. Poor compliance most of the time.
2. Frequently fail to keep clinic appointments, more often seen for emergency situations.
3. Meager and unreliable home records.
4. Glycosuria of varying degrees when urine specimens tested. More frequent and severe insulin reactions.
5. Delayed growth and maturation when accurate growth data are available.
6. High incidence of psychosocial problems.
7. Unstable family situation.

REFERENCES

Bilginturan, A.N., Jackson, R.L. and Ide, C.H. (1976). *Pediatrics (in press).*
Bloodworth, J.M.B., Jr. and Engerman, R.L. (1973). *Diabetes* **(Suppl.) 22**, 290.
Cahill, G.F. (1971). *Diabetes* **20**, 785.
Fajans, S.S., Williamson, J.R., Weissman, P.N., Vogler, N.J., Kilo, C. and Conn, J.W. (1973). "Early Diabetes Advances in Metabolic Disorders". Academic Press, New York.
Gabbay, K.H. (1973). *New Engl. J. Med.* **288**, 831.
Gabbay, K.H., Haney, D.N., Hasty, K., Gallop, P.M. and Bunn, H.F. (1976). *Diabetes* **(Suppl.) 24**, 335.
Jackson, R.L. and Kelly, H.G. (1946). *J. Pediat.* **29**, 316.
Jackson, R.L. and Guthrie, R.A. (1975). "The Child with Diabetes". Current Concept Series published by the Upjohn Company, Kalamazoo, Michigan.
Jackson, R.L., Hardin, R.C., Johnston, R.L. and Kelly, H.G. (1956). *Diabetes* **5**, 397.
Jackson, R.L., Onofiro, J., Waiches, H. and Guthrie, R.A. (1971). *Diabetes* **(Suppl.) 20**, 361.
Kilo, C., Vogler, N.,and Williamson, J.R. (1972). *Diabetes* **21**, 881.
Koening, R.J., Araiyo, D., and Cerami, A. (1976). *Diabetes* **25**, 1-5.
Mauer, S.M. (1976). *Diabetes* **(Suppl.) 25**, iv.
Monroe, L., Bryant, E. and Brewer, M.D. (1974). *ADA Forecast* Sept.–Oct.
Morrison, A.D. and Winegrad, A.I. (1972). *Diabetes* **21**, 330.
Osterby, R. (1973). *Diabetologia* **8**, 84.
Rosio, E.A., Morrison, A.D. and Winegrad, A.I. (1972). *Diabetes* **21**, 330.
Spiro, R.G. (1976). *Diabetologia* **12**, 1-14.
Spiro, R.G. and Spiro, M.J. (1971). *Diabetes* **20**, 641.
Williamson, J.R., Rowold, E., Hoffman, P. and Kilo, C. (1976). *Diabetes* **25**, 604.

GENETIC POLYMORPHISM IN JUVENILE-ONSET DIABETES

P. Lucarelli, R. Scacchi, R.M. Corbo, R. Palmerino, M. Orsini, L. Campea
E. Carapella and R. Pascone

National Research Council, Center for Evolutionary Genetics
(Department of Genetics, University of Rome, School of Science)
Department of Child Health, University of Rome, School of Medicine, Rome
Antidiabetic Center, Department of Pediatrics, University of Rome
School of Medicine, Rome
Pediatric "Diabetarium" E.N.A.M.S., Torre di Palidoro, Rome

Diabetes mellitus is one of the most common diseases in countries with an average to high standard of living and affects about 5% of the population: actually it is considered the third leading cause of death (Maugh, 1976).

The two fundamental types of diabetes are familiar, the insulin-dependent juvenile-onset kind and the maturity-onset kind. Hereditary factors appear to be of great importance in the aetiology of maturity-onset diabetes. On the contrary, the genetic contribution to classical juvenile-onset diabetes is much less clear: it is not unlikely that more genes at several loci may be involved in producing the genetic predisposition and that environmental factors operate to precipitate clinical disease. Recently, studies of histocompatibility antigens in patients with diabetes mellitus showed that the frequency of the antigens HL-A8 and W-15 is increased in insulin-dependent but not in maturity-onset diabetes (Nerup *et al.*, 1974; Cudworth and Woodrow, 1975).

In this investigation we report the results of a study of 9 genetic systems (ABO, Rh, MN, ACP_1, PGM_1, ADA, AK, G-6-PD) in a series of 138 patients, 71♂ and 67 ♀, affected by insulin-dependent juvenile-onset diabetes.

RESULTS

No significant differences were found with respect to phenotype and gene frequencies for PGM_1, ADA, AK, G-6-PD, Rh and Hp systems between patients and control groups.

Table I. Acid phosphatase system in diabetic patients and controls.

			Phenotypes							Alleles			
			A	B	C	BA	CB	CA	T	p^A	p^B	p^C	References
Patients	♂	obs.	4	35	—	25	1	3	68	36	96	4	
		%	5.88	51.47		36.76	1.47	4.41		0.265	0.706	0.029	
	♀	obs.	4	30	—	24	7	1	66	33	91	8	
		%	6.06	45.45		36.36	10.61	1.52		0.250	0.689	0.061	
	T	obs.	8	65	—	49	8	4	134	69	187	12	
		%	5.97	48.51		36.57	5.97	2.99		0.257	0.698	0.045	
Controls		obs.	36	183	1	132	51	14	417	218	549	67	G. Modiano
		%	8.63	43.88	0.24	31.65	12.23	3.36		0.261	0.658	0.080	*et al.* (1967)

Comparisons	All Phenotypes		CB *v.* Others	
	χ^2_{4df}	p	χ^2_{1df}	p
Patients *v.* Controls	6.105	ns	4.156	<.05
♂ *v.* ♀	5.876	ns	4.979	<.05
♂ *v.* Controls	8.415	.10< <.05	7.071	<.01
♀ *v.* Controls	1.663	ns	0.142	ns

Table II. ABO system in diabetic patients and controls.

			Phenotypes					Alleles			
			A	B	AB	O	T	I^A	I^B	i	References
Patients	♂	obs.	26	3	3	37	69	0.236	0.044	0.720	
		%	37.68	4.35	4.35	53.62	69				
	♀	obs.	20	14	1	30	65	0.179	0.124	0.697	
		%	30.77	21.54	1.54	46.15					
	T	obs.	46	17	4	67	134	0.208	0.082	0.710	
		%	34.33	12.69	2.98	50.00					
Controls		obs.	925	262	105	1130	2422	0.241	0.079	0.680	P. Fucci *et al.*
		%	38.19	10.82	4.33	46.66					(1956)

Comparisons	All Phenotypes		B *v.* Others	
	χ^2_{3df}	p	χ^2_{1df}	p
Patients *v.* Controls	1.751	ns	0.456	ns
♂ *v.* ♀	9.521	<.05	8.929	<.005
♂ *v.* Controls	3.339	ns	2.954	ns
♀ *v.* Controls	8.639	<.05	7.374	<.01

A significant deviation was noted for the erythrocyte acid phosphatase between males and controls (Table I): the phenotype CB is underrepresented in the diabetic males and differences with the control groups is statistically significant ($p < .01$). In the ABO blood groups (Table II) the phenotype frequencies showed marked differences between males and females ($p < .005$). Analysis showed that the groups of females differ significantly from controls, showing a marked excess in B phenotype ($p < .01$). For the MN system (Table III) the phenotype distribution showed some differences between patients and controls ($p < .05$). When the data were subdivided into sexes, analyses showed that only the group of males with an excess of the homozygotes MM and a defect of the

Table III. **MN system in diabetic patients and controls.**

			Phenotypes			Alleles	
		MM	MN	NN	T	L^M	References
Patients ♂	obs.	33	24	12	69	0.652	
	%	47.83	34.78	17.39			
♀	obs.	19	35	12	66	0.553	
	%	28.79	53.03	18.18			
T	obs.	52	59	24	135	0.604	
	%	38.52	43.70	17.78			
Controls	obs.	81	170	58	309	0.537	F. Vecchi
	%	26.21	55.02	18.77			*et al.* (1970)

	Comparisons					
	All Phenotypes		MM *v.* Others		MN *v.* Homozygotes	
	χ^2_{2df}	P	χ^2_{2df}	P	χ^2_{2df}	P
Patients *v.* Controls	7.130	.05	6.780	.01	4.814	.05
♂ *v.* ♀	5.756	.10 .05	5.153	.05	4.565	.05
♂ *v.* Controls	13.293	.005	12.508	.001	9.243	.005
♀ *v.* Controls	0.184	ns	0.184	ns	0.086	ns

heterozygotes MN, was significantly different from the controls.

DISCUSSION

The problem of the relationship between genetic polymorphisms, and in particular blood groups, and diabetes mellitus has been widely debated but results given in the literature are contradictory. From the data of Craig and Wang (1955), McConnel *et al.* (1956) and Zeytinoglu (1956/57) an excess of phenotype A is evident in diabetics with respect to the normal control, which concerns only males for the first, females for the second and subjects with renal lesions of a Kimmelsteil-Wilson type for the third. Tedeschi and Cavazzuti (1959) and Henry and Poon-King (1961) find instead an excess of phenotype B in diabetics with respect to the control. Andersen and Lauritzen (1960) report an increase in the frequency of the O group in males with respect to the control; Macafee (1964) and Berg *et al.* (1967) do not observe any difference in the frequency of the blood groups between diabetics and controls. Analysis of our data showed that the group of females differs significantly from the controls with a marked excess of B phenotype.

The authors who have dealt with the MN blood group system (McConnel *et al.*, 1956; Simpson *et al.*, 1962; Macafee, 1964) have found no differences between diabetic and controls. However, we have observed for the MN system significant differences in the distribution of phenotypes of males group with respect to the normal control. One of the causes of the contradictory results obtained for the ABO and for the MN system could be the clinical and genetic heterogeneity of the samples examined by some authors: in fact, contrary to the old idea that diabetes mellitus was a homogeneous disease transmitted as an autosomic recessive character, today it is widely accepted as a heterogeneous condition with a heterogeneous genetic background (Editorial of the Lancet, 1971).

Another fact which emerged from our investigation was the heterogeneity of the distribution of the phenotypes between males and females for the three genetic systems associated with diabetes mellitus. It is to be noted that the sex variable has already been found to be significant by other authors in previous researches (Rimoin, 1967; Maugh, 1975).

Lastly it seems to be interesting to note that the associations with insulin-dependent juvenile-onset diabetes mellitus shown up in this research specifically concern genetic markers which control structural components of the cell membrane. If it is taken into account that the cell surface is strictly involved in the processes of cell immunity, these results seem to be in favour of the hypothesis that more genes could be involved in the genetic predisposition – of an immunological nature – to the disease, on which exogenic factors, among which are probably some viruses, act to give rise to the clear form.

REFERENCES

Andersen, J. and Lauritzen, E. (1960). *Diabetes* **9**, 20-24.

Berg, K., Aarseth, S., Lundevall, J. and Reinskou, T. (1967). *Diabetologie* **3**, 30-34.

Craig, J. and Wang, I. (1955). *Glasgow Med. J.* **36**, 261-266.

Cudworth, A.G. and Woodrow, J.C. (1975). *Diabetes* **24**, 345-349.

Editorial (1971). *Lancet* **1**, 583-584.

Fucci, P. and Atella, P. (1956). *Policlinico, Sez. Prat.* **63**, 1096-1099.

Henry, M.U. and Poon-King, T. (1961). *W. Indian med. J.* **10**, 156-160.

Macafee, A.L. (1964). *J. clin. Path.* **17**, 39-41.

Maugh, T.H. (1975). *Science* **188**, 347-351.

Maugh, T.H. (1976). *Science* **191**, 272-274.

McConnell, R.B., Pyke, D.A. and Roberts, J.A.F. (1956). *Br. med. J.* **1**, 772-776.

Modiano, G., Filippi, G., Brunelli, F., Frattaroli, W., Siniscalco, M., Palmarino, R. and Santolamazza, C. (1967). *Acta gen. Stat. Med.* **17**, 17-28.

Nerup, J., Platz, P., Andersen Ortved, O., Christy, M., Lyngsøe, J., Poulsen, J.E., Ryder, L.P., Nielsen Staub, L., Thomsen, M. and Svejgaard, A. (1974). *Lancet* **II**, 864-866.

Rimoin, D.L. (1967). *Diabetes* **16**, 346-351.

Simpson, N.E., Gunson, H.H. and Smithies, O. (1962). *Diabetes* **11**, 329-333.

Tedeschi, G. and Cavazzuti, F. (1959). *Il progresso medico* **15**, 76-82.

Vecchi, F. and Purpura, M. (1970-71). *Rivista di Antropologia* **LVII**, 151-170.

Zeytinoglu, I. (1956/57). *Acta genet.* **6**, 564-566.

GROWTH AND MATURITY IN DIABETIC CHILDREN BEFORE PUBERTY

E. Vicens-Calvet, J. Sureda, M.G. Blanco and C. Pineda
Children's Hospital, Autonomous University of Barcelona, Spain

In spite of the efforts made in the last few years to obtain adequate treatment in the juvenile diabetic, recent publications (Bihrer, 1970; Craig, 1970; Pond, 1970; Evans, 1972; Jivani, 1973; Tattersall, 1973) indicate that diabetic children show an overall retardation of growth which signifies that the actual treatment is not able to assure them of a normal development.

MATERIALS AND METHODS

The study was performed in a group of 70 diabetic children aged between 1.025–11.930 years who attended our clinic from the onset of the illness, with the following characteristics:

1. All children had followed a normal diet according to their age, avoiding sweets and in general they received a daily injection in the morning of C.I. + I.P.Z. according to the results of the four daily checked urinary specimens.

   To obtain satisfactory results, the parents received instructions at the onset of the illness to understand the duties they had to perform. The method improved with later visits, and the intervals between them was up to 4 months.
2. All measurements were performed by the same team of anthropometrists with Holtain precision apparatus. Measurements were expressed in standard deviation score (S.D.S.) in relationship to a normal population (m = 0; S.D. = 1).

   The Tanner and Whitehouse charts model 38 × 30 cm were used because of their size, which enabled us to calculate the S.D. exactly.
3. In the bone-age study we used the Tanner and Whitehouse II method (20 bones and RUS). For the evaluation of the S.D. we used the charts model S.M.B. 32 and S.M.G. 33 from the same authors.
4. None of the children at the time of analysis showed any sign of puberty.

We performed the following studies:

1. At the onset of the illness a study of height was made in 70 patients (31 boys

and 39 girls). We considered "initial height" to be any measurement obtained during the first 3 months.

At the same time a study of weight at the onset of the illness was performed in 66 of the 70 test cases (31 boys and 35 girls). We considered "initial weight" to be the weight measured between the 6th and 9th months to correct the initial loss of weight at the onset of the illness.

2. A study of the height after a period of 3–8 years of the illness (mean = 4.679) was made. In this group there were 32 patients (16 girls and 16 boys) extracted from the initial 70 cases.

At the same time a study of weight was performed in the same patients.

3. A study of the evolution of the height every 6 months during the first four years was performed in the group of 32 patients (16 boys and 16 girls).

The initial and final weight was also studied in this group.

4. A maturity study was performed in a mixed group of 25 children at the onset and in another mixed group of 29 children after 3–8 years of evolution. All of them extracted from the initial 70 cases.

5. Finally we tried to find a correlation between height and bone age at the onset of the illness and at the time of analysis.

RESULTS

1. The distribution of height in the 70 test cases was normal at the onset (χ^2 test) (Fig.1). The mean height of 0.238 was higher than the normal population (m = 0; SD = 1) (see Table I, top) but did not reach a statistical significance ($0.06 > p > 0.05$). By sex, only boys were significantly taller ($p < 0.001$).

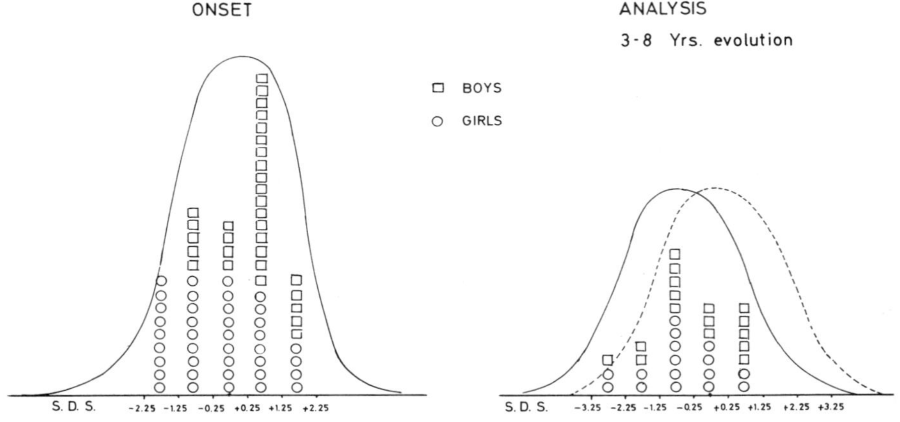

Fig. 1 **Observe the deviation of the diabetics to the left at the time of analysis although the distribution remains normal.**

2. After 3–8 years of evolution the distribution remained normal (Fig.1) but all of the mean heights were lower. In girls and in the total group they were significantly different from 0 ($0.01 > p > 0.001$ and $p = 0.001$).

The weight was normal at the onset (Table II, top) but had increased signi-

Table I. Height in diabetic children.

ONSET				ANALYSIS 3–8 YRS EVOLUTION			
Sex	N	S.D.S. Onset	p	Sex	N	S.D.S. Analysis	p
M	31	0.541	p < 0.001	M	16	–0.340	n.s., 0.2 > p > 0.1
F	39	–0.003	n.s.	F	16	–0.832	0.01 > p > 0.001
Total	70	0.238	0.06 > p > 0.05	Total	32	–0.586	p = 0.001

Sex	N	S.D.S. Onset	"t" test	p	S.D.S. Within patient basis	"t" test	p
M	16	0.628	3.49	0.01 > p > 0.001	–1.022	6.01	p < 0.001
F	16	0.071	0.24	n.s.	–0.893	6.85	p < 0.001
Total	32	0.349	2.02	n.s., 0.10 > p > 0.05	–0.957	9.03	p < 0.001

Table II. Weight in diabetic children.

ONSET				ANALYSIS 3–8 YRS EVOLUTION			
Sex	N	S.D.S. Onset	p	Sex	N	S.D.S. Analysis	p
M	31	0.085	n.s.	M	16	0.368	0.01 > p > 0.001
F	35	–0.214	n.s.	F	16	0.253	n.s.
Total	66	–0.076	n.s.	Total	32	0.310	p = 0.015

Sex	N	S.D.S. Onset	"t" test	p	S.D.S. Within patient basis	"t" test	p
M	16	0.264	2.19	0.05 < p < 0.02	0.103	0.84	n.s.
F	16	–0.322	–1.16	n.s.	0.576	2.33	0.05 > p > 0.02
Total	32	–0.029	–0.18	n.s.	0.340	2.39	0.05 > p > 0.02

ficantly at the time of analysis ($p = 0.015$).

3. When we studied the evolution of the height in the same group of 32 patients (Table I, bottom) we observed the same phenomenon at the onset but at the time of analysis the difference in S.D.S. from the onset was significant in all of them ($p < 0.001$).

In this group of 32 patients, weight was also normal at the onset (Table II, bottom) but had increased at the time of analysis which was due to the girls being heavier.

4. A 6-monthly study of the height during the first 4 years (Fig.2) showed a progressive decrease of the mean in both girls and boys. The difference between the initial and final mean was nearly the same in both (0.763 and 0.766) (Fig.2); the S.D. was always the same.

5. The bone age was normal at the onset (top of Table III) and it was significantly retarded at the time of analysis (Cochran test $0.01 > p > 0.001$ and $0.05 > p >$

EVOLUTION OF HEIGHT

(S. D. S.)

MONTHS		0	6	12	18	24	30	36	42	48
BOYS	m	0.628	0.408	0.274	0.285	0.183	0.071	0.000	-0.060	-0.135
	S.D.	0.718	0.768	0.738	0.780	0.772	0.809	0.778	0.724	0.774
GIRLS	m	0.071	-0.103	-0.260	-0.431	-0.542	-0.677	-0.596	-0.779	-0.695
	S.D.	1.140	1.067	1.089	1.103	1.198	1.229	1.111	1.137	0.980
TOTAL	m	0.349	0.142	0.010	-0.073	-0.179	-0.302	-0.298	-0.451	-0.450
	S.D.	0.979	0.980	0.964	1.027	1.056	1.092	0.991	1.030	0.943
16 BOYS 16 GIRLS	N	32	32	32	32	32	32	32	32	32

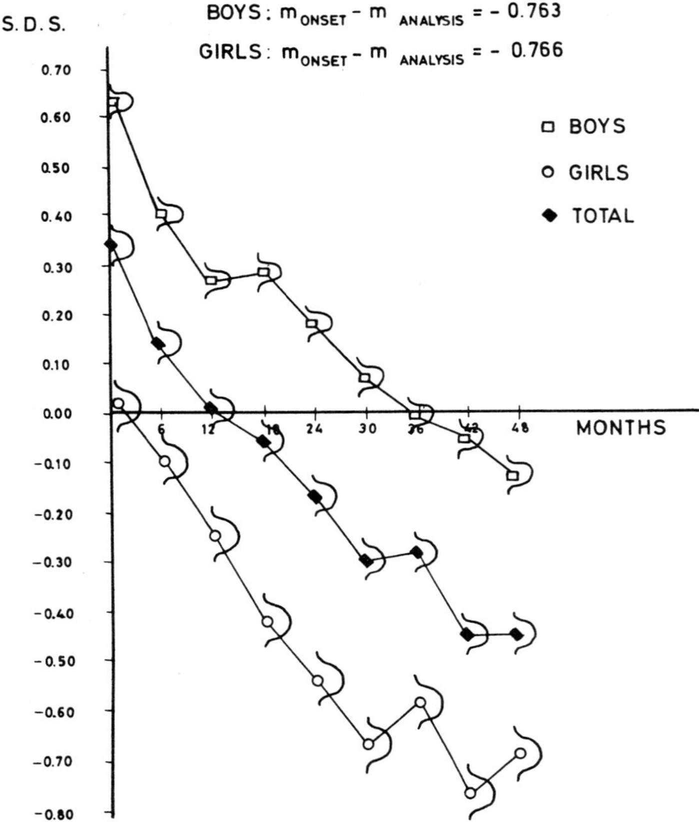

Fig. 2 (Top). In the six-monthly mean and S.D. of the group of 32 diabetics, the mean decreases progressively but the S.D. remains unchanged. (Bottom). A graphic representation of the same phenomenon.

Table III.

Maturity study in diabetic children.

	TW II Boys and Girls 20 Bones			TW II Boys and Girls RUS		
	Onset	Analysis	p Cochran Test	Onset	Analysis	p Cochran Test
m	−0.04	−0.93	$0.01 > p > 0.001$	−0.05	−0.73	$0.05 > p > 0.01$
s.d.	1.04	1.32	–	1.10	1.48	–
N	25	29	–	25	29	–

Linear regression: bone age – height

TW II Boys and Girls 20 Bones		TW II Boys and Girls RUS	
Onset	Analysis	Onset	Analysis
r = 0.252	r = 0.725	r = 0.180	r = 0.651

0.01). The correlation height to bone age increased with the evolution of the illness (bottom of Table III).

COMMENTS

The concept of the well-controlled diabetic child is nearly always subjective and it is difficult in the same way to classify diabetes into severe or mild forms except in extreme cases.

We considered our test group of children to be well-controlled because the parents had understood the treatment well and the daily routines they had to perform; the glycosuries in the patients were moderate, and severe hypoglycemia crises were rare, and after the onset of the illness there were no serious acidotic crises resulting in the readmission of the patient.

Obviously, we had to eliminate any cases that showed lack of good control. Most of these cases appeared at the bottom end of the socio-economic scale. At the onset of the illness some authors have found the heights in diabetic children to be normal (Jackson, 1946; Beal, 1948; Jivany, 1973), whereas others have found them to be taller than average (Craig, 1970; Pond, 1970). In our study group only boys were significantly taller than normal ($p < 0.001$) but the whole group just escapes statistical significance ($0.06 > p > 0.05$). All of these findings depend upon the types of reference charts used, the socio-economic level of the childrens' families, and the size of the group to be studied.

More important than the initial height is to observe its evolution during the course of the illness. In our study group, after a control period of three to eight years (32 from the initial 70 cases) the situation was that there was a difference in the S.D.S. from our initial findings. Both boys and girls had deviated to the lower end of the growth charts. In girls and the group as a whole the differences from the normal population with m = 0 and S.D. = 1 were significant. In boys the difference was not significant, as a result of their being taller at the beginning (Table I, top).

If we study the group of 32 children in which we know the initial and final heights, in the study period (Table I, bottom) their decrease in S.D.S. from the onset is statistically significant in all of them ($p < 0.001$) which indicates a very clear retardation of growth. Some authors have speculated that the short stature of juvenile diabetics is fundamentally due to a small pubertal spurt, and before puberty the height velocity is nearly normal (Jivani, 1973). In our group of 32 children who were measured every six months during the first four years (Fig.2) there is a progressive decrease in the mean value measured in S.D.S. in both boys and girls and we never observed any period of catch-up growth. The difference between initial mean and final mean is nearly identical in both sexes, which indicates a similar retardation in boys and girls, but other researchers have found a higher level of retardation in boys (Berquist, 1954; Sterky, 1967). So, as we have shown, we did not observe any period of catch-up growth in our controlled study group at the onset or during the illness which is contrary to earlier published observations (Jackson, 1946): rather, we found a progressive retardation which closely followed the evolution of the illness (Berquist, 1954; Knowles, 1965; Sterky, 1967; Pond, 1970; Craig, 1970; Tattersall, 1973).

The bone age (TW II 20 bones and RUS) in the mixed group was normal at the onset (Table III, top). When it was checked in another mixed group at the time of analysis (Table III, bottom), it was found to be retarded, which indicates a concurrent maturity retardation. Although we did not do initial bone age tests in the second group, we felt it safe to assume that they would have been the same as the first group at the onset of the illness. This progressive bone age retardation has been found by other authors (Craig, 1970). Surprisingly, though, Evans (1972) found an increase in bone maturity in boys at the onset.

It appears certain, then, that the juvenile diabetic will reach puberty with a marked retardation of growth and maturity. This retardation of maturity must offer the juvenile diabetic a much better prognosis for his adult stature, and it could be an explanation for their delayed puberty.

We have found the weight studies useful in checking nutrition throughout the illness. Along with other authors (Jackson, 1946; Sterky, 1967; Evans, 1972; Jivani, 1973) we found that girls have a tendency towards obesity.

Our studies have shown that there is only a small correlation between bone age and maturity at the onset (Table III) because there are numerous factors that influence both parameters, but at the time of analysis this correlation has increased, indicating that diabetes acts on both parameters resulting in a retardation of growth and maturity which has diminished the importance of the genetic, socio-economic factors, etc.. These other factors have more importance at the onset of the illness.

CONCLUSIONS

There is a progressive retardation of growth in the diabetic child from the onset of the illness which explains the retardation of the pubertal spurt despite normal nutrition using weight tests as guidelines. All of these findings indicate that the treatment is unable to assure the juvenile diabetic of a normal development.

REFERENCES

Beal, C.K. (1948). *J. Ped.* **32**, 170-179.
Berquist, N. (1954). *Acta endocr. (Copenh.)* **15**, 133-165.
Bihrer, R. (1970). *Helv. Paediat. Acta* **25**, 312-324.
Craig, J.O. (1970). *Postgrad. med. J.* **46**, 607-610.
Evans, N., Robinson, V.P. and Lister, J. (1972). *Archs. Dis. Childh.* **47**, 589-593.
Jackson, R.L. and Kelly, H.G. (1946). *J. Ped.* **29**, 316-328.
Jivani, S.K. and Rayner, P.H. (1973). *Archs. Dis. Childh.* **48**, 109-115.
Knowles, H.C., Guest, G.M., Lampe, J., Kessler, M. and Skillman, T. (1965). *Diabetes* **14**, 239-273.
Pond, H. (1970). *Postgrad. med. J.* **46**, 616-623.
Sterky, G. (1967). *Acta Paed. Scand.* **Suppl. 177**, 80-82.
Tattersall, R.B. and Pyke, D.A. (1973). *Lancet* **ii**, 1105-1109.

SUBJECT INDEX